THE C.I.A. DOCTORS
HUMAN RIGHTS VIOLATIONS BY AMERICAN PSYCHIATRISTS

COLIN A. ROSS, M.D.

MANITOU COMMUNICATIONS, INC.

ISBN-10: 0-9765508-0-6
ISBN-13: 978-0-9765508-0-6

Library of Congress Cataloging-in-Publication Data:

Ross, Colin A., M.D.

The C.I.A. Doctors: Human Rights Violations By American Psychiatrists

ISBN-10: 0-9765508-0-6
ISBN-13: 978-0-9765508-0-6

1. C.I.A. and Military Mind Control   2. Psychiatry   3. Human Rights Violations

Originally published as
BLUEBIRD: Deliberate Creation of Multiple Personality By Psychiatrists, 2000,
-ISBN 0-9704525-1-9.

Design by Deep River Design, LLC

Also By The Author

Northern Studies (1975)

Portrait of Norman Wells (1979)

Adenocarcinoma and Other Poems (1984)

Multiple Personality Disorder:
Diagnosis, Clinical Features, And Treatment (1989)

The Osiris Complex: Case Studies In Multiple Personality Disorder (1994)

Satanic Ritual Abuse: Principles Of Treatment (1995)

Pseudoscience In Biological Psychiatry (1995)

Dissociative Identity Disorder:
Diagnosis, Clinical Features, And Treatment Of Multiple Personality,
Second Edition (1997)

The Trauma Model:
A Solution To The Problem Of Comorbidity In Psychiatry (2000)

Spirit Power Drawings: The Foundation of a New Science (2004)

Songs For Two Children: On Dissociation and Human Energy Fields (2004)

Schizophrenia: Innovations in Diagnosis and Treatment (2004)

TABLE OF CONTENTS

KD2358LEB21891KIN203172QG50665TR7477QG411042

In working with individual subjects, special attention will be given to disassociative states, which tend to accompany spontaneous ESP experiences. Such states can be induced or controlled to some extent with hypnosis and drugs. . . The data used in this study will be obtained from group ESP experiments which have yielded significant results, high scoring subjects from special groups such as psychotics, children and mediums, and from psychological tests in which answers are of the multiple choice type. . . But the main consideration will be the attitude and general disposition of the subject. Wherever possible, every attempt will be made to tailor the tasks required to his preferences and his estimate of good working conditions. In one case the experimental procedure will be designed to achieve favorable motivation by such devices as instructing him that he is participating in a study of subception. In other cases drugs and psychological tricks will be used to modify his attitudes. The experimenters will be particularly interested in disassociative states, from the <u>abaissment de niveau mental</u> to multiple personality in so-called mediums, and an attempt will be made to induce a number of states of this kind, using hypnosis.

MKULTRA Subproject 136 Proposal, 30 May 1961, Experimental Analysis of Extrasensory Perception, approved by the Chief, Technical Services Division/Research Branch, Central Intelligence Agency, 23 August 1961, $8,579.00.

ACKNOWLEDGMENTS

I would like to thank the people who suggested books for me to read. During the thirteen years I have studied mind control, many people have provided me support and encouragement, in person, and through e-mail and correspondence. That helped a lot, especially when the disinformation campaign against me was taking its toll. Dale Reeves worked very hard making trips to TRIMS in Houston, Colgate College in New York, and other locations, and filing and organizing documents. Tere Kole worked equally as hard on the files and on preparation of the manuscript and the mechanics of publishing.

The CIA Doctors is based on 15,000 pages of documents obtained from the CIA through the Freedom of Information Act. Without this information, there would be no book. I want the reader to know that this book is not about the CIA nor the government. In my opinion, public scrutiny needs to be focused on the psychiatrists and medical schools. It was they who violated the Hippocratic Oath.

If the West had not won the Cold War, I would likely have died in Gulag many years ago. The CIA and military intelligence agencies are owed a personal debt by me on this count. I am not criticizing the CIA or the military in this book because I am not an expert on intelligence matters. I am a psychiatrist specializing in dissociative disorders, which include multiple personality disorder.

If I tried to write this book in Russia, I would be sent to Gulag. I would like to acknowledge the CIA for winning the Cold War, protecting democracy, and making my work possible. Many people have asked me if I am afraid of the CIA because of my investigation of mind control. I always tell them that the dangerous people, for me, are the psychiatrists.

Why do I admire the CIA? In part, because I admire its founder, William Donovan[43, 138, 302]. If Donovan had been in charge of U.S. foreign policy after World War II, there would not have been a Vietnam War. The true spirit of the CIA would have prevailed. Donovan was the head of the OSS during World War II. The OSS was disbanded in 1945, but resurrected as the CIA in 1947. During the Second World War France was occupied by the Nazis. The French were our allies and the OSS worked with the French resistance. During the Nazi occupation, the northern half of France was administered directly by the Nazis, while the southern half plus Algeria were administered on behalf of the Nazis by Frenchmen. This southern government was called the Vichy Government. Our allies the French were collaborating with our enemies the Germans. The Vichy Government hated our allies the British, and in fact the British attacked the Vichy naval fleet in July, 1940.

Around the other side of the world, our enemies the Japanese occupied what is now called Vietnam in September, 1940. At that time North Vietnam was called Tonkin and South Vietnam was called Cochin. In order to occupy Vietnam, the Japanese kicked out the French government which occupied the country before and after the Second World War. In Vietnam, the French were our allies and the Japanese were our enemies. Unfortunately, the French government kicked out of South Vietnam by the Japanese was a Vichy government; this Vichy government was an enemy of our allies the British.

Linked to this diplomatic mess was the situation in China. In July, 1942 the OSS set up guerrilla warfare unit in India for operations in southeast Asia and China. At the time, General Joseph Stilwell was U.S. Commander in China, Burma and India and also Chief of Staff to Chiang Kai-shek. The only American military force in China was an air force squadron called the Flying Tigers, headed up by General Claire Chennault. In 1947, Chennault became the head of Civil Air Transport, an airline owned and operated by the CIA.

In China, Chiang Kai-shek was enemies with Mao Tse-tung, so Mao Tse-tung should have been our enemy. On the other hand, Mao Tse-tung was aligned with our allies the Russians, so should have been our friend. The official American position was to be allies with Chiang Kai-shek, but the OSS trained about 25,000 of Mao's guerrillas and supplied them with 100,000 pistols.

Chiang Kai-shek's head of intelligence was a man called Tai Li. William Donovan met with Tai Li in person for various negotiations during the war. The British arrested Tai Li in Hong Kong in 1941 but he was released due to a personal intervention by Chiang Kai-shek.

In May, 1941 the Vietnamese, known at this time as the Annamites met in southern China, Chiang Kai-shek's territory, to set up a Vietnamese resistance organization. This organization was devoted to liberating Vietnam from Japanese occupation and establishing a free, democratic government aligned with the United States The OSS supported the resistance fighters in Vietnam just like it did those in France.

The leader of the Viet Minh, the name given to the resistance organization, was a man called Nguyen ai Qoc: this man was arrested and imprisoned by Tai Li's agents in August, 1942. He was not released until September, 1943, and then only because of a deal made with Chiang Kai-shek's government by a Chinese warlord. After his release Nguyen ai Qoc changed his name to Ho Chi Minh in order to avoid Tai Li's agents.

For the last two years of the Second World War, Ho Chi Minh was the leader of the Vietnamese resistance against the Japanese. He created an extensive underground network in Tonkin, supplied intelligence to U.S. forces, and aided in the rescue of downed Flying Tiger pilots. He had full OSS support.

Our allies, the French didn't like Ho Chi Minh because if he succeeded in liberating Vietnam from the Japanese, and established a free democratic government, the French would not be able to take over at the end of the war. The deal that ended up getting made between the Americans, British, French and Russians was that the French could have South Vietnam back. This meant that Ho Chi Minh had to be transformed into a communist enemy of democracy.

OSS support of Ho Chi Minh included an officer of the Chase Manhattan Bank who was parachuted into his camp, and an OSS medic named Paul Hoagland. Paul Hoagland saved Ho Chi Minh's life with quinine and sulfa drugs, otherwise he would have died of a combination of malaria, dysentery and other tropical diseases. The OSS also trained 200 elite troops of Ho Chi Minh's army commander, a man named Vo Nguyen Giap.

On August 17, 1945 Ho Chi Minh and the Viet Minh took control of Hanoi from the Japanese. Ho Chi Minh was accompanied on his march into Hanoi by Paul Hoagland and the rest of the OSS Deer team that had parachuted into his camp. On that day, August 17, 1945, Ho Chi Minh broadcast the following message in English to OSS headquarters:

> *National Liberation Committee on VML begs U.S. authorities to inform United Nations the following. We were fighting Japs on the side of the United Nations. Now Japs surrendered. We beg the United Nations to realize their solemn promise that all nationalities will be given democracy and independence. If United Nations forget their solemn promise and don't give Indochina full independence, we will keep fighting until we get it.*

On September 2, 1945 a band marched through Hanoi playing the Star Spangled Banner while OSS officer Colonel Archimedes Patti and Vo Nguyen Giap stood side by side, arms held in salute. The two men are shown in this stance in a photograph in Smith's book on the OSS[291]. Ho Chi Minh had declared that day Vietnam Independence Day, and he began his liberation speech with the words, *"All men are created equal."*

Ho Chi Minh, the hated Communist was originally a resistance fighter devoted to freedom and democracy, supported by William Donovan, the OSS and the American taxpayer in his fight against the Japanese. He was transformed into a Communist enemy because of the deal made between the British, Americans, French and Russians at the end of World War II. For several months after the end of the War, Donovan worked in Vietnam trying to rebuild the infrastructure, attract American capital to Vietnam, and establish a democracy lead by Ho Chi Minh. This effort was shut down for political reasons, and as a result the stage was set for American military involvement in Vietnam a decade later.

If the work of the OSS in Vietnam had continued under the CIA and William Donovan's leadership, there would have been no American casualties there in subsequent decades. Ho Chi Minh would have been the leader of a democracy aligned with the United States. But the true vision of the CIA did not prevail. I include this historical aside to show why I admire William Donovan, and to explain why I am not in any way a critic of the CIA.

My focus in *The CIA Doctors* is on the psychiatrists, not on the CIA. It is the psychiatrists who violated the Hippocratic Oath, and it is the psychiatrists who betrayed their patients' trust for career advancement funding, and academic promotions.

INTRODUCTION

The major goal of the Cold War mind control programs was to create dissociative symptoms and disorders, including full multiple personality disorder. The Manchurian Candidate[66] is fact, not fiction, and was created by the CIA in the 1950's under BLUEBIRD and ARTICHOKE mind control programs. Experiments with LSD, sensory deprivation, electro-convulsive treatment, brain electrode implants and hypnosis were designed to create amnesia, depersonalization, changes in identity and altered states of consciousness. One purpose of *The CIA Doctors: Human Rights Violations by American Psychiatrists* is to prove that the creation of controlled dissociation was a major goal of mind control research. Other authors, who are not specialists in dissociation [255-258], have failed to understand this fact. Multiple personality disorder is now classified by the American Psychiatric Association[12] as dissociative identity disorder.

The main purposes of this book are:

1. To document extensive human rights violations by American psychiatrists over the last 70 years.

2. To prove that these violations were pervasive, systematic and involved leading psychiatrists and medical schools.

3. To counter claims that the violations happened in an earlier time with different ethical standards – they violated the Hippocratic Oath and the Nuremberg Code.

4. To call for a systematic review of these violations by government and the profession of psychiatry.

Because the subject matter of this book is likely to provoke extreme reactions, I have taken great care to present only facts that are fully documented and based on objective, public domain information. Experiments to create Manchurian Candidate "super spies" must be understood in their social and historical context, which is one of pervasive, systematic mind control experimentation, not by a few isolated renegade doctors, but by the leaders of psychiatry and the major medical schools.

The literature on psychiatric participation in CIA and military mind control is incomplete. A systematic inventory of projects and investigators has never been attempted. Only one paper on the subject has been published in medical journals[248] and only one book was published by academic presses in the 1990's[313]. These treatments of the subject had a narrow focus. Other books and articles on the subject range from scholarly[277-278] to popular[301, 307, 333]. The last study of the subject with a broad perspective appeared almost two decades ago[184]. The medical schools and academia have been completely silent on psychiatric participation in mind control experimentation.

The participation of psychiatrists and medical schools in mind control research was not a matter of a few scattered doctors pursuing questionable lines of investigation. Nor did the experiments occur in a previous era governed by different ethical standards than those prevailing at the beginning of the twenty-first century. Rather, the mind control experimentation was systematic, organized, and involved many leading psychiatrists and medical schools. Many leading psychiatrists must have been directly aware of the Manchurian Candidate programs.

The mind control experiments were interwoven with radiation experiments, and research on chemical and biological weapons. The mind control work was funded by the CIA, Army, Navy and Air Force, and concurrently by other agencies including the Public Health Service and the Scottish Rite Foundation. The psychiatrists, psychologists, neurosurgeons and other contractors conducting the work were imbedded in a broad network of doctors and much of the research was published in medical journals.

Mind control contractors with TOP SECRET clearance included the American Psychological Association, Past Presidents of the American Psychiatric Association and the Society for Biological Psychiatry, and psychiatrists who have received awards from the American Psychological Association and the American Psychiatric Association. Many of the mind control doctors have been the subjects of obituaries in the American Journal of Psychiatry.

Clinical responsibility for the mind control experiments lies with the doctors, who should have been constrained by the Hippocratic Oath. National Security interests are the proper responsibility of the CIA, and the CIA is not governed by the Hippocratic Oath. That the CIA created Manchurian Candidates is a fact, but this book is not about the CIA, the military or the government. It is not based on conspiracy theory and it does not advance a conspiracy theory. I am not a critic of the CIA and I am not privy to the intelligence imperatives behind the Manchurian Candidate programs.

My focus in *The CIA Doctors: Human Rights Violations by American Psychiatrists* is on psychiatry and the dissociative disorders. My intent is to prove that the Manchurian Candidate is real, and to set the Manchurian Candidate programs in a historical and clinical context. *The CIA Doctors* documents extensive human rights violations by psychiatrists in North America in the second half of the twentieth century. Many thousands of prisoners and mental patients were subjected to unethical mind control experiments by leading psychiatrists and medical schools. Organized academic psychiatry has never acknowledged this history. The network of mind control doctors involved in BLUEBIRD, ARTICHOKE, MKULTRA and other mind control programs has done a great deal of harm to the field of psychiatry and to psychiatric patients. My goal is to break the ugly silence.

The CIA Doctors was originally published in the year 2000, with the title *BLUEBIRD: Deliberate Creation Of Multiple Personality By Psychiatrists*. I decided to change the title in this edition because potential readers might not know about BLUEBIRD, ARTICHOKE and other CIA mind control programs. Therefore it might be unclear to them what the book is about. I changed the subtitle in order to provide a clearer focus for the book. This edition contains no new references or documents. I have done some light revising and reorganizing and added some concluding comments about mind control programs that are ongoing in the twenty-first century.

I. Historical Background

To understand creation of Manchurian Candidates by CIA and military mind control doctors, it is necessary to have some historical background. The work of the mind control doctors did not occur in a vacuum. The importation of Nazi doctors to the United States through secret programs like PAPERCLIP is part of the context.

Likewise, the Tuskeegee Syphilis Study helps us understand how mind control experimentation was not only tolerated by medical professionals, but published in the peer-reviewed literature. Just as the results of the Tuskeegee Study were published in the medical literature[141, 253, 309] so was the mind control research condoned and tolerated via publication in psychiatric and medical journals. The climate was permissive, supportive and approving of mind control experimentation.

Radiation experiments conducted by doctors on behalf of the military, Atomic Energy Commission and other branches of government overlapped with biological and chemical weapons research and also with mind control. For instance, Dr. William Sweet participated in both brain electrode implant experiments and the injection of uranium into medical patients at Harvard University[89, 183]. The 925-page *Final Report. Advisory Committee on Human Radiation Experiments*[89] tells the story of the radiation experiments, and their linkage to mind control.

1
PROJECT PAPERCLIP

At the end of World War II, German scientists and technical experts were being held in a variety of detainment camps by the allies and Russians. The British, French, Americans and Russians became embroiled in highly competitive recruiting efforts to secure the services of these German specialists. Many of the scientists, however, could not qualify for immigration visas into the United States because they were war criminals or had actively served the Nazi cause. The prospect of losing the industrial and scientific services of these German experts lead to the creation of a series of secret programs including PAPERCLIP, PROJECT 63 and NATIONAL INTEREST[40, 135, 287, 288].

Through these programs, over 1000 German scientists and their families were secretly brought into the United States without State Department scrutiny or approval. Recruitment of German scientists through PAPERCLIP and related projects continued into the 1980's. The most famous individual brought over in this manner was Werner von Braun, the rocket scientist.

Von Braun was the head of the German V2 rocket program during World War II. The V2 rocket factory was the Mittlewerk, a site visited personally by von Braun. Labor for the factory was provided by the inmates of nearby Camp Dora. It is estimated that 20,000 inmates were worked to death at the Mittlewerk; 6000 bodies were found on the ground when American troops liberated the camp late in the War.

One of the survivors of Camp Dora, Yves Beon, said that workers were given one piece of bread and margarine per day. Despite these conditions, workers were able to sabotage some of the V2 rockets by tampering with parts or urinating on them. When sabotage was discovered, the prisoners were hanged in their work tunnels. Beatings by prison guards were routine.

Besides visiting the Mittlewerk personally, von Braun attended a meeting at which the Nazis discussed bringing French civilians in as slave labor for building rockets. At the Nuremberg trials, von Braun was said by a Nazi defendant to have worked closely with Dr. Albin Sawatzi. Camp Dora prisoners identified Sawatzi as being in charge of much of the deadly treatment they received, and as personally administering beatings.

A report by the Office of Military Government U.S., the *OMGUS Security Report*, listed von Braun as an ardent Nazi and a security threat to the United States, hence the need for routing through PAPERCLIP. Two weeks after the first U.S. moon landing, on August 2, 1969, von Braun wrote a letter to retired Major General Julius Klein on his Director of Marshall Space Flight Center stationery, in which he said, "It's true that I was a member of Hitler's elite SS. The columnist was correct. I would appreciate it if you would keep the information to yourself as any publicity would harm my work with NASA."

The NASA rockets that took Neil Armstrong to the moon were built by von Braun and his colleagues. When Armstrong stepped onto the surface of the moon, he did not realize that he was stepping on the ashes of 20,000 people who died at Camp Dora. Arthur Rudolph, head of production at the Mittlewerk, became the head of the U.S. Saturn V Rocket Program. Another Mittlewerk team member, Kurt Debus, became the first Director of the Kennedy Space Center.

Medical doctors also came over under PAPERCLIP. Dr. Albertus Strughold was named chief scientist of the Aerospace Medical Division of the U.S. Air Force in 1961. He is regarded as the father of aviation medicine. Strughold's first job in the U.S. was head of the Air Force School of Aviation Medicine at Randolph Field, Texas. In 1949 he took charge of the newly created Department of Space Medicine. Honors awarded Strughold included the Americanism Medal from the Daughters of the American Revolution. Also, June 15, 1985 was declared "Dr. Albertus Strughold Day" by the Texas Senate. The Aerospace Library at the School of Aerospace Medicine, Brooks Air Force Base, San Antonio, Texas is dedicated to Strughold.

An article in *The Dallas Morning News*, October 27, 1993 (page 8A) describes efforts by the Simon Weisenthal Center and other groups to have honors paid to Dr. Strughold, including the Library dedication, removed.

Strughold was head of the Luftwaffe Institute of Aviation Medicine in Berlin during the War. At the Nuremberg trials his military superiors, close associates and a subordinate were all tried for war crimes. Strughold, however, was never arrested, interrogated or called as a witness. Nuremberg investigator Herbert Meyer was given firsthand information about Strughold's direct involvement in war crimes for which people close to him were tried. Hermann Becker-Freysing, who gave this information to Meyer, was found guilty at Nuremberg and sentenced to twenty years in prison.

One study conducted by Nazi aviation doctors involved an attempt to ascertain the effects of ejecting from an airplane at high altitudes. Concentration camp prisoners were placed in a special chamber and the pressure would suddenly be dropped to the equivalent of 39,260 feet. One question addressed in the experiment was whether the decompression was more painful in the prone or sitting position. Some subjects went insane and some died.

At Dachau, Himmler personally approved the use of 200 prisoners (Jews, Russians, and members of the Polish resistance) in experiments by Dr. Sigmund Rascher. The experiments were expected to be fatal. Rascher went a step beyond prior research; he instantly decompressed subjects to the equivalent of 69,000 feet, which caused many to pull out their hair, tear their faces with their fingernails, and pound their heads on the wall.

Nearly eighty men died from being kept at simulated high altitude for up to thirty minutes. Others were taken out of the chamber alive, held under water till they drowned, then autopsied to determine the amount of air embolism in their brains. The reactions of the men inside the chambers were often filmed.

Karl Hoellenrainer was a gypsy prison-camp inmate who survived experiments at Dachau prison hospital conducted by Dr. Wilhelm Beigelboeck. Hoellenrainer was in Auschwitz briefly, where his own child, and his sister and her two children were killed. He was to have been transported from there to Buchenwald but was rerouted to Dachau. There, he and other subjects were starved then forced to drink putrid seawater, or seawater treated by one of two purification methods. Those who refused were tied up and force-fed by tubes.

Subjects in these experiments became violently ill, some went into coma, some were seriously wounded, and some died when their livers were punctured to drain off blood and water. The purpose of the experiments was to develop methods that would enable Nazi pilots downed at sea to survive by drinking seawater.

Besides strictly medical experiments, Dachau was also the site of mind control experiments involving the drug mescaline. Nazi doctors including Dr. Kurt Plotner administered mescaline to unwitting subjects by spiking prisoner's drinks[184]. During the same period, similar experiments involving mescaline, marijuana, barbiturates, and scopolamine were conducted by Dr. Winfred Overholser at St. Elizabeth's hospital in Washington, D.C.

The U.S. mind control experiments at St. Elizabeth's were conducted under the auspices of the Office of Strategic Services (OSS), the precursor of the CIA. A participant in the experiments, OSS officer George White, later became the contractor on the CIA's MKULTRA Subprojects 3, 14, 16, 42 and 149 that ran from 1953 to at least 1964.

An unanswered question is whether any Nazi psychiatrists or mind control experts were brought over under PAPERCLIP or related projects[156]. The full range of German scientific technical expertise was recruited through these programs including medical doctors, rocket scientists, propulsion experts, and experts in ball bearings, film, lubricants, jet engines and countless other areas of interest to the military. It seems unlikely that no psychiatrists were included in the recruitment programs, especially since the OSS was already testing and interested in the same mind control methods studied in the death camps.

It is not difficult to identify possible PAPERCLIP scientists in the medical literature. Theodore Wagner-Jauregg was a chemist born on May 2, 1903 in Vienna and educated in Munich and Vienna. He died on February 19, 1992. His father, Julius Wagner-Jauregg, won the Nobel Prize for Medicine in 1927 for research on syphilis[42].

Theodore Wagner-Jauregg worked at the Kaiser Wilhem Institute in Germany before the War and then worked at Edgware Arsenal from 1948 to 1955 before returning to Europe. Edgeware Arsenal was one of the key centers for CIA and Army LSD and mind control research during the 1950's and 1960's. In a paper on a defensive chemical weapon, an antidote to a class of drug called acetylcholinesterase inhibitors[104] the authors say in a footnote that, "The experimental results in this paper were obtained several years ago, but its publication has been delayed for various reasons."

Most likely, publication was delayed until the results of the work were declassified. Under the listing of authors, the paper is said to be, "From the Research Directorate, United States Army Chemical Research and Development Laboratories, Army Chemical Center, Maryland." Whether or not Wagner-Jauregg came over under PAPERCLIP is not the point; the point is that any psychiatrists brought over as mind control experts ought to be identifiable.

There was a round of declassification of mind control documents in the 1970's, which were the foundation of books published in the 1970's and 1980's[38, 65, 105, 158, 184, 278, 301]. These documents and books did not examine the possible role of German PAPERCLIP psychiatrists in mind control experimentation. The subject remains untouched by scholarly and investigative hands, but is an essential part of the historical background.

2
THE TUSKEEGEE SYPHILIS STUDY

Like the mind control research, the results of the Tuskeegee Syphilis Study were published in the peer-reviewed medical literature[309, 253]. The Tuskeegee Syphilis Study was clearly unethical and harmful to the subjects. The Study violated the 1943 Henderson Act, an Alabama public health statute for mandatory reporting of tuberculosis and venereal disease, and state health laws passed in 1927, 1957, and 1969[141]. In 1964 the World Health Organization issued the Helsinki Declaration, which provided ethical guidelines for medical research. The Tuskeegee Syphilis Study violated the Helsinki rule that research subjects must give informed consent.

The Study was started in Macon County, Alabama in 1932 as a spinoff from a 1930 project funded by the Rosenwald fund with a grant of $50,000.00. The study was run by the Public Health Service, which also co-funded mind control research after World War II. During its forty years, numerous accounts of the Study were published in medical journals including a 1964[253] paper in the *Archives of Internal Medicine* entitled, "The Tuskeegee Study of Untreated Syphilis: The 30th Year of Observation."

The paper begins, "The year 1963 marks the 30th year of the long-term evaluation of the effect of un-treated syphilis in the male Negro conducted by the Venereal Disease Branch, Communicable Disease Center, United States Public Health Service. This paper summarizes the information obtained in this study - well known as the "Tuskeegee Study" - from earlier publications."

People and organizations that knew about the Tuskeegee Study included the Surgeon General, the American Heart Association, the Macon County Medical Society, the Public Health Service, and the Center for Disease Control. The first recorded protest about Tuskeegee by a medical doctor did not occur until 1964, when Dr. Irwin J. Schatz, a staff member at Henry Ford Hospital in Detroit, wrote to the first author of a 1964 paper on the study.

Dr. Schatz's letter was referred to the Center for Disease Control where it was filed but not answered. A note by Dr. Anne R. Yobs, a coauthor of the 1964 paper, was stapled to Dr. Schatz's letter. It read, "This is the first letter of this type we have received. I do not plan to answer this letter."

Throughout its forty-year course, the Tuskeegee Study was praised and received various honors. Eunice Rivers, the black nurse who ran the study for decades, received the Oveta Culp Hobby Award for her work in the Study on April 18, 1958. This is the highest commendation the Department of Health, Education and Welfare can bestow on an employee.

What was the design of the Tuskeegee Syphilis Study? In 1932, 399 illiterate poor rural black men with syphilis were recruited as subjects, along with 201 controls without syphilis. The purpose of the Study was to make sure the 399 men never got treatment. They were followed up for decades to see how the syphilis affected them. Part of the purpose of the Study was to compare the results to a similar study done in Norway by Dr. Trygve Gjestland, who visited the Tuskeegee Study in November 1951.

The subjects and their families had no idea what the Study was all about. They weren't told they had syphilis and didn't know it was treatable. A black woman described in the book about Tuskeegee, *Bad Blood*[141], is quoted as saying that injections received at medical clinics were making women in Macon County pregnant. These people had no understanding of disease or modern medicine. *Bad blood* was a term used to describe all kinds of problems in the rural south, ranging from syphilis to pellagra to a general run down condition. The Tuskeegee subjects were told that they had *bad blood*.

In 1932, the standard treatment for syphilis was a combination of mercury, arsphenamine and neoarsphenamine. Although this treatment was primitive, it stopped the progression of the disease and made patients noninfectious. Public Health Service carried out large-scale screening, education and treatment programs for syphilis throughout the 1930's.

The cure for syphilis, penicillin, was introduced in the early 1940's. It was withheld from the Tuskeegee men for thirty years. If any of the men showed up at a non-Study clinic or doctor's office, the Study nurse would contact the staff and say, "He's under study and not to be treated."

The published results of the Study showed, as expected, that the men with untreated syphilis were sicker and died younger than controls. This is only part of the problem. How many acts of unprotected sexual intercourse did these 399 men engage in over forty years? How many women were infected with syphilis because these men were deliberately not treated? How many children were born with congenital syphilis because of the Study? It is a medical certainty that the Tuskeegee Syphilis Study resulted in preventable cases of congenital syphilis.

The contribution of the Tuskeegee men to medical science was recognized and rewarded. In 1958 a certificate bearing the Seal of the U.S. Public Health Service and the signature of the Surgeon General, Dr. Leroy E. Burney, was given to each surviving subject. The certificate read, "This certificate is awarded to _____ in grateful recognition of 25 years of active participation in the Tuskeegee medical research study."

The men were also given $25.00 each, one dollar for each year of participation. Study subject Herman Shaw testified at a Hearing of the Subcommittee on Health of the Committee on Labor and Public Welfare, United States Senate (1973). The Proceedings include a transcript of the following conversation between Mr. Shaw and Senator Edward Kennedy:

Senator KENNEDY:	*Did you feel during this period that you were being cured, that they were looking after your medical needs?*
Mr. SHAW:	*I just got a slap on the back and they said you are good for 100 years. That is all I ever had.*
Senator KENNEDY:	*How many years have they been slapping you on the back?*
Mr. SHAW:	*Forty years.*
Senator KENNEDY:	*You were in the study for forty years?*
Mr. SHAW:	*Yes, sir.*
Senator KENNEDY:	*Did they give you any kind of compensation while they were doing this study?*
Mr. SHAW:	*No sir, with the exception of a 25-year certificate.*

Senator KENNEDY:	Twenty-five year what?
Mr. SHAW:	Twenty-five year health certificate. They gave us a dollar a year, $25.00.
Senator KENNEDY:	A dollar a year?
Mr. SHAW:	Yes, sir. Up to that time, from 1932, up until the time the 25-year limit ran out.
Senator KENNEDY:	So the only compensation you received has been the $25.00?
Mr. SHAW:	That is right.
Senator KENNEDY:	What was the certificate of merit for?
Mr. SHAW:	I do not know, sir. It was for regular attendance, that is all I can figure.
Senator KENNEDY:	Do you think because you kept going back to the nurse or the doctor and letting them take your blood as they told you to do?
Mr. SHAW:	Yes, sir.
Senator KENNEDY:	When you were told to go back, did you think it was a check up and that since they didn't prescribe medication, that therefore you were healthy? What did you assume?
Mr. SHAW:	Every year they would give us a white tablet for pain and a little vial - I guess it was some type of tonic. Every year for forty years up to now, we had two different doctors. We would never get the same doctor back each time.
Senator KENNEDY:	Different doctors?
Mr. SHAW:	Different doctor every year.
Senator KENNEDY:	When was the last time you were at the clinic?
Mr. SHAW:	Last year.
Senator KENNEDY:	What did they tell you last year?
Mr. SHAW:	Slap on the back and said I was good for 100 years. I guess it was routine.

The Tuskeegee Syphilis Study was eventually shut down in 1972 because of the efforts of Peter Buxtun, an investigative journalist. There is no evidence to suggest that the government or the medical profession had any intention of closing the study as of 1972.

In December 1965 Buxtun was hired as a venereal disease investigator by the Public Health Service. As part of his job he began to hear about the Tuskeegee Syphilis Study. He wrote to the Center for Disease Control about it, and was brought to the Center at government expense in 1967. As a result of his visit a panel was convened by the Center for Disease Control on February 6, 1969. The panel, which consisted of five medical doctors, decided to continue the study, which by this time had been taken over by the Center for Disease Control.

Eventually, Buxtun talked about Tuskeegee with his longtime friend, Edith Lederer, an International Affairs reporter with Associated Press. She turned the story over to Jean Heller in Washington, D.C., who published it in the *Washington Post* on July 25, 1972.

Once the Tuskeegee Syphilis Study was in the media, official medical reaction condemned it, and it was shut down. On July 23, 1973 attorney Fred Gray filed a $1.8 billion class action suit in the United States District Court for the Middle District of Alabama. Defendants in the suit were the Department of Health, Education and Welfare, the U.S. Public Health Service, the Center for Disease Control, the State of Alabama, the State Board of Health for Alabama, and the Millbank Fund.

In December, 1974 the government agreed to an out-of-court settlement for $10 million. Cash payments were made as follows: $37,500.00 for every living subject; $15,000.00 to the heirs of deceased subjects; $16,000.00 to living control subjects; and $5,000.00 to the heirs of deceased controls. In May, 1997 President Clinton issued an official apology to the Tuskeegee subjects and their families.

The Tuskeegee Syphilis Study is relevant to mind control in several ways. It establishes that a large network of doctors and organizations were willing to participate in, fund and condone grossly unethical medical experimentation into the 1970's. This is the general setting for psychiatric participation in mind control and creation of the Manchurian Candidate. The Study proves that such experiments resulted in serious damage to study subjects and their children. Finally, the Tuskeegee Syphilis Study proves that considerable external pressure is often required before the medical profession takes the necessary action to terminate such experimentation.

The role of general medicine in Tuskeegee is the same as psychiatry's role in mind control.

3

RADIATION EXPERIMENTS

Unethical radiation experiments were conducted on about 600 subjects in the United States beginning in the 1940's and running into the 1970's [45, 89, 311]. These experiments overlapped with chemical and biological weapons research and mind control experimentation. The radiation experiments were funded by a variety of government agencies including the Department of Defense, the Department of Energy and the CIA. Subjects did not give meaningful informed consent.

As was true of mind control and biological weapons research, radiation experiments were conducted on children and unwitting civilians. Physicians were directly involved in administering the radiation and measuring its effects. The radiation experiments are part of the historical background of psychiatric participation in mind control.

President Clinton set up a Committee to look into radiation experiments after they were described in the media in late 1993. The information had been made public in a Senate Subcommittee report produced by Rep. Edward Markey of Massachusetts in 1986[311], but it didn't generate any public reaction at that time. The Advisory Committee on Human Radiation Experiments issued its *Final Report* in October, 1995.

An example of unethical radiation research is the experiment done on Ebb Cade, a 53-year old black man who was in a car accident on March 24, 1945. He was in treatment for fractures and other injuries at Oak Ridge Army Hospital when he was injected with 4.7 micrograms of plutonium on April 10, five days before his fractures were set. The experimental protocol was to sample his blood for four hours after injection, bone tissue ninety-six hours after, and bodily excretions for 40-60 days, all to measure the plutonium levels. Bone samples were taken when his fractures were set, and also some teeth were extracted for analysis.

Data on Mr. Cade were presented at a "Conference on Plutonium" in Chicago in May, 1945 by Wright Langham of the Los Alamos Laboratory's Health Division. Mr. Cade was given the subject number *HP-12* which stood for "human product", a code also used in radiation experiments at the University of Rochester. Ebb Cade died as a result of heart failure on April 13, 1953 in Greensboro, North Carolina.

Many people were injected with plutonium, x-rayed and exposed to other forms of radiation without their informed consent. Elmer Allen and his wife Fredna, a black couple, were pleased when, in 1973, doctors offered them a free trip to New York to study why he had survived bone cancer for so long (*The Dallas Morning News*, December 31, 1993, page 1A). As part of the trip they were picked up by limousine in Chicago and Mr. Allen was taken to the Argonne National Laboratory while his wife went sightseeing.

Doctors at the University of California in San Francisco injected Mr. Allen with plutonium on July 14, 1947, four days before his leg was amputated for bone cancer. Mr Allen and seventeen other patients were injected with plutonium in an experiment run by the MANHATTAN PROJECT.

John Simpson[311], a retired astrophysicist who worked for the MANHATTAN PROJECT commented on these plutonium injections by saying, "We should be extremely cautious about criticizing their work." He claimed that without such experiments, "radioactive dangers would be greater throughout the world today."

Although that claim is dubious, it misses the point even if accurate. The problem with the experiments is the lack of informed consent and the deceptive rationalizations of the physicians for their ongoing interest in Mr. Allen. These continued into the 1970's and are serious ethical violations even if there was no physical harm to Mr. Allen from the plutonium, and even if the experiments yielded valuable information.

Other subjects were financially compensated for their participation in radiation experiments. Prisoners in Washington and Oregon state prisons were paid to have their testicles irradiated; they got $5.00 a month for the irradiation, $10.00 each time a testicle was biopsied, and $100.00 for completing the experiment. According to project director Dr. Carl Heller, the prisoners received vasectomies "to avoid the possibility of contaminating the general population with irradiation-induced mutants."

Because of the need for vasectomies, Catholic prisoners were excluded from participating. During the experiment, which ran from 1963 to 1971, the subjects' testicles were exposed to 600 roentgen of radiation, which is 100 times the maximum recommended dose. In 1976 a group of subjects filed suit, as a result of which the Oregon State Legislature made an award of $2,215.00. This sum was split among nine men.

Other experiments were conducted at Los Alamos (site of the MANHATTAN PROJECT); Dugway Proving Ground, Utah (site of Army LSD experiments); Oak Ridge, Tennessee; and Hanford Nuclear Facility, Richmond, Washington from 1948 to 1952. Clouds of radioactive material were released into the atmosphere and tracked as they moved downwind, often through populated areas. In one experiment code-named GREEN RUN, radioactive iodine-131 was released from the Hanford Nuclear Facility and drifted over Spokane. The cloud contained hundreds and perhaps thousands as times as much radiation as was released accidentally at Three Mile Island in 1979.

Another project run jointly by Massachusetts General Hospital and the Health Physics Division of Oak Ridge National Laboratory was called the Boston Project. An investigator in this Project was Dr. William Sweet, a neurosurgeon whose brain electrode experiments will be discussed in a later chapter. In 1995 testimony to the Advisory Committee, Dr. Sweet claimed that all subjects injected with uranium in the Boston Project gave informed consent. However, Boston Project subject VI was injected after he arrived at the Emergency Ward unconscious, and he died of a subdural hematoma, without being identified and without regaining consciousness.

Chapter 7 of the *Final Report* is entitled "Nontherapeutic Research on Children." In 1961 researchers at Harvard Medical School, Massachusetts General Hospital and Boston University School of Medicine gave radioactive iodine to seventy retarded children at Wrentham State School. These institutions also received CIA mind control money through MKULTRA.

Other MKULTRA institutions that injected nontherapeutic radioactive materials into children included Johns Hopkins, the University of Minnesota and the Massachusetts Institute of Technology. MIT gave radioactive substances to children at the Fernald School by putting it in their food. The Advisory Committee notes that no risks of radioactivity were mentioned in the consent form signed by the parents. The consent form stated that the purpose of the experiments was "helping to improve the nutrition of our children."

The Advisory Committee says of the nutritional claim, "This was simply not true." (page 344).

In the 1940's, 751 women receiving prenatal care at Vanderbilt University in Tennessee were given experimental radiation doses. Several of the children of these pregnancies died of cancer. One died of leukemia at age 5.

The radiation experiments were interwoven with research on chemical and biological weapons, and infectious diseases[251]. As in the radiation experiments, children were the subjects of biological experiments. It is unknown how many mentally retarded children have been injected with viruses and bacteria in North America. Dr. Saul Krugman of New York University and his staff deliberately injected severely mentally retarded children at Willowbrook State School with hepatitis virus in the 1950's and 1960's[154].

Dr. Krugman's research was funded by the Army Medical Research and Development Command, Department of the Army under contract DA-49-193-MD-2331. It was also sponsored by the Commission on Viral Infections, Armed Forces Epidemiological Board, Office of the Surgeon General. Additionally, it was reviewed and approved by the New York University School of Medicine Committee on Human Experimentation and the New York State Department of Mental Hygiene. The ethics of Krugman's (1971) research were debated in *The Lancet* [107, 153, 282].

Dr. Krugman defended the morality of the project and said that it was scientifically justified. Although to date there has been no compensation for victims of unethical biological experiments, the federal government has officially disagreed with apologists for the radiation experiments. Energy Secretary Hazel O'Leary announced in New York on November 19, 1996 that twelve families of victims of radiation experiments were being compensated for a total of $4.8 million (*The Dallas Morning News*, November 20, 1996, page 6A). The only victim still alive to receive compensation directly was Mary Jean Connell, a 74-year old woman living in Avon, New York.

The radiation experiments are part of the cultural background of psychiatric participation in mind control. Many doctors and leading academic institutions participated directly in the research. The work was conducted in the absence of any public discussion, and without guidelines or monitoring from professional Associations. Informed consent was not obtained, funding sources were not revealed, and subjects were given disinformation about the intent of the experiments by doctors.

The participation of psychiatrists, other physicians and psychologists, and leading medical schools in mind control and radiation research was not an anomaly or aberration. It was not a matter of isolated rogue doctors and the experiments were not conducted during a period with different ethical standards. Much of the research was published in professional journals, though never with acknowledgement that experiments were funded by the CIA. The radiation experiments are part of the climate and historical background for mind control experimentation.

II. Cold War
Mind Control Experimentation

In this section, the major body of information about mind control and the creation of the Manchurian Candidate is presented. The experiments began during World War II and at least some elements of the programs, such as non-lethal weapons, have continued up to the present. Paranormal experiments under STARGATE continued until 1984, and Army doctors were actively involved in LSD testing at least until the late 1970's. Still-classified CIA mind control programs were operational at least into the early 1970's.

Subjects of LSD experiments included children as young as five years old, and brain electrodes were implanted in children as young as eleven years of age. Four of the CIA's MKULTRA Subprojects were on children, a fact that has not been publicly documented before.

The mind control experiments were conducted by a network of doctors that included the leaders of psychiatry and the major medical schools. The mind control doctors included Presidents of the American Psychiatric Association and psychiatrists who received full-page obituaries in *The American Journal of Psychiatry*. In this section of *The CIA Doctors*, extensive documentation of the interconnections between the mind control doctors and institutions is presented. The evidence refutes any claim that the mind control experiments involved only a few isolated renegades, or doctors practicing in an era with different ethical standards.

A number of individual mind control doctors are studied in detail because extensive information about them is available. All psychiatrists and medical schools are implicated because the network is so extensive. Responsibility for the unethical experimentation lies first with the individual doctors, but also collectively with the medical profession as a whole, and with academia as a whole. The Department of Psychiatry at Johns Hopkins University, for instance, may experience *blowback* resulting from decades of collusion, secrecy, and direct participation in mind control experimentation. Blowback is a CIA term for negative publicity resulting from clandestine operations[287]. Somewhere in this network of doctors and medical schools there are as-yet-unidentified creators of Manchurian Candidates.

4

BLUEBIRD AND ARTICHOKE

BLUEBIRD was approved by Roscoe Hillenkoetter, Director of the CIA, on April 20, 1950. In August 1951, the Project was renamed ARTICHOKE. The Korean War began in June, 1950. The CIA already had mind control programs in operation prior to the Korean War, therefore such programs were not a defensive reaction to the activities of the North Koreans, Russians, or Communist Chinese during the Korean War, as claimed by CIA career officer Edward Hunter[136]. BLUEBIRD and ARTICHOKE included a great deal of work on the creation of amnesia, hypnotic couriers and the Manchurian Candidate[66, 184].

The Manchurian Candidate is generally regarded as fiction. However, ARTICHOKE documents prove that hypnotic couriers functioned effectively in real-life simulations conducted by the CIA in the early 1950's. The degree to which such individuals were used in actual operations is still classified. Physicians were an integral part of the ARTICHOKE Team that conducted interrogations on U.S. soil. These interrogations were in part designed to detect mind-controlled agents of other Agencies and governments. The documents establish that Manchurian Candidate-related methods were part of CIA counter-intelligence work in the 1950's.

The basic premise of the book *The Manchurian Candidate*[66] is that a group of American POWs in the Korean War is brainwashed while crossing through Manchuria to freedom. They arrive back in the U.S. amnesic for the period of brainwashing and one of them has been programmed to be an assassin. His target is a candidate for President of the United States. His handlers at home control him with a hypnotically implanted trigger, a particular playing card.

A MEMORANDUM dated 15 July 1953 from the Chief, Bio-Chemistry & Pharmacology Branch, Medicine Division OSI [Office of Scientific

Intelligence] to the Chief, Technical Branch, SO [Special Operations] includes a paragraph summarizing discussions about recently returned Korean War POWs who had been brainwashed:

> *Following this [whited out] commented on the very interesting angle that interrogations of the individuals who had come out of North Korea across the Soviet Union to freedom recently had apparently had a "blank" period or period of disorientation while passing through a special zone in Manchuria. [Whited out] pointed out that this had occurred in all individuals in the party after they had had their first full meal and their first coffee on the way to freedom. [Whited out] pointed out that [whited out] was attempting to secure further confirmatory facts in this matter since drugging was indicated.*

In another memo dated 17 September 1953 the Scientific Adviser, Scientific Intelligence states that, "Detailed and valuable information has been obtained by [whited out] on "Big Switch" as a result of his interrogations of POW's on the return voyage from Korea." "Big Switch" was the code name for a prisoner exchange program during the Korean War; repatriated American prisoners of war released in Big Switch were interviewed by American psychiatrists including Robert Lifton[163]. Lifton[163] (p. 6) writes:

> *. . . I arrived in Hong Kong in late January, 1954. Just a few months before, I had taken part in the psychiatric evaluation of repatriated American prisoners of war during the exchange operations in Korea known as <u>Big Switch</u>; I had then accompanied a group of these men on the troopship back to the United States.*

It appears that American psychiatrists including or known to Robert Lifton, Louis Jolyon West and Margaret Singer must have been knowledgeable about the Chinese Manchurian Candidate program by 1953.

According to my definition, the Manchurian Candidate is an experimentally created dissociative identity disorder that meets the following four criteria:

> *1. Created deliberately*
> *2. A new identity is implanted*
> *3. Amnesia barriers are created*
> *4. Used in simulated or actual operations*

BLUEBIRD and ARTICHOKE were administered in a *compartmented* fashion. The details of the Programs were kept secret even from other personnel within the CIA. When asked why LSD research done under ARTICHOKE was hidden from the CIA Committee in charge of ARTICHOKE, Sydney Gottlieb (*Human Drug Testing by the CIA*, 1977, page 410), Chief, Medical Staff, Technical Services Division, CIA responded, "I imagine the only reason would have been concern for broadening awareness of its existence."

The creation of Manchurian Candidates by the CIA was probably not subject to the usual chain of operational command. Such breaches in the chain of command are an inherent structural risk of the *compartmented* nature of intelligence agencies. For security reasons, CIA operations including internal counter-intelligence investigations[182] are routinely kept secret from other divisions of the CIA. Although effective intelligence work could not be carried out without compartmentation, the structure makes it easier for CIA officers in charge of mind control to contract with unethical doctors.

Loss of central control occurred in the CIA's OPERATION CHAOS and probably in BLUEBIRD and ARTICHOKE. OPERATION CHAOS was a CIA program designed to collect information on foreign influence on student and civil unrest in the United States. It was created by the Director of the CIA in 1967 and ran until 1974. CHAOS developed files on 7,200 American citizens, and the files included mention of a total of 300,000 named U.S. citizens and organizations, all of which were entered into a computerized index (*The Nelson Rockefeller Report to the President by the Commission on CIA Activities*, 1975).

CHAOS intelligence generated 3,500 internal CIA memoranda, 3,000 memoranda for the FBI, and 37 for distribution to the White House and other top levels of government. The maximum CHAOS staff was 52 persons in 1971. Informants were recruited from student and dissident groups, and were instructed to infiltrate such groups in the United States.

According to *The Nelson Rockefeller Report to the President by the Commission on CIA Activities*:

> The isolation of Operation CHAOS within the CIA and its independence from supervision by the regular chain of command within the clandestine services made it possible for the activities of the Operation to stray over the bounds of the

Agency's authority without the knowledge of senior officials. The absence of any regular review of these activities prevented timely correction of such missteps as did occur.

In other instances, senior administrators within the CIA participated in plausible denial and other disinformation and cover-up strategies concerning CIA operations run on U.S. soil. Like the activities of the ARTICHOKE Team within the United States, such operations had to be kept secret because the CIA was prohibited by its Charter from carrying out operations in the United States.

In 1952, the CIA began to survey mail between the U.S. and the Soviet Union at a New York postal facility. In 1953 it began to open and read mail. The Program was approved by the Director of the CIA and at least three Postmasters General, Summerfield, Day, and Blount, as well as by Attorney General Mitchell. From 1958 to 1973, the FBI received 57,000 pieces of mail from the CIA in this Program. In the final year of the operation, out of 4,350,000 pieces of mail between the U.S. and Soviet Union, the CIA examined the outside of 2,300,000 pieces, photographed 33,000 and opened 8,700.

Smaller mail intercept operations were run in San Francisco from 1969 to 1971, in Hawaii from 1954 to 1955, and in New Orleans in 1957. The CIA's strategy for dealing with leaks about the Program is described in a February 1, 1962 memo sent from the Deputy Chief of Counterintelligence to the Director of Security:

Unless the charge is supported by the presentation of interior items from the project, it should be relatively easy to "hush up" the entire affair, or to explain that it consists of legal mail cover activities conducted by the Post Office at the request of authorized Federal Agencies. Under the most unfavorable circumstances, including the support of charges with interior items from the project it might become necessary, after the matter has cooled off during an extended period of investigation, to find a scapegoat to blame for unauthorized tampering with the mails.

The BLUEBIRD and ARTICHOKE documents available through the Freedom of Information Act, like all such documents, are heavily redacted. A great deal of text has been whited out, and other documents must still be entirely classified. Nevertheless, the available documents prove that ARTICHOKE operations involving physicians were carried out on U.S. soil at least until the mid-1950's.

A memo to the Director of Security of the CIA is entitled "report of ARTICHOKE Operations, 20 to 23 January, 1955" (see Appendix B). Paragraph two of the memo states that "these operations were the first ARTICHOKE operations undertaken in the United States."

The operation described in the memo involved the interrogation of a foreign national CIA agent who "speaks and understands English quite well." The Subject had previously provided high quality intelligence through penetration actions carried out in an unspecified country. The purpose of the ARTICHOKE Team's interrogation was to provide confirmation that the Subject was not a double agent.

The ARTICHOKE Team must have been under the command of James Angleton, who was Chief of the CIA Counterintelligence Staff from December 1954, until 1974. Angleton was also involved in MKULTRA, as described in an article in the February 18, 1979 *Wilmington Sunday News Journal* entitled "UD prof helps concoct 'mind control' potions." The article focuses on MKULTRA Subproject 51 contractor James Moore, a chemistry professor at the University of Delaware, but mentions Angleton's involvement in MKULTRA. Angleton's name appears in "a list of all persons who have been briefed on "Bluebird"," in a 2 July 1951 MEMORANDUM; the list also identifies three future Directors of the CIA, Allen Dulles, Richard Helms and William Webster.

The ARTICHOKE interrogation was conducted in a safe house in the remote countryside staffed by security-cleared personnel. It was conducted under medical cover of a routine physical and psychological assessment. The Subject was transported to the safe house in a "covert car" which picked him up at a secure location. At the safe house he was given a conventional interrogation and then some whiskey. This was followed by two grams of phenobarbital, which put him to sleep.

The next day a lie detector test was given, and the Subject was given intravenous chemicals. Following the chemically-assisted interrogation, according to CIA terminology, the "ARTICHOKE techniques were applied" in three stages:

1. *A false memory was introduced into the Subject's mind without his conscious control of the process, which took 15 to 20 minutes.*

2. *The procedure was repeated, this time taking 40 to 45 minutes.*

3. *The procedure was repeated again with interrogation added.*

The ARTICHOKE Team used medications including barbiturates, amphetamines and scopolamine, hypnosis, interrogation, and the deliberate introduction of false memories of the procedure. The Subject was told that part of what he remembered was actually a dream. The ARTICHOKE Team concluded that the procedure was successful; "the subject, although not having specific amnesia for the ARTICHOKE treatment, nevertheless was completely confused and memory was vague and faulty."

CIA career officer Edward Hunter [136] described the implantation of false memories by Chinese intelligence agencies in his book *Brain-Washing in Red China*. He wrote (page 11):

> *The Chinese masses were right in coining the phrases brain-washing and brain-changing There is a difference between the two. Brain-washing is indoctrination, a comparatively simple procedure, but brain-changing is immeasurably more sinister and complicated. Whereas you merely have to undergo a brain-cleansing to rid yourself of "imperialist poisons," in order to have a brain changing you must empty your mind of old ideas and recollections... in a brain-changing, a person's specific recollections of some past period in his life are wiped away, as completely as if they never happened. Then, to fill these gaps in memory, the ideas which the authorities want this person to "remember" are put into his brain. Hypnotism and drugs and cunning pressures that plague the body and do not necessarily require marked physical violence are required for a brain-changing. China evidently was not so "advanced" as yet. She was using brain-washing, and when that didn't work, resorted to the simpler purge system. But in time she will use the brain-changing system too.*

Since, according to Hunter, the Communist Chinese had not yet perfected the methods used by the CIA's ARTICHOKE Team, it is evident that his knowledge of these methods was derived from their use by American doctors.

An interrogation involving ARTICHOKE techniques and physicians was conducted on Russian defector Yuriy Nosenko under James Angleton's administration[182]. Angleton suspected Nosenko of being a triple agent. A triple agent is someone who pretends to be a defector or double agent but is actually working for his original, native country.

Nosenko was born in Nikolayev, Ukraine in 1927. He was trained by Russian Naval Intelligence before being transferred to MVD, the precursor of the KGB, in 1953. On June 5, 1962 Nosenko made secret contact with a U.S. State Department official in Geneva, a meeting that resulted in his being recruited by the CIA as a mole. Nosenko provided a rich fund of intelligence information to the CIA until he defected in February, 1964.

Angleton thought that Nosenko had been feeding the CIA a little bit of real information in order to cover up the fact that he was a triple agent. In late March, 1964 a decision was made to apply ARTICHOKE-like techniques to him. Whether these were administered under ARTICHOKE or some other still-classified cryptonym is unknown.

Nosenko was strip-searched, given a lie detector test and then placed in solitary confinement in a 10-foot by 10-foot cell in a safe house in Washington for sixteen months. One of his interrogators was Dr. John Gittinger, the lead psychologist for MKULTRA, who describes taking LSD himself in a documentary film[210]. From April 4, 1964 to August 13, 1965, Nosenko was held at the safe house and subjected to repeated interrogations.

From August 14, 1965 to October 28, 1967 Nosenko was held in solitary confinement in a tiny, windowless concrete cell at the CIA's training facility at Camp Peary, Virginia. He was subjected to sleep and food deprivation and there was neither heat nor air conditioning in his cell. He was monitored by closed-circuit television 24 hours a day.

In an interview with Tom Mangold [177] on June 12, 1990, John Gittinger described being asked by CIA personnel to administer LSD to Nosenko. Gittinger claimed he did not do so. Nosenko, however, described being drugged on a number of occasions at Camp Peary. Due to administrative changes inside the CIA, Nosenko was released from confinement in 1967 and later became a U.S. citizen.

Whoever the Nosenko interrogators were, and whatever cryptonym they worked under, it is clear that physicians and mind control specialists were directly involved. It is also clear that the actions of these physicians were unethical and inhumane. The BLUEBIRD and ARTICHOKE documents prove that the Nosenko interrogation was not an isolated incident. If such an interrogation was conducted by physicians in a third world country it would be decried as a human rights violation and a political abuse of psychiatry. We have been lax as a medical profession in applying the same standards at home.

The need for applying the ARTICHOKE technique to Nosenko can be inferred from an undated document entitled, "IMPLICATIONS OF SOVIET SUPPLEMENTS TO STANDARD PSYCHIATRIC INTERROGATION", which includes the statement that:

> _Hypnotism appears to have been used in some cases by the Soviet. It has the possibilities of (a) lowering resistance against telling the truth and (b) inducing specific action or behavior in the subject. In certain cases it would be possible for a skilled Russian operator to bring about condition (a) yet leave the subject with no specific recollection of having been interrogated. Under condition (b) it would be possible to brief an American, other prisoner or person, subsequently dispatch him on a mission, and successfully debrief him upon return home without his recollection of the briefing or debriefing._

Another undated document entitled, "DEFENSE AGAINST SOVIET MEDICAL INTERROGATION AND ESPIONAGE TECHNIQUES" echoes this point:

> _This proposed investigation appears to be more essential when documentary evidence leads to the belief that Russia has been conducting medical research on the subject, has actually used various techniques, and has made provision for large scale production of uncommon special drugs for their speech-producing effects on prisoners of war._
>
> _Adequate evidence is available to indicate that the Soviet has used physical duress and/or a large number of different drugs in their attempts to enhance results of standard psychiatric interrogation._

Evidence of subconscious isolation, amnesia, and destruction of mental function have been noted in some of the victims of Soviet methods.

All of these methods were also employed in experiments conducted under BLUEBIRD, ARTICHOKE, MKULTRA, MKSEARCH, MKNAOMI and other Programs.

ARTICHOKE operations involved detailed, systematic creation of specific amnesia barriers, new identities and hypnotically implanted codes and triggers. An untitled ARTICHOKE document dated 7 January 1953 with a section heading *Outline of Special H Cases* describes the experimental creation of multiple personality in two nineteen-year old girls by the CIA, in an extended series of hypnotic sessions beginning on January 9, 1952. "H" is used as shorthand for hypnotic, hypnotized or hypnotism in these documents:

In all of these cases, these subjects have clearly demonstrated that they can pass from a fully awake state to a deep H controlled state via the telephone, via some very subtle signal that cannot be detected by other persons in the room and without the other individual being able to note the change. It has been clearly shown that physically individuals can be induced into H by telephone, by receiving written matter, or by the use of code, signal, or words and that control of those hypnotized can be passed from one individual to another without great difficulty. It has also been shown by experimentation with these girls that they can act as unwilling couriers for information purposes and that they can be conditioned to a point where they believe a change in identity on their part even on the polygraph.

Another untitled ARTICHOKE document describes a series of cases of which the following, called "Analogous Case #3," is most compelling:

A CIA Security Office employee was hypnotized and given a false identity. She defended it hotly, denying her true name and rationalizing with conviction the possession of identity cards made out to her real self. Later, having had the false identity erased by suggestion, she was asked if she had ever heard of the name she had been defending as her own five minutes before. She thought, shook her head and said, "That's a pseudo if I ever heard one." Apparently she had a true amnesia for the entire episode.

The creation of new identities and the detection of foreign agents with hypnotically programmed new identities is mentioned in various locations in the BLUEBIRD and ARTICHOKE documents. As well, deconditioning of subjects is addressed. For instance, one document entitled, "CONDITIONING (& Deconditioning)" states:

Jones learns to respond to stimuli intended for a Smith, as though he were that Smith. He has been "conditioned" to Smith, "deconditioned" to Jones.

Such trainings are integrated on all levels, conscious and subconscious. <u>Hypnosis</u> can assist in establishing the desired conditioned responses.

A C.R. (condit. resp.) is meant to stick. It can be interfered with, or abolished, by new training in another direction, or back to the earlier state.

Deconditioning can probably be expedited by hypnotizing procedures. Also, a C.R. can be interfered with or abolished by violent physical shocks (e.g., electric shocks to the brain) although this reporter has not found a specific electric-shock procedure that would assuredly decondition any particular kind or number of C.R.'s.

Still problematic is the use of drugs for deconditioning. Chlorpromazine ought theoretically to have some value, and some deconditioning effect has been produced in laboratory animals. However, hospitalized patients taking daily doses of this drug seem to have been deconditioned only selectively; against certain psychotic behavior. It may be that this property is exactly what we are looking for; perhaps it could decondition an enemy agent out of his simulated personality and back to his real one.

It is evident from this passage that the CIA was seeking to improve its techniques for detecting and successfully penetrating the amnesia barriers of enemy Manchurian Candidates over five years before the book *The Manchurian Candidate*[66] was written.

A MEMORANDUM dated 25 January 1952 describes another case in which problems of reconditioning and the disposal of subjects arose:

On Friday, 25 January 1952, the writer was called to the office [whited out] for the purpose of a conference with one [whited out] concerning the instant case.

[Whited out] explained in substance the [whited out] case as follows: [whited out] (whose real name is [whited out], is a 29-year old [whited out] and was the head of a small political party based in [whited out] and ostensively working for [whited out] independence. [Whited out] was described by [whited out] as being young, ambitious, bright (elementary college education), a sort of "man-on-a-horse" type but a typical [whited out] politician. According to [whited out] our people discovered that [whited out] Intelligence Service were attempting to bribe [whited out] and make him a double agent and [whited out] was looking with favor upon the [whited out] offers. Accordingly, a plot was rigged in which [whited out] was told he was going to be assassinated and as a "protection", he was placed in custody of the [whited out] Police who threw [whited out] into a [whited out] prison. [Whited out] was held in the [whited out] prison for six months until the [whited out] authorities decided that [whited out] was a nuisance and they told our people to take him back. Since our people were unable to dispose of [whited out] they flew him to [whited out] where, through arrangement, he was placed in a [whited out] as a psychopathic patient. [Whited out] now has been in the [whited out] hospital for several months and the hospital authorities now want to get him out since he is causing a considerable trouble, bothering other patients, etc. [Whited out] is not a psychopathic personality.

[Whited out] explained that they can dispose of [whited out] by the simple process of sending him to a friend of his in [whited out], and as far as they are concerned, that type of disposal is perfectly o.k. However, because of his confinement in [whited out] prison and his stay in [whited out] hospital, [whited out] has become very hostile toward the [whited out] and our intelligence operations in particular. Hence [whited out] considering an "Artichoke" approach to [whited out] to see if it would be possible to re-orient [whited out] favorably toward us. This operation, which will necessarily involve the use of drugs is

being considered by [whited out] with a possibility that [whited out] will carry out the operation presumably at the [whited out] hospital in [whited out] Also involved in this would be a [whited out] interpreter who is a consultant to this Agency since neither [whited out].

[Whited out] pointed out to [whited out] that this type of operation could only be carried out with the authorization of Security and that, under no circumstances whatsoever, could anyone but an authorized M.D. administer drugs to any subject of this Agency of any type. [Whited out] pointed out that there was a strong possibility that the military authorities would not permit their hospital to be used for this type of work and also that a re-conditioning operation of this type might take 30-60 days. [Whited out] further pointed out that if such an operation were carried on, Security would have to be cognizant of it, would have to be co-ordinated into the organization and would possibly take over and run the operation themselves since this type of work is one which Security handles.

It was agreed between [whited out] and the writer that a conference would be laid on Monday afternoon when [whited out] representatives and the [whited out] interpreter return from [whited out] and their talk with [whited out] At which time, the angles would be explored and a dispatch would be forwarded to our people in [whited out] directing them to find out whether the [whited out] would permit such an operation and whether the [whited out] would allow the Agency to have the use of the necessary rooms, medical facilities, etc. as would be required for this type of operation. At this time, it was also to be determined whether the disposal of [whited out] could <u>in fact</u> be laid on.

Comment:

This particular operation was mentioned in general terms to the writer by [whited out] approximately thirty days ago on an informal basis but no significant details were given at this time.

While the technique that [whited out] are considering for use in this case is not known to the writer, the writer believes the approach will be made through the standard narco-hypnosis technique. Re-conditioning and re-orienting an individual in such a matter, in the opinion of the writer, cannot be accomplished easily and will require a great deal of time and the fact that an interpreter is necessary in the case complicates it considerably more. It is also believed that with our present knowledge, we would have no absolute guarantee that the subject in this case would maintain a positive friendly attitude toward us even though there is apparently a successful response to the treatment. The writer did not suggest to [whited out] that perhaps a total amnesia could be created by a series of electric shocks, but merely indicated that amnesias under drug treatments were not certain.

A document entitled, "Hypnotic Experimentation and Research, 10 February 1954" describes a simulation experiment of relevance to the creation of Manchurian Candidate assassins:

Miss [whited out] was then instructed (having previously expressed a fear of firearms in any fashion) that she would use every method at her disposal to awaken Miss [whited out] (now in a deep hypnotic sleep) and failing in this, she would pick up a pistol nearby and fire it at Miss [whited out]. She was instructed that her rage would be so great that she would not hesitate to "kill" [whited out] for failing to awaken. Miss [whited out] carried out these suggestions to the letter including firing the (unloaded pneumatic pistol) gun at [whited out] and then proceeding to fall into a deep sleep. After proper suggestions were made, both were awakened and expressed complete amnesia for the entire sequence. Miss [whited out] was again handed the gun, which she refused (in an awakened state) to pick up or accept from the operator. She expressed absolute denial that the foregoing sequence had happened.

In another experiment described in a document entitled "SI and H Experimentation (25 September 1951)," two of the female subjects took part in an exercise involving the planting of a bomb. SI means "Special Interrogations." Both Subjects performed perfectly and were fully amnesic for the exercise:

[Whited out] was instructed that upon awakening, she would proceed to [whited out] room where she would wait at the desk for a telephone call. Upon receiving the call, a person known as "Jim" would engage her in normal conversation. During

the course of the conversation, this individual would mention a code word to [whited out]. When she heard this code word she would pass into a SI trance state, but would not close her eyes and remain perfectly normal and continue the telephone conversation. She was told that thereafter upon conclusion of the telephone conversation, she would then carry out the following instructions:

[Whited out] being in a complete SI state at this time, was then told to open her eyes and was shown an electric timing device. She was informed that this timing device was an incendiary bomb and was then instructed how to attach and set the device. After [whited out] had indicated that she had learned how to set and attach the device, she was told to return to a sleep state and further instructed that upon concluding of the aforementioned conversation, she would take the timing device which was in a briefcase and proceed to the ladies room. In the ladies room, she would be met by a girl whom she had never seen who would identify herself by the code word "New York". After identifying herself, [whited out] was then to show this individual how to attach and set the timing device and further instructions would be given the individual by [whited out] that the timing device was to be carried in the briefcase to [whited out] room, placed in the nearest empty electric-light plug and concealed in the bottom, left-hand drawer of [whited out] desk, with the device set for 82 seconds and turned on. [Whited out] was further instructed to tell this other girl that as soon as the device had been set and turned on, she was to take the briefcase, leave [whited out] room, go to the operations room and go to the sofa and enter a deep sleep state. [Whited out] was further instructed that after completion of instructing the other girl and the transferring to the other girl of the incendiary bomb, she was to return at once to the operations room, sit on the sofa, and go into a deep sleep state.

Hypnosis was not the mind control doctors' only method for creation of controlled amnesia, however. Drugs, magnetic fields, sound waves, sleep deprivation, solitary confinement and many other methods were studied under BLUEBIRD and ARTICHOKE. The amnesia was often tested through memorization tasks of various kinds, and experiments were conducted to amplify subjects' memory for information hidden behind amnesia barriers. As well as being potential couriers and infiltration agents, the subjects could function in effect as hypnotically controlled cameras. They could enter a room or building, memorize materials quickly, leave the building, and then be amnesic for the entire episode. The memorized material could then be retrieved by a handler using a previously implanted code or signal, without the amnesia being disturbed. The research and its applications were both offensive and defensive, as evidenced by the following untitled and undated passage from the documents:

> For instance, Metrozal, which has been very useful in shock therapy, is no longer popular because, for one thing it produces feelings of overwhelming terror and doom prior to the convulsion.

> But terror, anxiety, worry would be valuable for many purposes from our point of view. We have some information (not in detail and not confirmed) that the Soviets and their satellites have used drugs which work along these lines. Therefore, this should be studied both from our use offensively and defensively and to find antidotes or counteracting agents.

The many different physical means for assisting interrogators were often combined with or amplified by hypnosis:

> Quite often amnesia occurs for events just prior to the convulsion, during the convulsion and during the post seizure state. It is possible that hypnosis or hypnotic activity induced during the post-seizure state might be lost in amnesia. This would be very valuable.

The fact that complex Manchurian Candidate experiments were conducted can be inferred from an untitled February 6, 1957 document in which the writer states that:

> Since the international situation is in its present state, I feel the need for positive action in the military application of hypnosis is imperative. In a field such as this you need an individual, such as myself, who has lived with the problems of hypnotism and its military applications for many years...

> Please look over the enclosed proposal and give me your reaction. The hypnotic messenger technique is relatively uncomplicated. There are several other projects which I could submit to you for

consideration which are, in my opinion, even more important than this but involve much more complicated techniques.

Similarly, a MEMORANDUM from the Chief, Security Research Staff to the Chief, Technical Branch dated 15 July 1954 states that:

The idea of a courier that has been hypnotized is not new and I am absolutely certain that [whited out] did not invent this idea. We ourselves have carried out much more complex problems than this and in a general sense I will agree that it is feasible...

[Whited out] proposal about using hypnotized individuals as counteragents is also not new and we, of course, have discussed this many times. Whether in fact it can be demonstrated we are not sure and it is hoped that the field tests we are working on may help us along these lines.

Yet another document entitled "STUDIES IN THE MILITARY APPLICATION OF HYPNOTISM: I. The Hypnotic Messenger" is a proposal for a grant of $10,000.00 to create hypnotic messengers out of twenty selected highly hypnotizable military personnel. The subjects would be sent to foreign countries to deliver their messages and then would be interrogated to determine if the amnesia barriers could be breached. Interrogation methods were to include "use of his wife, girl friend, alcohol, amytal or even physical duress."

Another prospective mind control doctor wrote a handwritten note to the CIA on a ruled notepad that has been labeled "A/B 5, 264/1" by hand by someone responsible for filing the document. "A/B" stands for ARTICHOKE/BLUEBIRD. The document reads:

I have developed a technic which is safe and secure (free from international censorship). It has to do with the conditioning of our own people. I can accomplish this as a one man job.

The method is the production of hypnosis by means of simple oral medication. Then (with no further medication) the hypnosis is re-enforced daily during the following three or four days.

Each individual is conditioned against revealing any information to an enemy, even though subjected to hypnosis or drugging.

If preferable, he may be conditioned to give _false_ information rather than _no_ information.

This should be repeated every six months in each case, in order to be sure that the suggestions established have not "worn off."

I would be glad to go anywhere in the world (including Korea) to accomplish this for you. I think that the greatest security would be in my travelling as a naval flight surgeon doing research in aviation medicine, especially with the project of "motion sickness" in mind.

Of course I would be willing to undertake more hazardous investigative methods if you should deem them advisable.

Another problem addressed repeatedly in the documents is called "The Problem of Disposal of Subjects." Several personnel recommended the use of lobotomies for this purpose, but according to the documents this was rejected as too unethical and too high a negative publicity risk for the CIA. Another document describes an alternative strategy for disposing of ARTICHOKE subjects:

Among the important security problems, which will be discussed in detail later and which are mentioned only briefly now for a matter of record, were the problems of disposal of subjects after Artichoke treatment and the important questions as to whether or not amnesias had been obtained. In connection with Case #1, in the professional opinion of [whited out] and as far as the writer is able to determine, a total amnesia was produced. Disposal of Case #1 (which was not a problem of the Artichoke team) was apparently handled as follows: Since the Artichoke technique had shown that, from an operational point of view the subject had no further value to the Agency, the subject was to be returned to [whited out] and after a period of time, removed from solitary and gradually permitted to mingle with larger and larger prison groups. Ultimately, and after a considerable lapse of time (perhaps as much as two years), the subject would be released. The Artichoke Team recommended some observation in this case with a later recheck on the amnesia, if possible.

In Case #2 on the first test, an almost total amnesia was reached with the exception of the last ten or twelve minutes of interrogation under the hypnotic technique. In the opinion of [whited out] and as far as the writer was able to determine, a total amnesia was produced at the end of the test on the second day after the Artichoke treatment of sodium pentothal and Desoxyn (full medication without hypnosis).

Again in so far as disposal of Case #2 was concerned (which was not a problem of the Artichoke Team), disposition was apparently to be made as follows: it had been decided that the subject would be moved as a prisoner to some place in [whited out] and held there until any possible usefulness to anyone had completely disappeared.

As noted above, both of the subjects were [whited out] speaking only and neither subject had any working knowledge of the English language. This, of course, involved the use of an interpreter and, in both cases, [whited out] the case officer involved in Case #1, acted as a general interpreter and [whited out] acted as a specific interpreter in the application of the hypnotic technique (under the direct guidance of [whited out] in hypnotic matters) and also acted as general interpreter in both cases.

Physicians including psychiatrists were directly involved in all of the ARTICHOKE team operations. Documents refer to psychiatrists "of considerable note" who were professors at prominent medical schools, who had TOP SECRET CIA clearance and who were involved as consultants on the development of the ARTICHOKE techniques. In summarizing the role of physicians in providing cover for ARTICHOKE interrogations, a writer stated that:

At the present time, the use of a carefully laid on medical cover to obtain either a narco-interrogation or narco-hypnotic interrogation appears to be the best weapon presently available. It is not necessary to go into detail as to how this is done but experience indicates it is our best technique.

The use of electric shock to the brain for creation of amnesia, and amplification of the amnesia with hypnosis were discussed by the author of an ARTICHOKE document dated 3 December 1951:

Immediately after the conference on Friday, 30 November 1951, [whited out] succeeded in finding [whited out] and [whited out], and the writer discussed electric-shock devices and certain related matters from about 3:30 to 4:45 with [whited out].

[Whited out] is reported to be an authority on electric shock. He is a professor at the Medical School of the [whited out] and, in addition, is a psychiatrist of considerable note. Pro-[whited out] is, in addition, a fully cleared Agency consultant.

[Whited out] explained that he felt that electric shock might be of considerable interest to the "Artichoke" type of work. He stated that the standard electric-shock machine (Reiter) could be used in two ways. One setting of this machine produced the normal electric-shock treatment (including convulsion) with amnesia after a number of treatments. He stated that using this machine as an electro-shock device with the convulsive treatment, he felt that he could guarantee amnesia for certain periods of time and particularly he could guarantee amnesia for any knowledge of use of the convulsive shock.

[Whited out] stated that the other or lower setting of the machine produced a different type of shock. He said that he could not explain it, but knew that when this lower current type of shock was applied without convulsion, it had the effect of making a man talk. He said, however, that the use of this type of shock was prohibited because it produced in the individual excruciating pain and he stated that there would be no question in his mind that the individual would be quite willing to give information if threatened with the use of this machine. He stated that this was a third-degree method but, undoubtedly, would be effective. [Whited out] stated that he had never had the device applied to himself, but he had talked with people who had been shocked in this manner and stated that they complained that their whole head was on fire and it was much too painful a treatment for any medical practice. He stated that the only way it was ever used was in connection with sedatives and even then it was extremely painful. The writer asked [whited out] whether or not in the "groggy" condition following the convulsion by the electro-shock machine anyone had attempted to obtain hypnotic control over the patient, since it occurred to the writer that it would be a good time to attempt to obtain hypnotic control. [Whited out] stated that, to his knowledge, it had never been done, but he could make this attempt in the near future at the [whited out] and he would see whether or not this could be done.

[Whited out] and [whited out], as well as all others present, discussed the use of electro shock at considerable length and it was [whited out] opinion that an individual could gradually be reduced through the use of electro-shock treatment to the vegetable level. He stated that, whereas amnesia could be guaranteed relative the actual use of the shock and the time element surrounding it, he said it would obtain perfect amnesia for periods further back. He stated several instances in which people who had been given the electro-shock treatment remembered some details of certain things and complete blanks in other ways.

[Whited out] said that a [whited out], who is practicing in [whited out] has perfected a battery-driven machine which, according to [whited out] is portable. [Whited out] said that the standard electro-shock machine is a very common machine in medical offices and in the major cities there must be several hundred of them in use at all times.

The use of electro-shock to produce amnesia was subsequently successfully demonstrated in a series of cases by Dr. Ewen Cameron at McGill, who received CIA money through MKULTRA Subproject 68 in 1957. Many of the discussions, literature reviews and experiments conducted under BLUEBIRD and ARTICHOKE were followed up on in MKULTRA and MKSEARCH.

The involvement of physicians including psychiatrists in BLUEBIRD and ARTICHOKE was extensive, systematic and fundamental to the Programs. The involvement included consultation, literature reviews, experimentation and direct participation in field operations. The full extent of this involvement is unknown because the names of the mind control doctors who created Manchurian Candidates are redacted from documents provided under the Freedom of Information Act, and because there are undoubtedly other documents which are still classified.

5
MKULTRA AND MKSEARCH

ARTICHOKE and BLUEBIRD were administratively rolled over into MKULTRA, which was created by the CIA on April 3, 1953. However, independent reports under ARTICHOKE continued into 1955. MKULTRA was in turn rolled over into MKSEARCH on June 7, 1964. MKSEARCH then ran until June, 1972, at which time extensive shredding of MKULTRA and MKSEARCH files was ordered by the Director of the CIA, Richard Helms. The surviving MKULTRA documents can be obtained from the CIA under the Freedom of Information Act, and MKSEARCH documents are in the process of being declassified. The four Directors of the CIA during MKULTRA and MKSEARCH were:

Allen W. Dulles	February 6, 1953 - November 29, 1961
John A. McCone	November 29, 1961 - April 28, 1965
William F. Raborn	April 28, 1965 - June 30, 1966
Richard Helms	June 30, 1966 - February 2, 1973

Like all other mind control materials, the MKULTRA documents are heavily redacted. All personal names are white out with two exceptions; that of the contractor for Subprojects 4, 15, 19 and 34, the magician John Mulholland, and that of Dr. Sidney Gottlieb, the CIA officer who ran MKULTRA from inside the CIA's Technical Services Division (TSD). TSD is also referred to as TSS in the documents. Administratively, TSS was part of the section of the CIA that ran spies and carried out clandestine operations. Other divisions were responsible for security, administration, and information gathering and analysis, but not field operations.

MKULTRA was divided into the 149 Subprojects listed in Appendix C. MKSEARCH consisted of the 7 Subprojects listed in Appendix D. Missing data in Appendices C and D is due to information still being classified and/or lack of success in piecing together identities and institutions from other sources and documents. These are by far the most systematic and comprehensive inventories of the MKULTRA and MKSEARCH Subprojects available to date. The clearance status of the individual investigators is left blank in the Appendices when it cannot be confirmed from the documents, even though in several instances other information sources lead to the conclusion that the investigator had TOP SECRET clearance. The clearance statuses listed in the Appendices are all definite and confirmed.

A typical MKULTRA file contains routine correspondence and internal CIA memos, financial audit information, copies of cancelled checks and invoices, and sometimes no material of any interest. Some Subproject files contain hundreds of pages, others only a dozen or two. Most contain a MEMORANDUM FOR THE RECORD like the ones for Subprojects 96, 103 and 142 (see Appendix C) which give the clearance status of the investigator, the amount of funding, the year of startup of the Subproject, and its basic purpose. Some files contain lengthy grant proposals and literature reviews by the investigators.

Additionally, the CIA will provide a list of INSTITUTIONAL NOTIFICATIONS, which list some but not all of the BLUEBIRD, ARTICHOKE, MKULTRA and MKSEARCH institutions. Many of the institution names are redacted. This material also lists which Subprojects were connected to which institution for MKULTRA and MKSEARCH.

Although the fact that the research was funded by the CIA was secret, much of it was published in the peer-reviewed literature. This material cannot be located unless one already knows the names of the contractors, or at least the year, institution and subject matter of the Subproject.

Another hurdle in completing Appendices C and D was explained by Dr. Robert Lashbrook, a CIA doctor involved in the death of Frank Olson. Olson was a Fort Detrick biological warfare expert who committed suicide after being given LSD hidden in Cointreau liqueur by Dr. Sidney Gottlieb, Director of MKULTRA. Olson's family determined that he had committed suicide subsequent to a bad LSD trip only after reading Nelson Rockefeller's 1975 Report on the CIA, published 22 years after Olson's death. They were given $750,000 in compensation by Congress. Dr. Lashbrook explained the CIA's filing system in Senate testimony transcribed in *Human Drug Testing by the CIA, 1977* (page 111):

Dr. LASHBROOK:　　All right. As I think I was intimating a little
　　　　　　　　　　bit before, I cannot make much sense out of
　　　　　　　　　　what you have read. It was intimated before,
　　　　　　　　　　I think, a large part of the documents you
　　　　　　　　　　have of this nature, are what we called
　　　　　　　　　　boilerplate -

Senator KENNEDY:　Excuse me?

Dr. LASHBROOK:　　Boilerplate. What was actually signed off on
　　　　　　　　　　was not the same as the actual proposal, or
　　　　　　　　　　actual project.

Senator KENNEDY:　How frequently do you use boilerplate?
　　　　　　　　　　Do you sign off on things that are not relevant
　　　　　　　　　　to what is happening?

Dr. LASHBROOK:　　You have both. You have what you sign
　　　　　　　　　　on, and the actual project, side by side.

Senator KENNEDY:　Who had got the real file?

Dr. LASHBROOK:　　TSS. [Technical Services Staff of the CIA].

Senator KENNEDY:　You mean this is not the real file. It is stamped
　　　　　　　　　　top secret.

Dr. LASHBROOK:　　It is a real file. It is the one which
　　　　　　　　　　goes through, receives the signatures,
　　　　　　　　　　and is then filed.

Senator KENNEDY:　It is what?

Dr. LASHBROOK:　　It is then filed?

Senator KENNEDY:　It is a real file, but does not mean anything, is
　　　　　　　　　　that about what you
　　　　　　　　　　are saying.

Dr. LASHBROOK:　　It has administrative value.

Senator KENNEDY:　It is not telling what the story is?

Dr. LASHBROOK:　　That is right. Not necessarily.

Senator KENNEDY:　Not necessarily?

Senator SCHWEIKER:　What is this, a cover file?
　　　　　　　　　　Do we have cover files? Is that what
　　　　　　　　　　we are dealing with?

Dr. LASHBROOK:　　In a sense, and in a sense it was done
　　　　　　　　　　for security. In other words, the files that
　　　　　　　　　　went through the system and ended up in the

*financial Section - obviously TSS lost control
of those files.*

*Senator SCHWEIKER: So the FBI had a "do not file" procedure
designed to handle this sort of thing, and
the CIA has a cover file system to handle it.
In this case, though, some of the cover files
contain pretty damaging information that
doesn't seem to reflect well on the Agency's
use of human subjects - I wonder what the
real files contain.*

A cover file system must have been used to handle Frank Olson's suicide. It is unknown whether Olson was involved in the CIA's biological warfare program MKNAOMI, or whether his death was more than a suicide. A cryptic document dated December 14, 1953 and titled CONVERSATION WITH GIBBONS was declassified by order of CIA Director William Colby on July 24, 1975; it reads in part:

1. Lovell has not heard anything from Gibbons.

*2. Lovell reported that Quarles and George Merck were about
to kill the Schwab activity at Detrick as "un-American".
Is it necessary to take action at a high place?*

*3. Lovell knew of Frank B. Olson. No inhibition. Baring of inner
man. Suicidal tendencies. Offensive usefullness? HMC told Shef
Edwards Saturday A.M. the 12th.*

Frank Olson committed suicide by jumping out the tenth floor window of a hotel room while Dr. Lashbrook was asleep in the room on November 28, 1953. Lovell must be Stanley Lovell, an OSS chemical warfare and mind control expert. Schwab is Dr. John Schwab who founded the Special Operations Division at Fort Detrick, which received CIA money through MKNAOMI, and where Dr. Olson worked. George Merck was a member of the Merck family that founded and owned a pharmaceutical company. He was also a consultant to the CIA.

George Merck is identified in *Biological Testing Involving the Department of Defense, 1977* as having been a consultant on biological warfare to the Secretary of Defense during the Second World War. Merck & Co. is listed as having received two contracts from Fort Detrick, one running from May, 1955 to December, 1956, and the other from April, 1960 to June, 1961.

Gibbons was the head of the CIA's Technical Services Division at the time of Olson's suicide. Edwards was the CIA's security officer for ARTICHOKE. I have not been able to identify Quarles.

In between taking LSD on November 19 and jumping through the glass window of his hotel room at 2:30 A.M. on November 28, 1953, Frank Olson was examined by Harold Abramson, M.D. In a CIA-sponsored LSD symposium some years later, Abramson[1] listened to a participant express concern about someone on LSD jumping out a window in Europe, but he did not comment on his own experience with Frank Olson.

An undated ARTICHOKE document entitled "D-Lysergic Acid Diethylamide (LSD-25)", probably written in 1952, describes the CIA's early concern about Russian efforts to buy huge quantities of LSD from Sandoz Ltd. of Switzerland, where LSD was first synthesized by Dr. Albert Hoffman in 1943. Sandoz held the patent for LSD and the CIA had no secure American source of large quantities of the compound:

> *Some of the more outstanding effects are the mental confusion, helplessness and extreme anxiety which are produced by minute doses of this substance. Based upon these reactions, its potential use in offensive psychological warfare and in interrogation is considerable and it may become one of the most important of the psychochemical agents. The mode of action, although not completely known to date, is believed to be due to an increased glycogen metabolism with a probably block of the hexoeamonophosphate catabolism. To date there is no known antidote.*

> *Great interest has been shown by the Soviet bloc countries in this compound and reports are available which indicate considerable traffic in this drug and the raw ergot from which it is prepared. One report indicates that sufficient material for 50,000,000 doses was purchased by the Soviets from Switzerland in 1951. Due to low potency of the ergot collected in East German rye fields, Mothes and co-workers have undertaken the cultivation of selected strains of ergot and the artificial infection of both rye and barley, the latter succeeding readily. Mothes also started experiments with biosynthesis of potent agents found in ergot. Manufacture of lysergic acid is controlled by SANDOZ Ltd. of Switzerland to whom the patent was issued.*

This company has a virtual monopoly on the purchase of ergot in this country. It is reported, however, that the [white out] is currently obtaining 10-12 tons of ergot each month from screened rye in Michigan. In the U.S. considerable interest has been aroused in psychochemical agents and particularly in lysergic acid. At present extensive research on this compound is being done by the [whited out]. Under this contract an attempt is being made to synthesize lysergic acid as well as many of its derivatives and analogues. Clinical evaluation of the effect of this compound has not yet been attempted. Admixtures containing lysergic acid diethylamide other than with barbiturates to shorten the period of apprehension have apparently not been tried. The biosynthesis of d-lysergic acid diethylamide has not been attempted in this country as far as we know.

The lack of a secure U.S. supplier of LSD was corrected by the CIA through MKULTRA Subproject 18. Under TOP SECRET clearance, Eli Lilly Company was given a $400,000.00 grant in 1953 to manufacture and supply LSD to the CIA. It is possible that the LSD which lead to Frank Olson's suicide was manufactured by Eli Lilly. At any rate, the first large-scale manufacturer of LSD in North America was Eli Lilly. The first suicide attributable to LSD was the death of Frank Olson, the LSD having been administered without consent by Dr. Sidney Gottlieb, the Director of MKULTRA. Dr. Abramson was the physician directly involved in the Olson case, and he participated in hiding the truth from his patient's family.

Unethical practice by physicians and the direct involvement of pharmaceutical companies are part of the early post-War history of hallucinogens. These facts have never been subject to ethical review or any policy or position statement by any medical organization.

Dr. Gottlieb (personal communication, October 8, 1994) stated n a telephone conversation with me that the overall scheme of MKULTRA had several components. One goal was to establish relationships with individual contractors so that they could be consulted or used in other ways in the future. In such cases, the content of the Subproject was not necessarily of direct interest to the CIA. According to Subproject 96 documents, Dr. George Kelly[147] provided a great deal of such service to the CIA prior to receiving funding through MKULTRA. In contrast, Martin Orne, M.D., provided consultation services to the CIA subsequent to receiving funding through MKULTRA Subproject 84, and did not receive TOP SECRET clearance from the CIA until after Subproject 84 was approved.

Another purpose of MKULTRA, according to Dr. Gottlieb, was to fund a broad range of exploratory research. Findings of interest could then be followed up on in subsequent research. It is evident from review of the Subproject files that another major purpose of MKULTRA was to obtain supplies of chemical and biological weapons from manufacturers. The Subprojects can be grouped into four categories.

A large number of Subprojects were for the procurement of drugs, chemicals and biological weapons, or for research directly related to field applications. The investigators for most of these projects are unknown. The Subprojects in this category are: 11, 13, 20, 30, 31, 37, 41, 50, 51, 52, 64, 78, 91, 93, 100, 101, 104, 105, 110, 113, 116, 118, 133, 139, 143, and 146. Much of the MKULTRA money went to research that was practical and designed for immediate operational use by the CIA.

Another group of Subprojects involved the development and testing of mind control drugs. The goal of these Subprojects was to identify compounds, used singly or in combination, which would assist in interrogation and in the creation of amnesia. This group of Subprojects overlaps with those on chemical warfare, therefore some Subprojects could be assigned to either category. Together the two categories account for about half of the MKULTRA Subprojects and apparently all of the MKSEARCH Subprojects. The mind control drug development was carried out under Subprojects 2, 3, 6-10, 14, 16-18, 22, 23, 26-28, 33, 35, 38-40, 42, 44-47, 53, 55, 56, 58, 59, 63, 66, 71, 72, 75, 80, 99, 109, 124, 125, 135, 140 and 147.

A third group of Subprojects consists of experiments and research on non-chemical mind control or psychological warfare techniques. These include studies of social psychology, group psychology, psychotherapy, hypnosis, sudden religious conversion, and sleep and sensory deprivation. This group of Subprojects is about one quarter of the total MKULTRA Subprojects. It involves most of the contractors with *unwitting* status. Unwitting contractors are ones who do not realize that the research money is from the CIA because it has been funneled through a *cutout* or front organization. These Subprojects are 5, 25, 29, 43, 48, 49, 57, 65, 68, 69, 73, 74, 76, 77, 81, 82, 84, 88-90, 95-98, 102, 103, 108, 111, 112, 114, 115, 117, 121, 123, 126-128, 130 and 134.

The remaining quarter of the MKULTRA Subprojects were miscellaneous in nature. By and large, the psychologists and sociologists were unwitting contractors, while the physicians, including the psychiatrists, the chemists and the biologists had TOP SECRET clearance and were aware that they were working for the CIA. In CIA terminology, these people were *witting*.

MKULTRA Subproject 35 involved funding the construction of the Gorman Annex at Georgetown University Hospital in Washington, D.C. The money was funneled through the Geschickter Foundation. Dr. Charles Geschickter, head of the Geschickter Foundation, conducted research on amnesia-producing drugs at Georgetown University Hospital under MKSEARCH through July, 1967. CIA Director Stansfield Turner could not determine whether this MKSEARCH work was done at the Gorman Annex, according to his 1977 Senate Testimony. Since Dr. Geschickter also testified at the same Senate Hearings transcribed in *Human Drug Testing by the CIA, 1977*, the only investigation required for Stansfield Turner to make this determination would have been to ask Dr. Geschickter directly.

The CIA funneled $375,000.00 of MKULTRA money through the Geschickter Foundation for construction of the Annex, which was then matched by federal funds. Federal matching funds were triggered because use of the Geschickter Foundation cutout made the money appear to be a grant from a private foundation. The total budget for the Annex of $1.25 million was to provide a hospital safe house for mind control research. Some subjects were terminal cancer patients. One sixth of the space was set aside for the CIA, which placed three biochemists there under cover.

In his testimony in *Human Drug Testing by the CIA, 1977*, Dr. Geschickter states that over thirteen years his foundation funded $1,030,000.00 of research at Georgetown and $2,088,600.00 at other universities. CIA money included the $375,000.00 for MKULTRA Subproject 35 and $535,000.00 for MKULTRA Subproject 45, meaning that most of the money awarded for research at Georgetown, if not all, was CIA money. Dr. Geschickter's testimony to the Senate Committee is a study in evasion, forgetfulness, doublespeak, and implausible denial. He claimed not to be able to remember many details he obviously would not have forgotten.

The medical profession and the leading academic institutions where mind control research was done have not yet provided a meaningful public accounting, financial or ethical, of this experimentation. This is one of the reasons that the entire medical profession and the entire academic community are implicated in the story.

Like the Tuskeegee Syphilis Study and the radiation research, MKULTRA involved direct experimentation on children without informed consent being given by their parents or guardians. In the case of the Tuskeegee Study, children were harmed by preventable congenital syphilis. In the radiation experiments they were harmed through direct exposure after birth or *in utero* exposure during experiments on their mothers.

Four of the MKULTRA Subprojects involved research on children; 102, 103, 112 and 117. Only one of these, Subproject 117, involved an investigator with TOP SECRET clearance. The fact that the CIA funded research on children has not been documented previously. Given that the mind control research declassified to date is certainly an incomplete account of everything done, it is unknown whether other mind control experimentation on children was unethical or harmful. An unanswered question is whether children were ever subjects in Manchurian Candidate experiments.

The four MKULTRA Subprojects on children were benign and did not involve unethical experiments. Subproject 102 was conducted by Muzafer Sherif of the University of Oklahoma. It involved studies of the social processes in teenage gangs in two cities. Subjects were 14 to 17 years of age and were studied by having social science students "hang out" with them. One student showed up at a basketball court with a new basketball and explained that he wanted to exercise to lose some weight. Observations were made about how group cohesiveness was maintained, how members were selected, status ranking of members, behavioral sanctions within the group, and similar matters. The CIA's interest in this Subproject is not stated in the documents, but one can assume it was relevant to understanding and manipulating social groups during psychological warfare and propaganda operations.

Subproject 103 was conducted by Robert Cormack and A.B. Kristofferson at the Children's International Summer Villages, Inc. in Maine. The subjects were 16 to 21 years of age and were there for a reunion; all had attended the camp in previous years as 11-year olds. The academic purpose of the project was to study how children communicate when they do not share a common language. The CIA was interested in the project as cover for establishing relationships with children from a variety of countries. Obviously, the intent was to recruit them as agents or assets. A MEMORANDUM FOR THE RECORD from the Subproject 103 documents dated 10 December 1959 states that:

It is felt that this project will support the [whited out] need for cover. In addition it will assist in the identification of promising young foreign nationals and U.S. nationals (many of whom are now in their late teens) who may at any time be of direct interest to the Agency. . . No cleared or witting persons are concerned with the conduct of this project.

The principal investigator for MKULTRA Subproject 112 was Melvin DeFleur of the University of Indiana. He studied perceptions of occupational roles in children from first to eighth grades. According to a MEMORANDUM FOR THE RECORD dated 24 March 1960, the CIA's "interest is connected with the current problems of vocational guidance with possible application to the selection of technical and scientific careers."

The materials for Subproject 117 have gone through many generations of photocopying and are very hard to read. The aim of the research was to study patterns of child discipline in families from a different culture. The CIA's interest in this Subproject is not clear but a MEMORANDUM FOR THE RECORD dated 10 May 1960 states that, "This Subproject was initiated at our request after consultation with chief, [whited out]."

Another example of an MKULTRA contract in which the CIA probably was not interested in the content of the research is Subproject 121. Dr. Raymond Prince[248] was unwitting of the fact that the grant he received from the Human Ecology Foundation was actually CIA money. In the only article on CIA and military mind control in the peer-reviewed medical literature, Prince[248] speculates that the CIA was not really interested in his research on Yoruba witchcraft, but used the Subproject as cover to make contact with Nigerians for other purposes. A similar purpose might have been behind Subproject 117.

MKULTRA Manchurian Candidate work on hypnotic couriers and hypnotic mind control was carried out by Alden Sears at the University of Denver and the University of Minnesota under Subprojects 5, 25, 29 and 49. Sears had TOP SECRET clearance and on September 8, 1954 he signed a CIA Secrecy Agreement. This document states that the legislation controlling the Agreement was the Espionage Act passed on June 15, 1917.

A MEMORANDUM FOR THE RECORD dated 28 May 1953 states that both Sears and the Head of the Department of Psychiatry at the University of Minnesota are "cleared through TOP SECRET and are aware of the real purposes of the project." The word "Minnesota" is redacted from the documents but Sidney Gottlieb's name is not. The fact that the Subproject was conducted at the University of Minnesota is proven by the listing in the INSTITUTIONAL NOTIFICATIONS provided by the CIA through the Freedom of Information Act.

Dr. Gottlieb describes a visit to Sears' office and laboratory on July 13, 1955 in a document dated July 15, 1955. In a MEMORANDUM FOR THE RECORD dated 20 April 1954 there is a description of direct observation by Dr. Gottlieb and a CIA officer with the rank of Major, of hypnosis experiments conducted by Sears in a hotel suite. On March 26, 1954 a demonstration of hypnosis was given by Sears for selected representatives of Senior Staffs and Area Divisions, according to the 20 April 1954 MEMORANDUM.

It appears that Alden Sears never created a full Manchurian Candidate under MKULTRA. However, in a proposal for work to be conducted from June 1, 1956 to May 31, 1957 under Subproject 49 Sears writes:

> *Since this research was started in September of 1952, work has been done on various projects which were outlined by the fund representative and myself. Some of these have been [white out] (These two have been published), [whited out] and various pilot studies concerning subconscious retention of material and ability to deliver same without the subject's knowing consciously that he had even had this material; i.e., an unwitting message carrier...*
>
> *In order to investigate the possibilities of hypnotic induction of non-willing subjects who have only a knowledge of some other language than that of the hypnotist....*
>
> *An investigation should be made into non-verbal induction techniques, such as long duration of monotonous audio or visual stimulation. A variation of this in which I am interested and in which I have done some work, a few pilot studies, is to use soft restful music in which my voice was also recorded at a subliminal level. With some subjects in the past this has been very effective...*
>
> *Can auto-hypnosis be taught so as to be as effective as hetero-hypnosis in the canceling out of pain or other stress conditions;*

i.e., if this can be done a person could create his own world and be happy in it even though he were actually confined in a very small place which was extremely filthy...

There are a great many areas which need investigation in the field of hypnosis. However, some of these (especially those connected with the use of drugs) could not be handled in the University situation.

Sears did some of his experiments at a CIA safe house that had to be "reasonably unobtrusive from public surveillance, and yet be capable of accommodating an increased number of people without causing suspicion or comment" (MEMORANDUM FOR Safehouse Procurement Officer, 3 June 1954).

Another MEMORANDUM dated 30 October 1956 is a request for a safe house under Subproject 49 for use from November 13 to December 12, 1956. The safe house was "so situated that both sides of the building are not easily subjected to eavesdropping. This safe site is to be used in connection with a conference pertaining to various aspects of MKULTRA." Sidney Gottlieb's name is at the bottom of the MEMORANDUM.

A list of equipment purchased under MKULTRA Subproject 49 includes "1 shock stimulator." Whether the shock stimulator was used as a conditioning tool, to check for hypnotic resistance to pain, or to determine whether a hypnotic subject can perform under stress, is unknown. The MKULTRA work conducted by Alden Sears demonstrates that hypnotic courier and Manchurian Candidate experiments and training were done by the CIA under a number of different Programs, and were contracted out to a number of different institutions and investigators.

In his MEMORANDUM of 11 May 1953 Sidney Gottlieb lists seven separate experiments conducted by Alden Sears, and gives the number of subjects for five of them, totaling 196 subjects. Experiments were concerned with:

Experiment 1 - N -18 Hypnotically induced anxieties to be completed by September 1.

Experiment 2 - N - 24 Hypnotically increasing ability to learn and recall complex written matter, to be completed by September 1.

Experiment 3 - N -30 Polygraph response under Hypnosis, to be completed by June 15.

Experiment 4 - N - 24 Hypnotically increasing ability to observe and recall a complex arrangement of physical objects.

Experiment 5 - N - 100 Relationship of personality to susceptibility to hypnosis.

Experiment 6 - The Morse code problem, with emphasis on relatively lower IQ subjects than found on University volunteers.

Experiment 7 - Recall of hypnotically acquired information by very specific signals.

Manchurian Candidate work was done under MKULTRA Subproject 136, which was approved for funding on August 23, 1961. The deliberate creation of multiple personality in children is an explicitly stated plan in the MKULTRA Subproject Proposal submitted for funding on May 30, 1961. TOP SECRET clearance status for the Principal Investigator on Subproject 136 had been initiated by the Technical Services Division of the CIA at the time the Subproject was approved. Quotations from the Subproject 136 documents appear immediately before the Introduction to *The CIA Doctors: Human Rights Violations By American Psychiatrists.*

Although MKULTRA has received the most public attention of any of the CIA and military mind control programs, most of its Subprojects were relatively benign compared to experiments carried out in PROJECT OFTEN and MKNAOMI. The declassified MKULTRA and MKSEARCH documents prove that systematic mind control experimentation involving physicians was ongoing at least until 1972. Like BLUEBIRD and ARTICHOKE, MKULTRA involved the creation of Manchurian Candidates. Most of the MKULTRA Subprojects involved study of subcomponents of the Manchurian Candidate construction process – without the BLUEBIRD and ARTICHOKE documents, it would be unclear if the mind control doctors ever created a full Manchurian Candidate. The BLUEBIRD/ ARTICHOKE materials establish conclusively that full Manchurian Candidates were created and tested successfully by physicians with TOP SECRET clearance from the CIA.

6
OTHER CIA
MIND CONTROL PROGRAMS

There is very little declassified information about other CIA mind control programs besides BLUEBIRD, ARTICHOKE, MKULTRA and MKSEARCH. Freedom of Information Act requests on them have not yielded any material beyond the documents on BLUEBIRD, ARTICHOKE, MKULTRA and MKSEARCH released by the CIA in the 1970's. These other programs also involved experiments by doctors on interrogation of subjects, creation of amnesia, detecting double agents, and mind control. The following summaries are mostly from *Project MKULTRA, the CIA's Program of Research in Behavioral Modification.*

PROJECT CHATTER

CHATTER was a Navy project begun in 1947 to test drugs that would make a subject talk during interrogation. The Air Force, Army, CIA, and FBI were also involved. One CHATTER contractor was Professor George Wendt of the University of Rochester. At one point, according to an undated memo from the Secretary of Defense, the funding for CHATTER was $100,000.00 a year, however in 1950 the Navy awarded Wendt a single grant of $300,000.00. The actual total amount of funding Dr. Wendt received is unknown.

QKHILLTOP

This project was begun in 1954 to study Communist Chinese brainwashing techniques. Most of the early studies were probably carried out by the Cornell Medical Human Ecology Program. QKHILLTOP was absorbed into MKULTRA, and ceased to exist as a separate program.

MKDELTA

MKDELTA was a special procedure designed by the CIA to oversee MKULTRA research conducted abroad in the 1950's. It involved the use of drugs in interrogation, therefore physicians, most likely psychiatrists, were direct participants. MKDELTA also funded research on the use of biological materials for "harassment, discrediting, or disabling purposes."

THIRD CHANCE

THIRD CHANCE is described in *Project MKULTRA, the CIA's Program of Research in Behavioral Modification* (p. 412). EA 1729 is LSD (see Appendix I for a listing of all mind control drugs tested by the Army up to 1973):

> *At the conclusion of the laboratory test phase of Material Testing Program EA 1729 in 1960, the Army Assistant Chief of Staff for Intelligence (ASCI) authorized operational field testing of LSD. The first field tests were conducted in Europe by an Army Special Purpose Team (SPT) during the period from May to August of 1961. These tests were known as Project THIRD CHANCE and involved eleven separate interrogations of ten subjects. None of the subjects were volunteers and none were aware that they were to receive LSD. All but one subject, a U.S. soldier implicated in the theft of classified documents, were alleged to be foreign intelligence sources or agents. While interrogations of these individuals were only moderately successful, at least one subject (the U.S. soldier) exhibited symptoms of severe paranoia while under the influence of the drug.*

In a report dated September 6, 12961, the following conclusions about the interrogation of the U.S. soldier were presented (p. 415):

> *(1) This case demonstrated the ability to interrogate a subject profitably throughout a highly sustained and almost incapacitating reaction to EA 1729.*
>
> *(2) The apparent value of bringing the subject into the EA 1729 situation in a highly stressed state was indicated.*
>
> *(3) The usefulness of employing as a stress factor the device of inviting the subject's attention to his EA 1729-influenced state and threatening to extend this state indefinitely even to a*

permanent condition of insanity, or to bring it to an end at the discretion of the interrogators was shown to be effective.

(4) The need for preplanned precautions against extreme paranoiac reaction to EA 1729 was indicated.

(5) It was brought to attention by this case that where subject has undergone extended intensive interrogation prior to the EA 1729 episode and has persisted in a version repeatedly during conventional interrogation, adherence to the same version while under EA 1729 influence, however extreme the reaction, may not necessarily be evidence of truth but merely the ability to adhere to a well rehearsed story.

The trip report also stated that, "The interrogation results were deemed by the local operational authority satisfactory evidence of Subject's claim of innocence in regard to espionage intent."

DERBY HAT

DERBY HAT was the Far eastern equivalent of THIRD CHANCE. In one experiment a suspected Asian agent was given 6 micrograms of LSD per kilogram of body weight and interrogated for seventeen and one-half hours. At one point he was semicomatose and was described as "shocky."

OFTEN/CHICKWIT

A CIA program divided into two subcomponents was begun at Edgeware Arsenal in 1967. Testing on human subjects continued until at least 1973. Project OFTEN was designed to test the behavioral effects of drugs on animals and humans, while CHICKWIT was created to gather intelligence on new drug development in Europe and the Orient. One of the drugs tested in Project OFTEN was a hallucinogen called EA6167. It caused psychosis with subsequent amnesia lasting three to four days. According to the document in Appendix K, "Patients would see and hear persons not there and speak to them. Frequent complaints were bright lights or objects on the wall and roaches or flying insects in the room."

Attempts were made under Project OFTEN to develop a "compound that could simulate a heart attack or stroke in the targeted individual, or perhaps a new hallucinogen to cause the targeted individual to act bizarrely." Subjects in OFTEN testing were soldiers and prisoners, two groups that can be compelled to participate without true informed consent being given.

STARGATE

In cooperation with the military, the CIA ran a project called STARGATE that stopped in 1984. At least $20 million was spent on remote viewing and other paranormal methods of spying. Much of the work was done at the Stanford Research Institute. Major contractors included Edwin May, Hal Puthoff and Russell Targ[280]. Early work on STARGATE subject matter was done as far back as BLUEBIRD and ARTICHOKE; scattered discussion of paranormal phenomena can be found in those documents. MKULTRA Subproject 136 involved an $8,579.00 grant to an unwitting investigator in 1961 for an experimental analysis of extrasensory perception.

The CIA funded work on extrasensory perception and paranormal phenomena through a variety of different programs from the early 1950's until at least 1984. In STARGATE, remote viewers would leave their bodies and travel to remote locations to do surveillance. STARGATE documents have not yet been released through the Freedom of Information Act. STARGATE remote viewing is described by David Morehouse[197], who was himself a remote viewer, in his book *Psychic Warrior*.

Technically, STARGATE was not a mind control program in the usual sense, although it involved controlling certain properties of the human mind. It perhaps could be better described as a program that tapped certain powers of the mind. There is no evidence that any STARGATE activities violated medical ethics. The remote viewing was conducted under a series of cryptonyms including STARGATE and GRILL FLAME. Remote viewing work was being done in the private sector into the 1990s, with medical oversight by MKULTRA contractor, Dr. Louis Jolyon West[280].

MKNAOMI

MKNAOMI was a joint project of the CIA and the Army's Special Operations Division in Fort Detrick, Maryland. It ran from 1953 to 1970. MKNAOMI involved "developing, testing, and maintaining biological agents and delivery systems for use against humans as well as against animals and crops." The number of human subjects who participated in MKNAOMI, and the complete list of chemical agents used, is unknown. MKNAOMI received CIA money through MKULTRA Subprojects 13, 30 and 50 (see Appendix C for Subproject 50 document).

Additional information on MKNAOMI is available in *Biological Testing Involving Human Subjects By the Department of Defense, 1977*. This is a transcript of Senate Committee hearings chaired by Edward Kennedy on March 8 and May 23, 1977. MKNAOMI dealt mainly with biological and chemical warfare. It also solidified a relationship between the CIA and the Special Operations Division at Camp Detrick that included hallucinogen and mind control research.

OTHER PROGRAMS

William Sinclair Augerson, M.D., testified to a Senate Committee about Army LSD research that was ongoing in 1977, when LSD was a controlled substance. Dr. Augerson obtained his M.D. at Cornell in 1955 and worked as a physician at Walter Reed Army Institute of Research and in NASA's Project Mercury. In August, 1976 he became Commander of the U.S. Army Medical Research and Development Command. Dr. Augerson testified that (*Biological Testing Involving Human Subjects By the Department of Defense, 1977*, p. 238):

> *The LSD follow-up study has moved slower than we wished, due to the problems of organizing a control group, as well as the persistent problem of constrained clinical resources. We will complete the matched study of 50 controls, 50 LSD subjects in midsummer. When that study is complete, we should be able to move faster on the remaining subjects.*

Dr. Augerson stated that the LSD research was being done at Edgeware Arsenal, located at Camp Detrick. His testimony proves that Army LSD experiments continued at least into the late 1970's, well after the termination of MKSEARCH in 1972.

Biological warfare (BW) and chemical warfare (CW) research was run out of Edgeware Arsenal but also involved testing in many other locations including Dugway Proving Ground, Utah. As in the radiation experiments described in an earlier chapter, BW/CW research involved releasing bacteria, fungi and viruses into general population areas. The bacterium *Serratia marascens* was released in many locations including New York (June 7-10, 1966), San Francisco (September, 1950), and Pennsylvania State Highway #16 westward for one mile from Benchmark #193 (January 7, 1955). Other infectious agents released into civilian populations included *Aspergillus fumigatus* and *Bacillus globigii*.

Dr. Wheat and coauthors[332] published a paper in the *Archives of Internal Medicine* describing eleven *Serratia marascens* infections observed in one San Francisco Hospital between September 1950 and February 1951. The paper was published because *Serratia marascens* infections are very rare.

In its submission to Senator Kennedy's committee hearing entitled *U.S. Army Activity in the U.S. Biological Warfare Programs, Volume 11, 24 February 1977 Unclassified*, the Army denied a causal relationship between its secret experiments and the civilian infections reported by Dr. Wheat.

The Chief, Chemical Division, TSS wrote a memo to the Deputy Director of Security of the CIA on 18 May 1953 in which he stated his concern that a chemical weapon might have been tested on unwitting civilians in Gallup, New Mexico:

> *Reference is made to our conversation concerning the attached newspaper article which appeared in the 14 May issue of the Washington Star. Please note the report from Gallup, New Mexico reported by doctors that residents of that city have been bothered by a wave of nausea and lightheadedness. Although the possibility is remote, it may be that "seranim" could be involved and it is suggested that a routine inquiry, through Public Health, be made as to the facts of the case.*

The chemical identity of the compound "seranim" is unknown, although the spelling of the name and the effects of the compound suggest that it could be *sarin* or a related nerve gas.

A number of committees oversaw the CW/BW research including the Interagency Survey Committee Chaired in 1959 by David E. Price, Chief, Bureau of State Services, U.S. Public Health Services. The committee included representation from the Johns Hopkins Hospital. A similar committee, the Ad Hoc Committee for Dugway Proving Ground, was chaired by Leonard A. Scheele, M.D., Surgeon General in 1953; membership on that committee included the Operations Research Office and the Johns Hopkins University. In 1961 Johns Hopkins was represented on the Board of the CIA mind control cutout, The Human Ecology Foundation, by Dr. John Whitehorn, Chairman of the Department of Psychiatry, Johns Hopkins. A Johns Hopkins researcher received money through MKULTRA Subproject 87 in 1958.

MKULTRA and MKSEARCH Institutions listed by the U.S. Army as having received BW/CW contracts from Fort Detrick include Columbia University, Cornell University, Emory University, Florida State University, University of Illinois, University of Indiana, Johns Hopkins University, University of Maryland, University of Minnesota, Montana State University, University of Pennsylvania, Stanford, University of Texas, Yale University, and the Worcester Foundation for Experimental Biology (see chapter on G.H. Estabrooks).

The CIA maintained its relationship with this network of BW/CW and mind control contractors through MKULTRA, MKSEARCH and MKNAOMI, which provided funding of the Special Operations Division at Fort Detrick. In 1963 the CIA's Inspector General estimated that the annual transfer of funds from the Technical Services Division of the CIA (which ran MKULTRA and MKNAOMI) to Fort Detrick at $90,000.00.

A memo from Thomas H. Karamessines, Deputy Director for Plans, CIA, to Richard Helms, Director of the CIA declassified on September 15, 1975 describes ten chemical warfare agents and six toxins stored at Fort Detrick for the CIA:

Agents:

1. *Bacillus anthracis (anthrax) - 100 grams*

2. *Pasturella tularensis (tularemia) - 20 grams*

3. *Venezuelan Equine Encephalomyelitis virus (encephalitis) - 20 grams*

4. *Cocccidiodes imnitis (valley fever) - 20 grams*

5. *Brucella suis (brucellosis) - 2 to 3 grams*

6. *Brucella melitensis (brucellosis) - 2 to 3 grams*

7. *Mycobacterium tuberculosis (tuberculosis) - 5 grams*

8. *Salmonella typhimurium (food poisoning) - 10 grams*

9. *Salmonella typhimurium (chlorine resistant) (food poisoning)- 3 grams*

10. *Variola virus (small pox) - 50 grams*

Toxins:

1. *Staphylococcal Enterotoxin (food poisoning) - 10 grams*

2. *Clostridium botulinum Type A (lethal food poisoning) - 5 grams*

3. *Paralytic Shellfish Poison - 5.193 grams*

4. *Bungarus Candidis Venom (Krait) (lethal snake venom) -*
   2 grams

5. *Microcystis aeruginosa toxin (intestinal flu) - 25 mg.*

6. *Toxiferine (paralyic effect) - 100 mg*

Several of these materials were also the subject of MKULTRA contracts. The only field use of these materials described by the CIA was hand-launched darts taken on a mission to bug a North Vietnamese embassy in a southeast Asian country. The darts were to deliver an incapacitant to the guard dogs. They were unnecessary because the dogs accepted meat laced with the incapacitant.

The CIA also described a successful biological warfare mission carried out by the OSS against Hjalmar Schacht, a German economist. He was unable to speak at an economic conference because he was given staphylococcus enterotoxin food poisoning by the OSS.

The MKULTRA Subprojects by magician John Mulholland involved teaching the CIA methods of clandestine delivery of materials in the field. They are linked to the MKNAOMI BW/ CW materials. Offensive use of BW/CW weapons by the United States was banned by President Nixon on November 26, 1969.

A research program called PROJECT WHITECOAT began in 1959. It involved an agreement between the U.S. Army and the Seventh Day Adventist Church by which 2200 conscientious objectors were recruited at Fort Sam Houston to serve as research subjects. Another 800 Seventh Day Adventist personnel served as technicians and ward attendants. All these individuals received non-combatant, or I-A-O, draft status. WHITECOAT continued until 1973. Subjects were studied at Walter Reed Army Medical Center and were immunized against and infected with dozens of different viruses and bacteria, all listed by the Army in detail.

After termination of PROJECT WHITECOAT, volunteers for medical experiments were recruited at Fort Sam Houston through Provision AR 601-210, under the enlistment status of Medical Research Volunteer Subject. The Army reported that 76

MRVS subjects were enlisted at Fort Sam Houston in 1976, and two further individuals in January and February, 1977.

AR 601-210 was necessary because conscientious objectors could not enlist as medical experiment volunteers when there was no active draft program, according to prior Army regulations. This meant that the supply of WHITECOAT volunteers was cut off at the end of the Vietnam War.

Mind control research took place in a broad network of BW/CW research, chemical development, and radiation experiments. Physicians including psychiatrists were involved in an extensive, systematic way in this network of contractors, and they also participated in reviewing and allocating grant money to investigators with TOP SECRET clearance. Subjects in the experiments were sometimes unwitting civilians. At other times they were soldiers, prisoners, mental patients, sex offenders, cancer patients and other individuals who were unwitting, or who could not give meaningful informed consent.

7
LSD EXPERIMENTS

LSD was discovered accidentally in 1943 by Dr. Albert Hoffman, a chemist working on ergot alkaloids at Sandoz Laboratories in Switzerland. He accidentally ingested some of the compound and then had the first LSD-induced psychedelic experience. Sandoz became the major supplier of LSD in the world for several decades. The CIA obtained a secure North American supply of LSD from Eli Lilly in 1953 through MKULTRA Subproject 18, a TOP SECRET grant for $400,000.00. Through this Subproject, Eli Lilly became the first North American manufacturer and distributor of LSD.

No-one knows the exact number of mind control subjects who received LSD from the CIA and the military. In a U.S. Army memorandum dated July 15, 1975 Kenneth R. Dirks, M.D., Brigadier General, MC, Assistant Surgeon General for Research and Development, U.S. Army estimated that at least 1500 soldiers were given LSD without informed consent as part of Army mind control experiments. Review of the list of drugs tested by the U.S. Army up until 1973 included in Appendix I, and the fact that there are three branches of the military plus the CIA, leads to the conclusion that a large number of people received mind control drugs without giving true informed consent.

Many leading figures in American psychiatry in the second half of the twentieth century were among the first people to take LSD in North America. These ingestions began in the late 1940's and continued to be discussed in public into the 1960's. The CIA sponsored LSD research through MKULTRA and it also financed LSD conferences and books. In one of these books[1], major figures in psychiatry discuss their own experiences with LSD and how they obtained the drug. The book, published by CIA cutout, The Josiah Macy, Jr. Foundation, is the proceedings of a conference held on April 22-24, 1959 with financial support from Sandoz Pharmaceuticals (see Appendix J). The doctors state:

Charles Savage (p. 9): In 1949, under Navy auspices, I was looking for improved methods of inducing psychocatharsis and facilitating psychotherapy, as I had found sodium amytal and pentothal disappointing. I ran through the gamut of alkaloids, from mescaline and cannabis, through harmine, harmaline, scopolamine, and cocaine. I was primarily interested in mescaline, but was disappointed by the intense nausea it produced in both me and my patients.

Gregory Bateson (p. 10): My interest in LSD began when Dr. Abramson gave me 35 ug., about two years ago, and was revived the other day by the study just mentioned by Dr. Savage, in which Dr. Abramson gave me 100 ug.

Sidney Cohen (p. 11): I work at the Neuropsychiatric Hospital, Veterans Administration, in Los Angeles... It was an easy jump from the examination of toxic psychoses to my own provocation of these states with LSD.

My first subject was myself, and I was taken by surprise. This was no confused, disoriented delirium, but something quite different.

Louis Jolyon West (p. 12): I am a clinical psychiatrist and became interested in LSD while I was in the Air Force. Many Air Force prisoners of war were subjected by their Communist captors to various kinds of stress, sufficient to cause them to sign confessions of germ warfare, in which, in fact, they had <u>not</u> been engaging. At that time, many of us concerned with this problem were considering the possibility that special drugs, hyposis, Pavlovian conditioning, or what not, were being used to elicit these confessions.

T.T. Peck, Jr. (p. 13): From the peyote buttons, then, I became interested in these drugs that could promote physical as well as mental health. I made some studies among the Hopi Indians in Arizona, and then went into Mexico after Dr. Wasson's trip down there [MKULTRA Subproject 58], and ate some of the mushrooms; and I also tried peyote.... When LSD came out, with Sandoz's help, we used that.

C.H. Van Rhijn (p. 14): *I had a vision, and I still have a vision, of mass therapy: institutions in which every patient with a neurosis could get LSD treatment and work out his problems largely by himself. Classical psychotherapy or psychoanalytical therapy is, of course, a costly procedure, and most people do not have enough money to undertake it; nor do we have health benefits to pay for individual psychotherapy. I hope that there will eventually be health insurance funds to pay for LSD therapy.*

Ronald Sandison (p. 14): *The introduction of LSD has transformed the situation, as we are now able to deal with these patients. It has done more than that: It has transformed the entire hospital, because the whole atmosphere engendered by LSD has spread throughout the hospital and, in fact, forms an essential part of the hospital culture.*

Betty G. Eisner (p. 15): *I first read about LSD in* Life. *Then I heard that a friend of mine was to do an experiment with LSD. I offered to help, with the provision that I be one of the subjects. The experience so impressed me that I felt LSD had therapeutic possibilities, and so I tried it therapeutically on myself, with such extraordinary results that Dr. Cohen and I felt a therapeutic study should be done.*

Keith S. Ditman (p. 16): *I am a research psychiatrist in the Department of Psychiatry at UCLA. . . But after experiencing LSD, which I had done under Dr. Cholden's supervision, I was impressed that here was something, at least, that had some effect.*

Sidney Malitz (p. 19): *I joined the team, which included Dr. Hoch, Dr. Pennes, and Dr. Cattell. As I worked very closely and directly with the patients, I learned much about mescaline, LSD, and psychosurgery.*

Arthur A. Chandler (p. 20): *In taking the drugs ourselves [mescaline, ibogaine, amphetamines], we followed two general principles: (a). Nearly everything I see down in there is me, or some aspect of me; even if it looks like mother or father, there are many of my projections on it. (b). There is nothing I find in any of my patients that in some way is not also in me. If I cannot find it down in my subconscious, it must be blocking somewhere. On these principles, and with some prolonged treatment, we felt that we had explored our own and other people's subconscious rather deeply.*

Mortimer A. Hartman (p. 20): *About a year and a half ago, Dr. Wesley told me that Dr. Cohen and Dr. Eisner had achieved some spectacular results with an hallucinating agent called LSD, and I joined Dr. Wesley in some research on it. When I took the drug myself, I found I was suffering from the delusion that I had been psychoanalyzed. I had spent seven and a half years on the couch and over $20,000.00, and so I thought I had been psychoanalyzed. But a few sessions with LSD convinced me otherwise.*

Charles Savage (p. 30): *The first time my wife ever took LSD, she noticed how dirty the ceilings were and got after me to repaint them.*

Harold Abramson (p. 33): *In my experience, the use of LSD seemed to introduce a new era, a new search for magic. It had a glamorous appeal. Magazine articles distorted the situation very much. I, and I am sure many of you, have been besieged by people who wanted to take the drug, who wanted to experience the LSD reaction. This reaction produced anxiety in many of us and in many others connected with research in the field.*

Abram Hoffer (p. 41): *Dr. Abramson, in my statement about being unable to detect the effect of 100 ug., the subject was a psychiatrist who had probably taken it a hundred times.*

Louis Jolyon West (p. 46): *To what extent does the subjective experience of the therapist or the observer, who almost inevitably has taken LSD himself, influence the results he finds in therapy?*

Charles Savage (p. 56): *. . . the effects with the doses you are using may be quite different from those with the doses of 400 or 500 ug which Dr. Hoch is using.*

Arthur A. Chandler (p. 60): *There is a case I have heard about in Europe, where a person was given it without knowledge and jumped out of a window. We have to be careful about this sort of thing.*

Abram Hoffer (p. 89): *How many months gestation?*

T.T. Peck Jr.: *Five and a half months. She was gravida III, had had previous shock therapy, and had been under psychiatric care for a long time. . . she was very apathetic, wanted to die, wanted to kill the baby. She had been taking pills and barbiturates by the handful. She was given about 175 ug of LSD. . . We also gave LSD to a deaf girl during her first pregnancy, and to two other women, one 3-months pregnant and another a little over 6-months pregnant.*

Robert C. Murphy, Jr. (p. 91): *I treated three children with LSD over a period of several months. One eight-year old boy made a good recovery. That was completed nearly three years ago...*

Louis Jolyon West (p. 101): *With small doses, this is the case; in larger doses the other phenomenon occurs. This would fit in nicely with Marrazzi's ideas however.*

Louis Jolyon West (p. 131): *If the hypnotic experience is a* <u>controlled</u> *dissociated state or reaction, what is seen in the subjects under LSD are* <u>spontaneous</u> *dissociative reactions, in which all sorts of dissociative phenomena occur.*

C.H. Van Rhijn (p. 172): *The male nurse is 55 years old, married, and has observed a great deal of psychiatric treatment.*

Arthur L. Chandler: *Has he ever taken LSD himself?*

C.H. Van Rhijn: *No, not yet, but he should.*

There is a large psychiatric literature on LSD psychotherapy from the 1950's and 1960's[1, 2, 158]. Many psychiatrists gave highly positive reports about curing alcoholism, homosexuality (which they considered to be a perversion) and other illnesses with LSD. Dr. Sidney Malitz[1], the current archivist-historian of The American College of Psychiatrists, describes being introduced to LSD research by his mentor, Dr. Paul Hoch[130].

In his obituary in *The American Journal of Psychiatry*, Dr. Hoch[179] is eulogized by Dr. Malitz[178] as a great leader in American psychiatry. The obituary omits the fact that Dr. Hoch killed tennis pro, Harold Blauer with an injection of Army mescaline on January 8, 1953, at the New York State Psychiatric Institute. The family was told that Harold Blauer died as a result of a reaction to a drug given for diagnostic or therapeutic purposes, but this was a lie. A settlement for $18,000.00 was approved by the New York Court of Claims on June 17, 1955. Dr. Hoch's partner in mescaline research, Dr. James Cattell[131] is quoted[184] as having told Army investigators into Blauer's death, "we didn't know if it was dog piss or what it was we were giving him."

Another psychiatrist whose obituary appeared in *The American Journal of Psychiatry*[57], was child psychiatrist Dr. Lauretta Bender. Faretra and Bender[91] describe an experiment in which they gave LSD or psilocybin to 50 boys age 7 to 15. The children took these hallucinogens daily for weeks or months at a time. The dosage of LSD was 150 micrograms, a hallucinogenic dosage level of the drug equivalent to a strong adult street dose. In another study, children given LSD were 6 to 12 years old[32]. Some of Dr. Bender's child subjects received LSD daily for a year or longer[31].

Dr. Bender's experiments were conducted on the Children's Unit of Creedmore State Hospital, Queen's Village, New York. There is no evidence that Dr. Bender was funded directly by the CIA or military, however her LSD experiments on children demonstrate that the climate for such work was highly permissive. Her experiments were discussed at meetings of the Society for Biological Psychiatry and published in the medical literature.

On May 8-10, 1965 *The Second International Conference on the Use of LSD in Psychotherapy and Alcoholism* was held under the auspices of South Oaks Psychiatric Hospital in Amityville, New York. MKULTRA contractor and Director of CIA cutout, The Human Ecology Foundation, Dr. Harold Abramson was Director of Research at South Oaks Hospital and edited the proceedings of the conference[2]. He and Dr. Frank Fremont-Smith, former Medical Director of CIA cutout, The Josiah Macy, Jr. Foundation were co-organizers of the conference.

Attendees at the 1965 conference overlapped with those in the first conference and are listed in Appendix J. MKULTRA contractor, Dr. Louis Jolyon West attended the first conference while Josiah Macy, Jr. Foundation consultant, Dr. Daniel X. Freedman attended the second. Dr. West and Dr. Freedman Co-Chaired a session at the Meeting of the Society for Biological Psychiatry entitled, "Session IV. CLINICAL CONSIDERATIONS: a. Model Psychosis b. Therapeutic Use and Therapeutic Potential" in which Morris A. Lipton[172] presented a paper entitled, "The Relevance of Chemically-Induced Psychoses to Schizophrenia." In that paper, Dr. Lipton states that:

> *A few reports of the accidental ingestion of LSD by children and anecdotal reports of people who took LSD without knowing it suggest that it is a terrifying experience that might closely resemble an acute schizophrenic reaction. There are also persistent rumors that psychotomimetics have been administered to naïve troops in the Army with devastating results. Whether or not this is the case remains a military secret.*

Dr. Lipton was the subject of an obituary in *The American Journal of Psychiatry*, written by his co-author, Dr. Charles Nemeroff[211, 245]. Dr. Nemeroff states that, "One of my most vivid memories of Morrie was sitting in his office one summer day when he related his idea that hallucinogenic drugs, if proved safe, could be used to provide impoverished adults with a choice for a "vacation" or "a trip." Even when discussing psychopharmacology, he was always a humanitarian."

Dr. Freedman was the Editor of the most prestigious psychiatric journal in the world, *Archives of General Psychiatry* from 1970 till his death in 1993, according to his obituaries in *The American Journal of Psychiatry*[14] and the *Archives of General Psychiatry*[314]. Besides working for the Josiah Macy, Jr. Foundation, Dr. Freedman published research on LSD[96-98]. He was also a discussant of many presentations on LSD at meetings of the Society for Biological Psychiatry.

Among his numerous appointments, Dr. Freedman was at the U.S. Army Chemical Center from 1965 to 1967. From 1983 to 1984, he was on the Research Advisory Committee of the Texas Research Institute for Mental Sciences (TRIMS) which received funding from the CIA, Army, Navy, NASA and Air Force (see Chapter Thirteen). In 1972 Dr. Freedman was appointed to the Scientific Advisory Board of the Scottish Rite Foundation Schizophrenia Research Foundation. The Scottish Rite Foundation funded a great deal of hallucinogen research, sometimes concurrently with MKULTRA and MKSEARCH funding. Dr. Freedman was also President of the American Psychiatric Association, the American College of Neuropsychopharmacology, and the Society for Biological Psychiatry.

The interlocking academic relationships of the mind control doctors involved the most influential figures in American psychiatry in the second half of the twentieth century. Not every doctor in the network was directly funded by the CIA or military, and some, like Dr. Morris A. Lipton, were genuinely unaware of the scope of psychiatric participation in CIA and military mind control. Others, like Dr. Louis Jolyon West, who killed an elephant with LSD at Oklahoma City Zoo, had TOP SECRET clearance with the CIA and branches of the military.

One of the attendees at the May 8-10, 1965 LSD Conference was Dr. John Lilly[169], who described giving LSD to dolphins. In another paper, MacLean, MacDonald, Ogden and Wilby[174] describe LSD treatment at Hollywood Hospital in Vancouver; the paper includes a Table describing 338 patients who received LSD. Dr. James Tyhurst, a psychiatrist who attended BLUEBIRD and ARTICHOKE oversight meetings in Montreal in 195[105], practiced at Hollywood Hospital for a period of time and also received funding from Canada's Defense Research Board[304].

In the same volume Dr. Abram Hoffer[132] describes LSD treatment he conducted in Saskatchewan in partnership with Humphry Osmond[133] before Osmond[226] moved to Princeton, New Jersey to become the Director, Bureau of Neurology and Psychiatry, New Jersey Neuropsychiatric Institute. The Institute was the site of hallucinogen experiments by Dr. Carl Pfeiffer funded through MKULTRA and MKSEARCH. Along with John Smythies, Carl Pfeiffer was the Editor of *International Review of Neurobiology*[238]. Dr. Smythies was from the Worcester Foundation for Experimental Biology, site of MKULTRA Subproject 8. Contributors to the volume included Dr. Robert Heath, who received CIA and military money for hallucinogen and brain electrode implant research at Tulane University (see next Chapter). Associate Editors of the volume included Dr. Hoffer, Dr. Heath and the British psychologist, Dr. H.J. Eysenck, the contractor on MKULTRA Subproject 111.

An article in the February 12, 1996 *Sunday Times* and another in the October 11, 1995 *The Guardian* indicate that LSD was widely used in England from 1952 to 1972. At least 4,500 National Health Service patients were given LSD by 74 different doctors. The main hospitals included Powick, in Malvern, Worcestershire; Marlborough day hospital, in Wiltshire; Clifton Hospital, in York; and Roffey Park, in Lincolnshire. The *Times* article says that LSD was also given at a private hospital in New South Wales, Australia. How much of this LSD was given under military contracts is unknown.

By 1965 the American mind control doctors were having difficulty obtaining LSD. The Federal Drug Administration was starting to limit the supply of LSD and was about to make it illegal. How did the mind control doctors react? They lamented the move towards criminalization of LSD and saw it as uninformed and anti-scientific. In the Preface to *The Use of LSD in Psychotherapy and Alcoholism* Dr. Frank Fremont-Smith[99] says:

> *Since the Second International Conference on the Use of LSD in Psychotherapy was held, in May 1965, there has been a flood of highly emotional and often ill-considered discussion of LSD and the possible dangers inherent in its use. The article on LSD in the March 25, 1966, issue of Life is probably the most widely noted example.*

> *Certain university health officials have been troubled by the extremes to which "far out" groups of students are likely to go in personal experimentation, and have been aroused to action by the understandable concern of parents who feared for their children. Such officials have issued grave warnings about LSD that have caused serious alarm. One would wish that these officials would be equally diligent in trying to eradicate the genuinely harmful use of alcohol and cigarettes.*

> *Most statements which have appeared in the press are based principally upon the undesirable experiences of a limited number of people who have bought LSD on the black market and administered it to themselves without medical supervision. The unfortunate publicity which ensued has resulted in violent attacks against LSD itself, even when used by physicians, in careful studies carried out in psychotherapeutically oriented medical research and treatment. The federal government, in response to this ill-advised criticism on the part of unqualified individuals, has placed severe restrictions upon the availability of LSD to the medical profession. In some instances, these regulations have halted research on the value of LSD in the treatment of severe neurotic behavior patterns being conducted*

by precisely those physicians with the most extensive experience in the clinical and experimental use of LSD, leaving LSD research to the hostile and the ignorant.

On December 22, 1965, <u>The New England Journal of Medicine</u>, one of the most respected medical publications in the country, published an editorial under the title, "LSD - A Dangerous Drug." This editorial ignored the entire body of published data, including the report published by the Josiah Macy, Jr. Foundation on the First International Conference on LSD, "The Use of LSD in Psychotherapy," in stating ". . . today. There is no published evidence that further experimentation is likely to yield invaluable data." (Emphasis mine). Such unwarranted denigration is almost the ultimate expression of an anti-scientific attitude.

The network of LSD experimentalists regarded the criminalization of LSD as "hostile, ignorant and anti-scientific." There are only two possibilities; 1) LSD is a safe and effective adjunct to psychotherapy, and 2) LSD is a dangerous drug. If the first proposition is correct, current psychiatrists who regard LSD as a dangerous drug are hostile, ignorant and anti-scientific. If the second proposition is correct, then psychiatrists like Lauretta Bender did a great deal of harm to research subjects.

The 1960's slogan of *better living through chemistry*[158] was a guiding premise of the LSD psychotherapists, a group which included academic psychiatrists and CIA mind control contractors. The premise was shared by flower children who were fans of the rock group, The Animals; in the 1960's, The Animals produced a song about LSD entitled, "A Girl Named Sandoz." Current attitudes towards LSD of psychiatrists specializing in substance abuse are diametrically opposed to the teachings of the previous generation of specialists in LSD. Many leading psychiatrists in the 1960's dated the girl named Sandoz.

The shift from LSD as prescribed medication to LSD as substance of abuse is part of the history of CIA mind control and its effects on society at large. The medical professionals who consider LSD to be a dangerous drug in the 1990's are separated by one generation from the psychiatrists who introduced LSD into North America, took it recreationally under cover of supervised medical usage, distributed it in North America, and endorsed it as an aid to better psychological adjustment.

Like the Tuskeege Syphilis Study and the radiation experiments, the LSD research violated the requirements for informed consent that had been in place since the Nuremberg trials. At Nuremberg, Nazi doctors who experimented with mescaline in the death camps were regarded as war criminals. A decade later, such research was conducted by the leading figures in academic psychiatry in North America, and published in the leading medical journals.

8

BRAIN ELECTRODE IMPLANTS

Dr. Harold Wolff, a Professor of Medicine at Cornell, was a Director of the CIA cutout, The Human Ecology Foundation, and the investigator on MKULTRA Subproject 61. He treated the son of CIA Director, Allen Dulles for a combat-acquired head injury received during the Korean War. His published research includes a paper on Hungarian refugees coauthored with Human Ecology Foundation Director, Lawrence Hinkle[127]. Hungarian refugees were also studied under MKULTRA Subproject 89. In a footnote to his paper on Hungarian refugees, Dr. Wolff states that, "Among those who participated in these studies were Eva Bene, Ph.D., Sandor Borsiczy, M.D., George Devereux, Ph.D., William J. Grace, M.D., Ari Kiev, Maria H. Nagy, Ph.D., Thomas J. O'Grady, Jay Schulman, M.A., Richard M. Stephenson, Ph.D., and William N. Thetford, Ph.D.

William Thetford was the contractor on MKULTRA Subproject 130 with TOP SECRET clearance; Stephenson and Schulman were the contractors on MKULTRA Subproject 69 (their security status is not stated in the documents); and George Devereux's *Transcultural Psychiatric Research Review* at McGill received money from the Human Ecology Foundation (see Chapter 12).

Another publication on LSD and mescaline[34] demonstrates the overlap between hallucinogen experiments and other aspects of mind control. Another paper by Wolff includes Dr. John Gittinger, the lead psychologist for MKULTRA, as a coauthor along with William Thetford and Lawrence Hinkle[228].

In his obituary in *The Journal of Nervous and Mental Disease*[244] Dr. Wolff's accomplishments are listed at length. They include being

President of the American Neurological Association in 1960-61 and editor of the *Archives of Neurology*. He was a consultant for the Department of Defense and the Veterans Administration.

In one of the MKULTRA Subproject 61 documents, Dr. Wolff defines the historical context for the CIA's interest in mind control in general, which is also the context and motive for military funding of brain electrode implant experiments:

> *The investigations of the highest integrative functions are fundamentally aimed at increasing our understanding of the functions of the human cerebral hemispheres in overall adaptive behavior. They arose out of our laboratory and clinical experience during the past twenty years, and especially out of our interest in the phenomena exhibited by men exposed to extremely threatening life situations; and they were initiated during the period when we were investigating the untoward effects of Communist police procedures.*

When Dr. Wolff [126] refers to "communist police procedures," he means the brainwashing of American POWs during the Korean War (see Chapter 4), which probably included the creation of Manchurian Candidates. Another MKULTRA Subproject related to the goal of "increasing our understanding of the human cerebral hemispheres" was Subproject 129, which was entitled, "Computer Analysis of Bioelectric Response Patterns." This was a TOP SECRET cleared project conducted at George Washington University and Leler University of Georgia.

MKULTRA Subproject 94 involved placing electrodes into the brains of animals in order to control their behavior. By using a remote transmitter, the doctors could control the animals' movements and use them for delivery of bombs and biological and chemical weapons. A CIA MEMORANDUM FOR THE RECORD dated 18 October 1960 describes the research:

> *The purpose of this Subproject is to provide for a continuation of investigations on the remote directional control of activities in selected species of animals. Miniaturized stimulating electrode implants in specific brain center areas will be utilized... The ultimate objective of this research is to provide an understanding of the mechanisms involved in the directional control of animals and to provide practical systems for [whited out] application.*

The document describes Subproject 94 as a fine-tuning of extensive prior successful research.

A CIA memorandum for MKULTRA Subproject 142 is included in Appendix C. It describes the use of animals for delivery of biological and chemical weapons, and the control of animals through stimulation of brain electrodes. Various aspects of the overall research program were parceled out via different Subprojects and under other cryptonyms besides MKULTRA, but the overall goal was clear; to control the mind and behavior and to create dissociation, through a combination of drugs, sensory isolation, hypnosis, brain electrode implants, electric shock and beaming different kinds of energy at the brain. The ability to create limited, controlled amnesia through a variety of methods was a primary goal of the mind control programs.

A MEMORANDUM FOR THE RECORD for MKULTRA Subproject 142 dated 22 May 1962 states:

> *The reason for separating this work financially from the other efforts of [whited out] in the Agency's behalf is to allow him to engage in some very practical experiments at some point in the work which would present security problems if this effort were handled in the usual way. Some of the uses proposed for these particular animals would involve possible delivery systems for BW/CW agents or for direct executive action type operations as distinguished from the eavesdropping application of [whited out].*

"Executive action type operations" means human assassination. Brain electrode experiments were also conducted in humans, but there is no declassified documentation of the use of the human subjects in field-testing or in actual operations.

Dr. Jose Delgado, a neurosurgeon and professor at Yale, received funding from the Office of Naval Research, the Air Force 657 1st Aeromedical Research Laboratory (Grant Number F29600-67-C-0058) and the Public Health Service for brain electrode research on children and adults[69, 70, 71, 72, 73, 75, 76, 261].

Dr. Delgado's research grants from the Office of Naval Research included:

Year	Amount	Subject
1954	$7,950.00	Neurological mechanisms in epilepsy
1955	$9,610.00	Neurological behavior in epilepsy and in group behavior
1956	$9,610.00	Neurological behavior in epilepsy and in group behavior
1960	$10,000.00	Neurological mechanisms in epilepsy and behavior

Mark and Ervin [183] describe one of their brain electrode patients at Massachusetts General Hospital:

> G.C. This 14-year old Negro girl was brought up in a foster home and was of borderline intelligence. On two separate occasions her violent behavior resulted in the death of a young foster sibling, and she subsequently assaulted a 7-year old child at the state hospital where she was confined. . . Depth electrodes were placed in each amygdala through the posterior approach.

Dr. Delgado did similar research in monkeys and cats and in one paper describes the cats as "mechanical toys." He was able to control the movements of his animal and human subjects by pushing buttons on a remote transmitter box. Another case involved an 11-year old boy who under went a partial change of identity upon remote stimulation of his brain electrode[67]:

> In the same patient electrical stimulation of the superior temporal convolution induced the appearance of feminine striving and confusion about his own sexual identity. These effects were specific, reliable, and statistically significant. For example, the patient, who was an 11-year old boy, said, "I was thinking whether I was a boy or a girl, which one I'd like to be," and "I'd like to be a girl." After one of the stimulations the patient suddenly began to discuss his desire to get married, expressing then a wish to marry the male interviewer. In two adult female patients stimulation of the same region was also followed by discussion of marriage and expression of a wish to marry the therapist. Temporal-lobe stimulation produced in another patient open manifestations and declarations of pleasure, accompanied by giggles and joking with the therapist.

Dr. Delgado[75] wrote a book entitled *Physical Control of the Mind: Toward a Psychocivilized Society*. In it he described his vision of evolution. Delgado believed that control of the human brain through remote stimulation of implanted electrodes offered man another step up the evolutionary ladder. With this technology, man could directly control his own mind, mood and behavior.

Brain electrode research was also conducted independently at Harvard by Dr. Delgado's coauthors, Drs. Vernon Mark, Frank Ervin and William Sweet (see Chapter 3 for Radiation Committee testimony of Dr. Sweet). Dr. Delgado supplied brain electrodes to the Harvard team through an Office of Naval Research contract. Frank Ervin, the psychiatrist on the team, was trained at Tulane by brain electrode specialist, Dr. Robert Heath. He was later recruited by Dr. Louis Jolyon West to join the UCLA Violence Center (see Chapter 10). One of the plans for the Center was to control criminals through brain electrode implants. The Harvard work was described in Mark and Ervin's[183] book *Violence and the Brain*; in that book, the authors describe the potential use of brain electrodes for controlling urban violence. They suggest that this technology might have been useful in controlling black riots in Watts, California during the 1960's.

Mark and Ervin[183] describe implanting brain electrodes in a large number of patients at Harvard hospitals including a 25-year old man named Fred who had received a head injury while in the Navy. According to their description, Fred appeared to suffer from organic seizures, however, he also had a dissociative disorder which they did not recognize (p. 129):

> *On one occasion when he was driving a large trailer truck, Fred blacked out in the middle of Los Angeles and did not come to until he was on the outskirts of Reno. He had a similar experience while riding a motorcycle. Although nothing untoward happened during either of these two episodes, another time he did kill someone in a head-on collision.*

It is impossible to drive a truck from Los Angeles to Reno, a distance of 470 miles, while having a seizure. With absolute certainty this was an episode of dissociative amnesia. Instead of providing psychotherapy for their patient's dissociative disorder, Drs. Mark and Ervin attributed his amnesia to epilepsy and treated it with electrical stimulation of implanted brain electrodes.

Another patient named Jennie was 14 years old when Drs. Mark and Ervin[183] put electrodes in her brain. She appears to be the same patient described in Delgado, Mark, Sweet, Ervin, Weiss, Bach-y-Rita and Hagiwara[76]; one of the other four patients described in that paper appears to be the patient, Fred from *Violence and the Brain*.

Mark and Ervin[183] observed that "a baby's cry was a able to provoke an extreme behavioral change in Jennie." They played a tape of a baby crying while taking EEG readings from Jennie's brain electrodes. She was then transferred to a state hospital and Mark and Ervin were unable to "keep on with what we believed was necessary medical treatment." According to Mark and Ervin, it was epileptic discharges in her brain that caused Jennie to murder her two younger stepsisters. An alternative theory of the case based on chronic, severe psychological trauma, posttraumatic stress disorder and dissociative symptoms in Jennie, would lead to a psychotherapeutic treatment plan. The mind control doctors saw their patients as biological machines, a view which made them sub-human and therefore easier to abuse in mind control experiments.

Another patient in *Violence and the Brain*, 18-year old Julia, may also have had an undiagnosed, psychologically-based dissociative disorder. Photographs in the book show her smiling, angry, or pounding the wall depending on which button is being pushed on the transmitter box sending signals to her brain electrodes.

Theresa L., a 38-year old patient of Drs. Mark and Ervin, was regarded as a candidate for brain electrode implants because she masturbated compulsively 18 to 20 times per day, had sex with female prostitutes, had sex with more than one man at a time, was abusive and assaultive towards other patients, and had attempted to castrate her husband with a broken bottle. There is no mention of whether she was sexually abused as a child or physically abused by her husband. Theresa L. was given the anticonvulsant, phenytoin, which decreased her sex drive, but she would not take it regularly and did not receive further treatment.

Mark and Ervin describe psychosurgery being conducted for violent behavior in Japan, India, Mexico, France and Denmark. They mention a 1965 paper from Japan by a Dr. Narabyashi in which the amygdala was destroyed in 98 "mentally defective" patients, of whom 85 were children. Screening of these psychosurgery patients for childhood trauma, posttraumatic stress disorder and dissociative disorders was non-existent.

The percentage of patients who were candidates for psychotherapy is unknown, but unlikely to be zero.

Dr. Ervin's residency supervisor, Dr. Robert G. Heath, was Chairman of the Department of Psychiatry and Neurology at Tulane University in New Orleans from 1949 to 1980. He became the President of the Society for Biological Psychiatry at its 23rd annual convention on June 16, 1968. Born in Pittsburgh on May 9, 1915, Dr. Heath received his M.D. from the University of Pittsburgh in 1938 and his Board certification in Psychiatry and Neurology in 1946. His curriculum vitae list 13 different awards, and 49 teaching, hospital and professional appointments. Dr. Heath's military and government service included being assigned to the Navy as a P.A. Surgeon; working at the Merchant Marine Rest Center, Long Island, New York; Chief Psychiatrist, U.S. Marine Hospital, New York; and Chief Psychiatrist, U.S. Penitentiary, Lewisburg, Pennsylvania.

Dr. Heath was a member of the American Psychiatric Association Task Force on Medical Research Involving Human Subjects from 1966 to 1968. Four years later he published a brain electrode paper entitled, "Septal Stimulation for the Initiation of Heterosexual Activity in a Homosexual Male"[193].

Dr. Heath was a member of the Drug Abuse Research Advisory Committee, Food and Drug Administration from 1975 to 1977; a member of the Scientific Advisory Board of the American Council on Marijuana from 1980 to at least 1985; Chairman and Member of the Scientific Advisory Board of the American Council for Drug Education from 1983 to at least 1985; and a member of the Scientific Committee of the National Foundation of Parents for Drug Free Youth.

Dr. Heath did extensive research in which subjects with implanted brain electrodes in place had hallucinogens introduced directly into their brains. Subjects were monitored by EEG, self-report and clinical observation for their reactions. The hallucinogenic drugs he introduced into patients' brains in this manner included LSD, mescaline, psilocybin and a substance he called taraxein which he extracted from the blood of patients diagnosed with schizophrenia[123, 124, 194, 286].

Dr. Heath's work was described in Senate testimony given on September 10, 1975 by Charles D. Abelard, General Counsel, Department of the Army (*Biomedical and Behavioral Research*, p. 156):

Turning to some of the other contracts involving research on hallucinogenic drugs, we have learned of a 1955 contract with Tulane University which involved the administration of LSD, Mescaline, and other drugs to mental patients who had theretofore had electrodes implanted in their brains as part of their medical treatment unrelated to an Army contract. The electrodes were utilized to study the effects of the drugs on the brain's functioning. The methodology used might be subject to some criticism on the ground that a range of compounds was administered to at least one patient without apparent relation to therapy or diagnosis. However, work on the brain chemistry of mental illness was still pioneering work in 1955, and perhaps it is not surprising that in the cool light of analysis 20 years later that some of the techniques employed now seem less than perfect.

In his 1975 testimony, Mr. Abelard refers to Dr. Heath's "less than perfect" experiments as being twenty years old. A paper on electrical self-stimulation of the brain was published in 1963[116]; another paper on brain electrode recordings in patients given acetylcholine and gamma aminobutyric acid was published by Dr. Heath in 1965[120]; one on brain electrode recordings during orgasm in 1972[118]; another on brain electrodes in man in 1976[121]; one entitled, "Modulation of emotion with a brain pacemaker: Treatment for intractable mental illness" in 1977[119]; and one on electrode responses to marijuana in the monkey brain in 1979[208].

One of the ways to produce a psychocivilized society would be to treat the DSM-III psychiatric disorder of *ego-dystonic homosexuality* (American Psychiatric Association, 1980) with brain electrode implants. Dr. Heath made this attempt. He placed brain electrodes in a young homosexual man and fitted him with a box; a button on the box could be used to electrically stimulate an electrode implanted in the septal region of his brain, a pleasure center. Sometimes the electrode was stimulated by Dr. Heath, sometimes by his colleagues, and sometimes the subject was allowed to press the button himself. During one three-hour period, the patient, referred to as B-19, stimulated himself 1500 times. Dr. Heath describes the case as follows[193]:

During these sessions, B-19 stimulated himself to a point that, both behaviorally and introspectively, he was experiencing an almost overwhelming euphoria and elation and had to be disconnected, despite his vigorous protests. His post stimulation EEGs were unremarkable. Over the next 4 days there was no septal stimulation, either passive or self because of an intervening weekend and other of the patient's commitments. However, during this time B-19 did show a notable improvement in disposition and behavior, was less recalcitrant and more cooperative both at the laboratory and his hospital ward, and reported increasing interest in female personnel and feelings of sexual arousal with a compulsion to masturbate. The next afternoon he agreed without reluctance to re-view the stag film and during its showing became sexually aroused, had an erection, and masturbated to orgasm. At the conclusion of this session the patient stated that he "felt great" and was highly pleased with himself. EEG immediately before the movie was not unusual; and no specific activity was later present to be linked with any events during the film. The behavior of the patient over the ensuing 4 days showed increased self-satisfaction, preoccupation with sex, and a continued growing interest in women. At this time, and throughout all phases of the present procedure, no attempt was made to instigate any formal psychotherapeutic program. The patient was, however, given encouragement and support in the development of heterosexual interest and was directly counseled when he solicited information regarding sexual technique and behavior.

Stimulation was resumed with passive activation of various combinations of electrodes at several sites within the septal region (Table 1). It resulted in the patient reporting feelings of alertness, elation and being quite "high." Consequent self-stimulation through other septal electrode combinations (Table 1) produced an experience of warmth, a flushing sensation, and sexual arousal.

At this time, the patient was maintaining an active interest in females, culminating in an expressed desire to attempt heterosexual activity in the near future. Therefore, arrangements were made for a 21-year old prostitute to spend 2 hours with him in a laboratory specially prepared to afford complete privacy. B-19 was receptive to the plan, and the woman agreed after being apprised of the circumstances. On the afternoon of their meeting, the patient's electrodes were attached to an electroencephalograph via an extension cord for increased mobility, and recordings were obtained for 45 minutes with an interruption for delivery of passive stimulation of the septal region for 20 seconds (Table 1). B-19 was then introduced to the prostitute, and EEG's were obtained throughout his relationship with her.

Separate interviews with the patient and the prostitute provided information about their time spent together. Both reported that B-19 was initially anxious and reluctant when they were left alone, though his apprehension gradually subsided. The first hour of the session was essentially spent in conversation about the patient's experiences with drugs, his homosexuality and his personal shortcomings and negative qualities. Such material was seemingly presented as a defense on his part against progressing too far too quickly. During this time, his partner was most accepting and reassuring and gradually moved closer to him in an attempt to arouse his interest in her. He responded by trying to avoid eye contact, but at no time did he move away or express a desire to discontinue. She proceeded to remove her dress, but not her underclothing. B-19 did not respond with any advance though he did report feelings of interest and sexual arousal. As the second hour began, she relates that his attitude took an even more positive shift to which she reacted by removing her bra and panties and lying down next to him. Then, in a patient and supportive manner, she encouraged him to spend some time in a manual exploration and examination of her body, directing him to areas which were particularly sensitive and assisting him in the initial manipulation of her genitalia and breasts. At times, the patient would ask questions and seek reinforcement regarding his performance and progress, to which she would respond directly and informatively. After about 20 min of such interaction she began to mount him, and though he was somewhat reticent he did achieve penetration. Active intercourse followed during which she had an orgasm that he was apparently able to sense. He became very excited at this and suggested that they turn over in order that he might assume the initiative. In this position he often paused to delay orgasm and to increase the duration of the pleasurable experience. Then despite the milieu and the encumbrance of the electrode wires, he successfully ejaculated. Subsequently, he expressed how much he had enjoyed her and how he hoped that he would have sex with her again in the future.

During this session, EEG recordings from the deep leads indicated that delta waves appeared at several of these sites as sexual arousal increased and that immediately prior to orgasm striking changes in recordings from septal leads occurred resembling epileptiform discharge. These changes were characterized by spike and slow wave activity with considerable numbers of superimposed fast frequencies. This pattern was essentially unchanged at the moment of orgasm.

During 11 months of follow-up, B-19 maintained a primarily heterosexual orientation.

Dr Heath also brought women to orgasm by electrical stimulation of electrodes he had implanted in their brains. One experimental subject was a 34-year old woman of "borderline defective intelligence" who had a sixth grade education. She had been married three times when electrodes were implanted in her brain in 1960. She is called B-5 in a paper entitled "Pleasure and Brain Activity in Man"[118].

B-5 received injections of acetylcholine and levterenol into the septal region in combination with electrical stimulation of electrodes:

The degree of change was dependent on the patient's condition at the time the stimulus was given; if she had been in a low mood, the change was dramatic, whereas if she had already been feeling pleasant at the onset of treatment, the change was less profound. The patient became more attuned to her environment, answered questions more rapidly and accurately, and solved simple mathematical problems with more ease. The elevation in mood and heightened awareness involved development of a sexual motive state and in most instances, within another 5 to 10 minutes, this culminated in repetitive orgasms. Not only did the patient describe the response when questioned, but her sensuous appearance and movements offered confirmation.

Another paper[117] describes brain electrode research conducted on three groups of subjects; prisoners at Louisiana State Penitentiary, schizophrenics and rhesus monkeys. Table 1 in the paper lists 50 different drugs Dr. Heath tested, including those he injected into the brain of subject B-5.

One of the discussants for this paper[117] was Hudson Hoagland, Ph.D., Executive Director, the Worcester Foundation for Experimental Biology, Shrewsbury, Massachusetts. Hoagland was directly recommended to J. Edgar Hoover by G.H. Estabrooks (see Chapter 14). The Worcester Foundation received funding through MKULTRA Subproject 8; chief investigator Dr. Robert Hyde had TOP SECRET clearance with the CIA.

The second discussant for Dr. Heath's paper was Frank R. Ervin, M.D., Director, Stanley Coob Laboratories for Psychiatric Research, Harvard Medical School. Dr. Ervin did brain electrode implant experiments at Harvard (see Chapter 8) and was recruited for the UCLA Violence project by MKULTRA Subproject 43 contractor, Dr. Louis Jolyon West (see Chapter 10). It is evident that the brain electrode doctors knew each other well.

Dr. Heath acknowledged receiving money from the CIA in an interview by my research assistant on September 21, 1995. He also described being asked by Dr. Amedeo Marrazzi (see Chapter 17) to do LSD research on humans for the U.S. Army, but declined.

In April, 1973 a patient identified in legal documents as John Doe, a 36-year old male, was freed from eighteen years of confinement in state mental hospitals as a result of the court's decision in Kaimowitz v. Department of Mental Health[103]. John Doe was a patient in Ionia State Hospital at the time of his release. On March 23, 1973 the court held that the criminal sexual psychopath statute under which he was being held in hospital was unconstitutional.

Ionia State Hospital was the site of MKULTRA Subproject 39, in which investigators cleared at TOP SECRET received $30,000.00 in 1955 for drug testing on prisoners and sexual psychopaths including interrogation with hypnosis, LSD and marijuana. John Doe was committed to Ionia State Hospital in 1955 for the alleged rape and murder of a student nurse.

MKULTRA Subproject 39 documents include a description of four psychiatrists, a psychologist and a physician who participated in the Subproject. The Director of the hospital was also witting; the documents include six signed Secrecy Agreement forms with names whited out. One of the psychiatrists is described as follows: "As a Navy psychiatrist he has had extensive experience in [whited out] in the field of eastern cultures, Oriental psychiatry, brainwashing, etc. He has also done drug interrogation with criminals and has engaged in narcoanalysis and hypnoanalysis."

A Subproject 39 MEMORANDUM FOR THE RECORD dated 9 December 1954 states that:

> This project is designed to exploit the research potential that is represented by a group of 142 criminal-sexual psychopaths confined in the [whited out]. Several materials and techniques will be assessed for their information-eliciting properties on these individuals. It is thought that these individuals have the kind of motivation for withholding certain information that is comparable to operational interrogation situations in the field.

The Research Plan submitted by the investigators specifies that, "Subjects will be selected who have denied allegations of various kinds that can be checked or strongly assumed on the basis of previously established records."

A CIA Trip Report on Subproject 39 dated 7 April 1958 states that:

> It is apparent that [whited out] is so involved in the administrative problems of the project that he is not paying any attention to the results. Since to date only 4 cases have been transcribed there is no way of telling what is coming out of it. I assume there were no dramatic reactions, because the interviewers would have let him know about them had they emerged. It is possible, however, that our own analysis of the data may dredge up something of value, although I am dubious on this point.
>
> [Whited out] gave me his usual long involved talk on the difficulties he had encountered which account for the delays. He also talked at some length about his "experiments" with hypnosis, some aspects of which are mildly hair-raising. Finally he made quite a pitch for continuing some such project as this next year, "with realistic, specific deadlines." I told him we would discuss possibilities after the present project was completed and we had a chance to closely examine the take.

The Kaimowitz v. Department of Mental Health court case arose because Dr. Ernst Rodin, a neurologist, and Dr. Jacques S. Gottlieb, a psychiatrist wanted to implant brain electrodes in John Doe. A psychiatric resident at the Lafayette Clinic at Wayne State University College of Medicine in Detroit, where Dr. Jacques Gottlieb (who is not the same individual as Sidney Gottlieb, the Director of MKULTRA) worked as Director, was uncomfortable about the ethics and procedures in the Clinic's aggression project. He brought his concerns to Gabe Kaimowitz, an attorney for the Michigan Medical Committee for Human Rights, who filed an action.

The "Proposal for the Study of the Treatment of Uncontrolled Aggression at Lafayette Clinic" was stimulated by Dr. Rodin and Dr. Jacques Gottlieb's reading of *Violence and the Brain*[189]. Dr. Rodin met with Drs. Vernon Mark and Jose Delgado as part of his development of the Michigan brain electrode project.

Dr. Jacques Gottlieb received funding for research on schizophrenia from the Scottish Rite Committee for Research on Schizophrenia, as did MKULTRA and MKSEARCH contractor Dr. Carl Pfeiffer. One paper by Dr. Gottlieb entitled, "Steps Towards Isolation of a Serum Factor in Schizophrenia"[100] deals with taraxein, the substance Dr. Heath believed he had discovered in the blood of schizophrenics. Another paper is entitled, "Sensory Isolation: Hallucinogenic Effects of a Brief Procedure"[63]. In this experiment, subjects were placed in sensory isolation wearing blackened-out, or white or red-frosted goggles.

Another Gottlieb paper is entitled "Combined Sernyl and Sensory Deprivation"[61]. In another study entitled "Comparison of Phencyclidine Hydrochloride (Sernyl) with Other Drugs"[64], the authors thank Parke, Davis & Company, the pharmaceutical firm, for supplying the phencyclidine and "subsidizing the normal controls." Subjects were schizophrenic patients and normal controls. They were given LSD, phencyclidine or sodium amytal, then tested for their cognitive abilities.

Phencyclidine known on the street as PCP or "angel dust" causes delusions, hallucinations, paranoia, amnesia, and agitation. In overdose it causes seizures, coma and death. There is a diagnostic category in DSM-IV[12] called "Phencyclidine Intoxication" that describes the symptoms caused by the drug. Use of PCP as a street drug was first reported by medical professionals in Los Angeles in 1965. As for LSD, it was doctors in the mind control network who first distributed PCP in North America. The drug was first developed as a general anaesthetic in the 1950's but is now a controlled substance, like LSD. A milder drug with similar action is currently marketed under the trade name Ketamine.

When the John Doe case appeared in the *Detroit Free Press* on January 7, 1973, there was an immediate negative public reaction. As a result, the Michigan State Department of Health terminated its support of the Lafeyette Clinic aggression project and withdrew a pending budget approved for $172,995.00. John Doe was released without having been psychocivilized.

The history of the termination of the Lafeyette Clinic brain electrode project parallels the demise of the Tuskeegee Syphilis Study in several ways: it was initiated by a single individual; the involved doctors were prepared to continue; and public funding was withdrawn only in response to negative publicity. The same is true for Dr. Louis Jolyon West's UCLA Violence Center (see Chapter 10). These facts illustrate how the history of the different elements of mind control, biological and chemical weapons development, radiation testing, and the creation of Manchurian Candidates are intertwined and part of the same historical period.

9
<u>NON-LETHAL WEAPONS</u>

The network of mind control doctors, as it existed in the 1950's and 1960's, included specialists in non-lethal weapons. *Non-lethal weapons* is a broad category which includes devices for beaming various kinds of energy at human targets in order to temporarily incapacitate them, or to control or affect their behavior. Non-lethal weapons research has been conducted at universities in the United States on contract to the CIA, and has overlapped with research on hallucinogens and brain electrode implants. Funding of the experiments began in MKULTRA.

MKULTRA and MKSEARCH contractor Dr. Charles Geschickter described some of the early non-lethal weapons research in Senate testimony transcribed in *Human Drug Testing by the CIA, 1977* (p. 90.):

Senator KENNEDY:	*Was the NIH [National Institute of Health] involved in any of the research projects?*
Dr. GESCHICKTER:	*There was NIH involvement.*
Senator KENNEDY:	*Could you tell us the nature of that involvement?*
Dr. GESCHICKTER:	*I can tell you the nature of it accurately. One was on studies on concussion in which they rocked the heads of animals back and forth to try to cause them amnesia by concussion of the brain. And that was for $100,000.*
	The other, which was funded through this later business [Dr. Geschickter being used to funnel CIA money to other researchers through separate bank accounts] was the use of radar to put monkeys to sleep,

> *to see if they could be, should I say,*
> *instead of Mickey Finn, they could put*
> *them under with radar directed towards*
> *the monkey's brain.*

Senator SCHWEIKER: Could they?

Dr. GESCHICKTER: Did they go to sleep?

Senator SCHWEIKER: Yes.

Dr. GESCHICKTER: Yes, sir. But, Senator, it showed if you got
> *into too deep a sleep, you injured the heat*
> *center of the brain the way you cook meat,*
> *and there was a borderline there that made*
> *it dangerous.*

The research described by Dr. Geschickter is MKULTRA Subproject 62, conducted at the National Institutes of Health by Dr. Maitland Baldwin[24], a neurosurgeon. Subproject 62 documents describe Dr. Baldwin's interest in sensory isolation experiments, and a Subproject status report states that, "certain kinds of radio frequency energy have been found to effect reversible neurological changes in chimpanzees."

In the publication resulting from Subproject 62, entitled, "Effects of radio-frequency energy on primate cerebral activity," Baldwin, Bach and Lewis[25] thank the Naval Research Laboratory and Rome Air Force Base for supplying equipment used to generate the radio waves.

Dr. Baldwin also did a study in which he gave LSD to monkeys[25]. In the experiment, control monkeys were compared to monkeys who had had their temporal lobes removed surgically. Based on the responses of the two groups of monkeys to LSD, Dr. Baldwin concluded that the temporal lobes must be in place for monkeys to experience the effect of LSD. The LSD used by Dr. Baldwin was supplied by Sandoz Laboratories.

Li and Baldwin[160] described a technique for implanting electrodes in the human brain; at that point in time they had implanted electrodes in the brains of 30 people over a five-year period. Penfield and Baldwin[234] performed a series of temporal lobectomies at the Montreal Neurological Institute and McGill University during the same time period that Dr. Ewen Cameron (contractor on MKULTRA Subproject 68) was the Chairman of the Department of Psychiatry at McGill, and Dr. James Tyhurst of McGill was attending BLUEBIRD and ARTICHOKE meetings in Montreal (see Chapter 12 for information on other CIA and military contracts at McGill).

MKSEARCH Subproject 1 documents, for which Dr. Baldwin was the investigator, have not yet been released by the CIA. Baldwin was a Lieutenant in the Navy from 1944 to 1947 and joined the Naval Reserve in 1957.

Through MKULTRA Subproject 54, the CIA gave $62,400.00 to the Office of Naval Research in 1955. The researcher funded in this project was studying how to produce concussions from a distance using mechanical blast waves propagated through the air. Under a heading of "POTENTIAL APPLICATIONS OF THE RESEARCH FINDINGS," the contractor says that such concussion "is always followed by amnesia for the actual moment of the accident." He also states:

> *The blast duration would be in the order of a tenth of a second.*
> *Masking of a noise of this duration should not be difficult.*
> *It would be advantageous to establish the effectiveness of both of*
> *the above methods as a tool in brain-wash therapy.*

MKULTRA Subproject 119 was a literature review that included a summary of existing information on "Techniques of activation of the human organism by remote electronic means."

This early experimental and scholarly research under MKULTRA was the foundation of non-lethal weapons programs that are currently active. According to a report in *Defense Electronics*[299], consideration was given to using non-lethal weapons technology on David Koresh during the Branch Davidian siege in the spring of 1993.

A Russian expert on non-lethal weapons, Dr. Igor Smirnov, was brought to the United States for a series of meetings in northern Virginia that began on March 17, 1993. The meetings were attended by representatives of the CIA, the Defense Intelligence Agency, the FBI, and the Advanced Research Projects Agency. Civilian attendees included Dr. Richard Nakamura of the National Institute of Mental Health and Dr. Christopher Green, Director of Biomedical Research at General Motors Corp.

According to the article, the device was not used on David Koresh because of software incompatibility problems. Smirnov could not guarantee its safety. A firm called Psychotechnologies Corp, based in Richmond, Virginia entered into an agreement with the Russians to share and develop this technology for American use.

Pasternak[233] described non-lethal weapons research in the 1990's in an article in *U.S. News and World Report*. According to the article, acoustic weapons research is ongoing at Scientific Applications & Research Associates, Inc. in Huntington Beach, California, with testing at nearby Camp Pendleton Marine Corps Base; Mission Research Corps in Albuquerque, New Mexico; and the Armstrong Laboratory at Brooks Air Force Base, San Antonio, Texas. From 1980 to 1983, according to Pasternak, the Marine Corps Nonlethal Electromagnetic Weapons project was run by a man named Eldon Byrd, who did work at the Armed Forces Radiobiology Research Institute in Bethesda, Maryland. Bethesda is the location of the National Institute of Mental Health, a representative of which attended the meetings with Dr. Igor Smirnov in 1993.

There is abundant evidence in the public domain[233] that non-lethal weapons research is ongoing and funded annually in the tens of millions of dollars, or more. Given the fact that chemical and biological weapons, mind control drugs and radiation have been tested on unwitting civilian populations, it is possible that non-lethal weapons have also been tested on unwitting civilians.

As is true for mind control experimentation, physicians must be involved in non-lethal weapons programs. Non-lethal weapons programs therefore pose a problem in medical ethics and require official policies and guidelines from the American Medical Association and the American Psychiatric Association. To date, organized, academic medicine has acted as if non-lethal weapons do not exist.

10
DR. LOUIS JOLYON WEST

Dr. Louis Jolyon "Jolly" West was born in New York City on October 6, 1924. He died of cancer on January 2, 1999. Dr. West served in the U.S. Army during World War II and received his M.D. from the University of Minnesota in 1948, prior to Air Force LSD and MKULTRA contracts carried out there. He did his psychiatry residency from 1949 to 1952 at Cornell (an MKULTRA Institution and site of the MKULTRA cutout The Human Ecology Foundation). From 1948 to 1956 he was Chief, Psychiatry Service, 3700th USAF Hospital, Lackland Air Force Base, San Antonio, Texas. This base is not far from Brooks Air Force Base in San Antonio, which houses the Albertus Strughold Library (see Chapter 1).

While at Lackland Air Force Base, Dr. West examined Air Force pilots who had been converted to Communism while held as POWs in the Korean War. Based on this experience he published a paper[315] entitled, "United States Air Force prisoners of the Chinese Communists. Methods of Forceful Indoctrination: Observations and Interviews."

Other papers published by Dr. West were entitled: "Sleep deprivation"[41] "Lysergic acid diethylamide: Its effects on the male asiatic elephant"[330] "Brainwashing"[316] "Hypnosis and experimental psychopathology"[68]; "Sensory isolation"[317]; "Monkeys and brainwashing"[319]; "Psychiatry, brainwashing, and the American character"[320]; "Brainwashing, conditioning, and ddd (debility, dependency, and dread)"[90]; "Dissociative reaction"[321]; "Hallucinogens"[181]; "Psychobiology of racial violence"[322]; "Flight from violence: Hippies and the green rebellion"[10]; "Hippie culture"[327]; "Campus unrest and the counter culture"[323]; "Contemporary cults:

Utopian images, internal reality"[324] "Cults, liberty, and mind control"[325]; and "Persuasive techniques in contemporary cults"[326].

A list of Dr. West's military appointments obtained from his curriculum vitae is included in Appendix G. His curriculum vitae does not mention that he received TOP SECRET clearance from the CIA as the contractor on MKULTRA Subproject 43. This was a $20,800.00 grant given to Dr. West in 1956 while he was Chairman of the Department of Psychiatry at the University of Oklahoma. The Subproject proposal submitted to the CIA by Dr. West is entitled, "PSYCHOPHYSIOLOGICAL STUDIES OF HYPNOSIS AND SUGGESTIBILITY" and an accompanying document is entitled "STUDIES OF DISSOCIATIVE STATES." This latter document reads:

> *An examination of current descriptions of dissociative reactions reveals a rather stereotyped concept, differing little from [whited out] original one, and offering limited definition of the dissociative mechanisms and their role in normal and abnormal psychological functions. The literature concerning clinical entities ordinarily considered to constitute the dissociative reactions is fairly well limited to case-studies of patients with fugues, amnesia, somnambulisms, and multiple personalities.*
>
> *Unpublished studies by the writer have led him to a greatly expanded concept of dissociation. Dissociative phenomena are found in everyday life. Such manifestations include "highway hypnosis", states of "fascination" in flyers, hypnagogic and phantasy hallucinations, transient anaesthesias, and many other examples. These reactions have many features in common with a variety of clinical disorders including "sleep paralysis", trance states, Gilles de la Tourette's disease, latah, "Arctic hysteria", and a number of other disturbances in addition to the well-known dissociative reactions of the text-books.*
>
> *There is considerable experimental evidence pointing to the significant role played by dissociative mechanisms in the production of the various phenomena of hypnosis. In fact, hypnosis may be considered to be a pure-culture, laboratory controlled dissociative reaction. Of the entire phenomenology of the various states described above, there is not one single manifestation which cannot be produced experimentally in the hypnotic subject. Thus, through the use of hypnosis as*

a laboratory device, the dissociative mechanisms can be studied with a high degree of objectivity.

Of increasing interest at the present time are the actions of a variety of new drugs which alter the state of psychological functioning. Some of these agents produce disturbances of perception and integration (mescaline, lysergic acid, etc.). Others produce alterations of autonomic reactivity through inhibition of central (hypothalamic?) functions, so that "emotional responsiveness" is diminished (reserpine, chlorpromazine, etc.). The effects of these agents upon the production, maintenance, and manifestations of dissociated states have never been studied.

Only the first page of this document, stamped "<u>WARNING NOTICE SENSITIVE INTELLIGENCE SOURCES AND METHODS INVOLVED</u>", and reproduced in its entirety above, is available under the Freedom of Information Act. That Dr. West continued to study dissociation intensively into the 1960's is demonstrated by the fact that he wrote the section entitled "Dissociative Reactions" in the major textbook of psychiatry in North America[321].

In 1980, Dr. West co-authored a chapter in the next edition of this textbook, *The Comprehensive Textbook of Psychiatry*, with Dr. Margaret Singer[329] entitled, "Cults, quacks, and nonprofessional psychotherapies." Dr. Singer[289] thanks, among others, Richard Ofshe and Louis Jolyon West for support of her work in the Acknowledgements to her book *Cults in Our Midst*[289, 290]. In the Introduction she writes:

After a number of years at the University of Colorado School of Medicine, Department of Psychiatry, I went to Washington, D.C., as a senior psychologist in the laboratory of psychology at the Walter Reed Army Institute of Research. There, among other things, I worked with people who were studying prisoners of war from the Korean War. I became knowledgeable about, and intrigued with, the forms of coercive persuasion, or thought-reform programs, that not only prisoners of war but also civilians in a variety of milieus had been exposed to in the Far East. I also interviewed a number of Jesuit priests who had been exposed to thought-reform processes while imprisoned in Mainland China.

In his MKULTRA Subproject 43 proposal, Dr. West describes a research plan that involved many of the mind control techniques of both the Communist Chinese and leaders of destructive cults:

> *It is proposed that the experiments begun during 1955-56 involving hypnotizability, suggestibility, and the role of certain drugs in altering these attributes, be continued and extended during 1956-57. . . Experiments involving altered personality function as a result of environmental manipulation (chiefly sensory isolation) have yielded promising leads in terms of suggestibility and the production of trance-like states. There is reason to believe that environmental manipulations can affect the tendencies for dissociative phenomena to occur. Isolation, in particular, can markedly change the individual's response to suggestion in the form of verbal communication. . .*
>
> *All of the above-recommended experimental procedures will require special equipment, special methodologies, and special skills. In order to make possible a continuing research program in this area, a psychophysiological research team is being developed at the [whited out]. Facilities of the [whited out], and the [whited out] are available. However, within the overall framework of these facilities, a unique laboratory must be organized and constructed. This laboratory will include a special chamber, in which all psychologically significant aspects of the environment can be controlled. This chamber will contain, among other things, a broad-spectrum polygraph for simultaneous recordings of a variety of psychophysiological reactions of the individual being studied. In this setting the various hypnotic, pharmacologic, and sensory-environmental variables will be manipulated in a controlled fashion and quantitative recordings of the reactions of the experimental subjects will be made.*

Dr. West devoted four decades to study, writing and experimentation on dissociation, hypnosis, Communist mind control, hallucinogens, sensory deprivation, and methods of social influence; he concluded that the methods used by destructive cults result in the creation of new identities and dissociated states[328]. The same methods, when applied to experimental subjects under BLUEBIRD, ARTICHOKE and MKULTRA, also resulted in the creation of amnesia, new identities and dissociated states. This was the Manchurian Candidate program.

In his Chapter on destructive cults in the *Comprehensive Textbook of Psychiatry*[329], Dr. West writes disparagingly of psychiatrists who are interested in parapsychology and hallucinogens:

> *In the past few years some psychiatrists have shown a growing and unabashed interest in parapsychology, including telepathy, psychokinesis, clairvoyance, and presience. A distinguished psychiatrist (Stevenson, 1966) has written on reincarnation, another (Eisenbud, 1967) on mediums, a third (Ullman, 1973) on thought transference in dreams. Experiences with hallucinogenic drugs have led some behavioral scientists, such as Castaneda (1968) to formulate different, even mystical, ways of knowing reality. However, even the biological scientist (Lilly, 1972) and the astronaut (Mitchell, 1974) are no longer hesitant about involving themselves in experiments and self-revelations that would have seemed outrageously mystical 20 years ago but that are now taken as a matter of course.*

> *Astrology and prophecy seem to be as much in vogue today as they were in the 16th century. Many citizens eagerly accept the idea that the earth is being visited regularly by benign denizens of other solar systems who are ferried by spacecraft seen as unidentified flying objects (UFO's).*

ESP research was conducted at UCLA's Neuropsychiatric Institute by CIA consultant, Dr. Thelma Moss while Dr. West was the Director. The CIA funded paranormal research through STARGATE and MKULTRA; Dr. West himself obtained research funds through MKULTRA. Dr. Moss was an Assistant Professor at the Neuropsychiatric Institute beginning in 1966; her curriculum vitae lists 43 publications from 1961 to 1973, many of which are on ESP and the paranormal.

A paper by Ditman, Moss, Forgy, Zunin, Lynch and Funk[78] was entitled, "Dimensions of the LSD, Methylphenidate and Chlordiazepoxide Experiences." First author Keith Ditman, Research Psychiatrist, Neuropsychiatric Institute, UCLA, first took LSD himself when it was supplied to him by his colleague, Dr. Cholden[1] (see Chapter 7). Fourth author, Leonard M. Zunin, is described in a footnote as Assistant Chief, Neuropsychiatry, Naval Hospital, Camp Pendelton, California.

In the paper, Ditman et al.[78] reference MKULTRA Subcontractor Harold Abramson's[2] edited book on the second CIA-sponsored LSD symposium, and LSD papers by Drs. Savage[275] and Malitz[177], who attended the first CIA-sponsored LSD symposium.

Dr. Moss consulted to NASA, the Rand Corporation (contractor on MKULTRA Subproject 79), ARPA (The Defense Department's Advanced Research Projects Agency) and the CIA on radiation photography, also known as Kirlian photography, according to her curriculum vitae. One of her papers[200], published in the *Journal of Parapsychology* was entitled "ESP Effects in "Artists" Contrasted with "Non-Artists."" Other papers included "Quantitative Investigation of a "Haunted House"[204]; "ESP Over Long Distance"[199]; "Telepathy in the Waking State"[201]; "Hypnosis and ESP: A Controlled Experiment"[206]; "The Effect of Belief on ESP Success"[202]; "Skin Vision and Telepathy in a Blind Subject"[205]; and "Is There An Energy Body?"[203].

Dr. Moss' curriculum vitae lists numerous presentations on ESP including to the UCLA medical students and psychiatry residents. She was also interviewed by newspapers many times and appeared on many television programs including *60 Minutes*. There would appear to be a contradiction between Dr. Moss' career at UCLA's Neuropsychiatric Institute, which began in 1966, Dr. West being Director of the Neuropsychiatric Institute from 1969 to 1989, and Dr. West and Singer's 1980 statement that research such as hers "would have seemed outrageously mystical 20 years ago."

Files for MKULTRA Subproject 43, for which Dr. West was the contractor with TOP SECRET clearance, contain a letter to an unidentified Major dated 18 April 1955. The letter states that:

> *Due to circumstances beyond our control, our channel of communication has been changed. Beginning upon receipt of this letter, all mail will be addressed to the following location: [whited out]*
>
> *The instructions listed below must be followed implicitly:*
>
> *1. All communications MUST BE double enveloped.*
>
> *2. The outer envelope MUST BE addressed as indicated above.*
>
> *3. All mail MUST BE transmitted as first class mail, registered, return receipt requested.*
>
> *4. True or full names MUST NOT appear in any of the correspondence. Reference to our personnel may be made*

by first name and last initial or to the individual's assigned nom de plume.

5. Be sure that ALL persons responsible for preparing or transmitting correspondence to us are properly advised of this change of address and ALL instructions are understood. Should any questions arise incident to this change, please let us know immediately.

The fact that Dr. West was the contractor on MKULTRA Subproject 43 is proven by a letter dated 29 February 1956 from "[whited out], M.D., Professor of Psychiatry, Head of Department." The INSTITUTIONAL NOTIFICATIONS provided by the CIA under the Freedom of Information Act indicate that the University of Oklahoma was the site of MKULTRA Subproject 43, and Dr. West's curriculum vitae indicates that he was "Professor and Head" of the Department of Psychiatry at the University of Oklahoma from 1954 to 1969.

A letter from Dr. West to Sidney Gottlieb dated 29 February 1956 states:

Up to today I have been working very hard on my assigned investigation of POW problems for the Air Force. Some interesting things have turned up in the process of this study, bearing upon potential research issues of material interest to all concerned.

It is possible that I may be in Washington again in the very near future. [Whited out] will know about it before I will; if you want to see me, get in touch with him and find out whether the Surgeon General is going to be calling me up there next week.

Dr. West was co-editor of a book entitled *Hallucinations. Behavior, Experience, and Theory*[285]. One of the contributors to this book, Theodore Sarbin, Ph.D., is a member of the Scientific and Professional Advisory Board of the False Memory Syndrome Foundation (FMSF). Other members of the FMSF Board include Dr. Martin Orne, Dr. Margaret Singer, Dr. Richard Ofshe, Dr. Paul McHugh, Dr. David Dinges, Dr. Harold Lief, Emily Carota Orne, and Dr. Michael Persinger. The connections of these individuals to the mind control network are analyzed in this and the next two chapters.

Dr. Sarbin[272] (see Ross, 1997) believes that multiple personality disorder is almost always a therapist-created artifact and does not exist as a naturally-occurring disorder, a view adhered to by Dr. McHugh[188, 189], Dr. Ofshe[213] and other members of the FMSF Board[191, 243]. Dr. Ofshe is a colleague and co-author of Dr. Singer[214], who is in turn a colleague and co-author of Dr. West[329]. Denial of the reality of multiple personality by these doctors in the mind control network, who are also on the FMSF Scientific and Professional Advisory Board, could be disinformation. The disinformation could be amplified by attacks on specialists in multiple personality as CIA conspiracy lunatics[3, 79, 191, 213].

The FMSF is the only organization in the world that has attacked the reality of multiple personality in an organized, systematic fashion. FMSF Scientific and Professional Advisory Board Members publish most of the articles and letters to editors of psychiatry journals hostile to multiple personality disorder. They claim that most if not all cases have been created unwittingly by therapists, using the same techniques of mind control employed by destructive cults. Is this honest academic opinion, or disinformation? If any of the FMSF Scientific and Professional Advisory Board Members are attacking multiple personality disorder for disinformation purposes, this is itself a violation of professional and medical ethics.

Another of Dr. West's[318] publications is a chapter entitled "Hypnosis in Medical Practice" in a book edited by Dr. Harold Lief. Dr. Lief is a Member of the FMSF Board and a coauthor of Tulane brain electrode specialist and CIA contractor, Dr. Robert Heath[121, 161]. Dr. Lief has also functioned as the personal treating psychiatrist for Dr. Peter Freyd, husband of Dr. Pamela Freyd, Executive Director of the FMSF.

Dr. Michael Persinger[235], another FSMF Board Member, is the author of a paper entitled "Elicitation of 'Childhood Memories' in Hypnosis-Like Settings Is Associated With Complex Partial Epileptic-Like Signs For Women But Not for Men: Implications for the False Memory Syndrome." In the paper, Dr. Persinger writes:

> *On the day of the experiment each subject (not more than two were tested per day) was asked to sit quietly in an acoustic chamber and was told that the procedure was an experiment in relaxation. The subject wore goggles and a modified motorcycle helmet through which 10-milligauss (1 microTesla) magnetic fields were applied through the temporal plane. Except for a weak red (photographic developing) light, the room was dark.*

Dr. Persinger's research on the ability of magnetic fields to facilitate the creation of false memories and altered states of consciousness is apparently funded by the Defense Intelligence Agency through the project cryptonym SLEEPING BEAUTY. Freedom of Information Act requests concerning SLEEPING BEAUTY with a number of different intelligence agencies including the CIA and DIA has yielded denial that such a program exists. Certainly, such work would be of direct interest to BLUEBIRD, ARTICHOKE, MKULTRA and other non-lethal weapons programs.

Schnabel[280] lists Dr. Persinger as an Interview Source in his book on remote viewing operations conducted under Stargate, Grill Flame and other cryptonyms at Fort Meade and on contract to the Stanford Research Institute. Schnabel states (p. 220) that, "As one of the Pentagon's top scientists, Vorona was privy to some of the strangest, most secret research projects ever conceived. Grill Flame was just one. Another was code-named Sleeping Beauty; it was a Defense Department study of remote microwave mind-influencing techniques…"

It appears from Schnabel's well-documented investigations that Sleeping Beauty is a real, but still classified mind control program. Schnabel[280] lists Dr. West as an Interview Source and says that West was a, "Member of medical oversight board for Science Applications International Corp. remote-viewing research in early 1990s."

Brain research related to the work by Dr. Persinger was conducted at UCLA by Dr. William Ross Adey, who was born in Australia on January 31, 1922. Dr. Adey had already published in Australia before moving to California in 1954. His research at UCLA has been funded by the Office of Naval Research [ONR Contract 233 (91)], the Air Force Office of Scientific Research (Contract AF 49 (638)-1387) and NASA (Contract 9-1970).

Dr. Adey's work involved putting brain electrodes in cats and monkeys and giving the cats LSD and psilocybin[7]; these experiments were funded by "grant AF49 (638)-686 from the Office of Scientific Research of the U.S. Air Force and grant B-1883 from the U.S. Public Health Service." The drugs were supplied by Sandoz Pharmaceuticals.

A 1969 research project, also funded by the Air Force and the Public Health Service[110] describes using EEG telemetry equipment on a 10-year old girl. The girl slept at home with external EEG leads on her head (not electrodes implanted in her brain), and the EEG signals were transmitted from the electrodes to a radio receiver, then fed into the phone line and transmitted to Dr. Adey's lab two miles away. The EEG printout was read easily by laboratory personnel.

In September, 1965, Dr. Adey attended a conference in Hakone, Japan. Dr. Adey and Dr. T. Tokizane[6] edited the proceedings. In this volume, brain research funding is acknowledged as coming from the U.S. Army Research and Development Group (Far East), the Office of Naval Research, NASA, the U.S. Air Force and the Army Chemical Corp. Presenters included Dr. Jose Delgado[74], the brain electrode specialist from Yale whose paper includes photographs of monkeys running frantically in their cages because their brain electrodes are being stimulated by a remote transmitter.

Like Dr. Persinger, Dr. Adey[4] also did experiments in which subjects' heads were placed in electromagnetic fields. This work was funded by U.S. Air Force Contract F44620-70-C-0017. Other papers of his were entitled "Prolonged Effects of LSD on EEG Records During Discriminative Performance in Cat: Evaluation by Computer Analysis"[8] and "Autonomic Responses During A Replicable Interrogation"[33]; the latter research was funded by the Office of Naval Research.

Dr. Adey was a member of the MIT Neurosciences Research Program and edited a volume for them entitled *Brain Interaction with Weak Electric and Magnetic Fields*[5]. Another 1977 volume in the same series was edited by Dr. Robert D. Hall of the Worcester Foundation for Experimental Biology (site of MKULTRA Subproject 8).

Dr. Adey worked as a consultant for NASA, the Department of Energy and the Veterans Administration. He was the project leader for the Medical Hazards of Microwaves Exposure, US/USSR Exchange Program beginning in 1976. In the same year he became a member of the National Academy of Sciences panel on biosphere effects of extremely low frequency radiation. Both of these subjects are of direct relevance to non-lethal weapons programs.

Other related brain work was to have been done at the UCLA Violence Project, which was to have been headed by Dr. Louis Jolyon West. Dr. West[173] describes the demise of the Project prior to startup in a chapter entitled "Research on Violence: The Ethical Equation." The book was edited by CIA contractor, Dr. Neil Burch (see Chapter 14). Other contributors to the volume include Dr. Frank Ervin from the Harvard brain electrode team, and doctors from Walter Reed Army Institute of Research, the Navy Medical Neuropsychiatric Research Unit, San Diego and the Veterans Administration Hospital, Salt Lake City. Dr. West writes:

> *Actually Ervin was never involved with the CSRV [UCLA Center for the Study and Reduction of Violence] and had no part in its planning or development. Nevertheless, a radical students organization called Students for a Democratic Society (SDS) pounced on the "UCLA psychosurgery project" in wildly accusatory articles in the <u>Daily Bruin</u> and the underground press. Politically activist students suddenly began to picket with signs denouncing "A Clockwork Orange at UCLA", "Stop Psychosurgery at UCLA", "Fire Frank Ervin", "Drive West into the Sea" and the like.*
>
> *At first the staff assumed that the sudden hostile attack on the yet unfunded center was essentially political. The theme seemed to be, "If Governor Reagan is for it, we are against it." However, a small group of much more sophisticated political radicals, including two or three psychiatrists, took over the fight against the establishment of the CSRV. They went to many community groups and organizations, ranging from the American Civil Liberties Union to the Black Panther Party, and persuaded them that the proposed center was in fact racist, sexist, and dangerous to human rights; in fact, nothing less than a government-sponsored program for mind control.*

Funding for the UCLA Violence Project had been approved by Ronald Reagan but was withdrawn in response to public protest. The Project was to have been housed at a used Nike missile site outside Los Angeles. Dr. West states in a footnote to his chapter on the Project, that Dr. Frank Ervin had recently been recruited to the Department of Psychiatry at UCLA.

Another California project cancelled due to public protest was a proposal to implant brain electrodes in prisoners at Vacaville State Prison, site of CIA mind control experiments on the drug pemoline under MKSEARCH[103, 278]. The prisoners were to be monitored by remote tracking technology post-discharge. If they entered a restricted area or exhibited sexual arousal patterns on remote EEG telemetry, a signal would be sent to their brain electrodes immobilizing them, and law enforcement personnel would be dispatched to apprehend them.

Dr. Lois Jolyon West was cleared at TOP SECRET for his work on MKULTRA. His numerous connections to the mind control network illustrate how the network was maintained; not through any central conspiracy, but by an interlocking network of academic relationships, grants, conferences, and military appointments. Some doctors in the network were not funded directly by the CIA or military, but their work was of direct relevance to mind control, non-lethal weapons development, and the creation of controlled dissociation and Manchurian Candidates.

11

DR. MARTIN ORNE

Martin Orne was born in Vienna on October 16, 1927. He died on February 11, 2000. Dr. Orne immigrated to the United States with his family in 1938, studied psychology at Harvard and then went to medical school, receiving his M.D. from Tufts University Medical School in 1955. He received his Ph.D. in psychology from Harvard in 1958 while in his first year of training in psychiatry. He received CIA money through MKULTRA Subproject 84 in 1958; Subproject documents indicate that he received TOP SECRET clearance from the CIA in 1960.

In 1962, Dr. Orne founded the Institute for Experimental Psychiatry and married Emily Farrell Carota. Both he and his wife are on the Advisory Board of the False Memory Syndrome Foundation (FMSF). In 1964, Orne was recruited to the Institute of the Pennsylvania Hospital, where he remained until its closing over thirty years later. For about thirty years, he was the editor of *The International Journal of Clinical and Experimental Hypnosis.*

Martin Orne is one of the leading experts on hypnosis of the twentieth century. He is referenced throughout the hypnosis literature and received the Distinguished Scientific Award from the American Psychological Association in 1986. His curriculum vitae lists numerous awards, grants, publications and appointments including research grants from many military intelligence agencies (see Appendix F). His curriculum vitae does not list his MKULTRA contract nor his work for the National Security Agency. A reliable physician described to me Dr. Orne's stopping off at a National Security Agency building while they were on a trip together to another location.

Dr. Orne's publications include a 1980 report[223] with his wife, D.F. Dinges (a FMSF Board Member) and F.J. Evans entitled "Voluntary self-control of sleep to facilitate quasi-continuous performance. Fort Detrick, MD: U.S. Army Medical Research and Development Command. (NTIS No AD-A102264)." A book chapter[215] is entitled "The Potential Uses of Hypnosis in Interrogation." Dr. Orne[216, 217] also published chapters in books edited by G.H. Estabrooks and Louis Jolyon West.

Dr. Orne received research money from the CIA, Army, Navy and Air Force. He published many papers relevant to the creation of amnesia and Manchurian Candidates including one entitled "Can a hypnotized subject be compelled to carry out otherwise unacceptable behavior?"[218]. Another example is a paper entitled "Attempting to breach posthypnotic amnesia"[224]. Coauthor on that paper, Dr. John Kihlstrom is on the Advisory Board of the False Memory Syndrome Foundation.

Dr. Orne also studied the cueing and triggering phenomena developed in BLUEBIRD and ARTICHOKE as a method of programming Manchurian Candidates. One paper was entitled "The significance of unwitting cues for experimental outcomes: Toward a pragmatic approach"[220] and another "Restricted use of success cues in retrieval during posthypnotic amnesia"[225]. He said of Dr. Louis Jolyon West[221]:

> As one reviews Jolly West's contributions, his depth and breadth are unique, ranging from brainwashing to sleep deprivation, from cults to psychotherapy, from hallucinations to dissociative reactions.

Dr. Orne was also interested in hallucinations, brainwashing, psychotherapy, and dissociation, as was the CIA, which funded research on each of those topics through MKULTRA. Dr. Orne[217] wrote a chapter entitled "Hypnotically Induced Hallucinations" in a book edited by Dr. West. Other books to which he contributed chapters included one[219] edited by Dr. Daniel X. Freedman, who worked for CIA cutout The Josiah Macy, Jr. Foundation.

An MKULTRA Subproject 84 MEMORANDUM FOR THE RECORD dated 17 August 1960 states that, "it is contemplated that Dr. [whited out] will be made witting of sponsorship and purpose on or about 1 September 1960 in order to guide his project along lines that will further Agency operational needs." Dr. Orne's proposal in the MKULTRA Subproject 84 file mentions a study on sensory deprivation he had completed and concludes with the statement:

Finally, the controversial question of anti-social behavior in hypnosis will be re-evaluated experimentally. It is hoped to be able to shed considerable light on the limitations of hypnosis as a technique of controlling behavior in this manner. A paper has been written, in part under the auspices of [whited out] dealing with the potential uses of hypnosis in interrogation and is to be published [whited out].

A March, 1996 letter from Dr. Orne to the CIA explains that he has not yet spent all his MKULTRA money. Dr. Orne says that he understands there is no time limitation on spending the remaining funds. The reason the CIA was not anxious to see the completion of any particular piece of research by Dr. Orne is explained in a MEMORANDUM FOR THE RECORD dated 27 July 1960; "No special direction will be given to [whited out] research since virtually every problem he has set for himself has a bearing upon Agency interests."

The total of $30,000.00 provided to Dr. Orne through MKULTRA Subproject 84 was not subject to the usual reporting and accounting procedures required for almost all other MKULTRA Subprojects. A 1961 CIA document entitled CERTIFICATION states that, "it is therefore requested that the unexpended portion of the original grant ($20,507.55) be written off based on services being received in the form of research reports."

In an interview with John Marks[184], unidentified CIA personnel explained that Dr. Orne was one of a handful of informal consultants the CIA used on a regular basis. Another was MKULTRA Subproject 96 contractor, Dr. George Kelley, who also had TOP SECRET clearance. The purpose of the money funded through MKULTRA Subproject 84 was to establish a relationship, more than to support any specific piece of work.

Dr. Martin Orne is one of two psychiatrists professionally active into the late 1990's who is a documented CIA mind control contractor, along with Dr. Louis Jolyon West. Both men were lifelong students of dissociation, amnesia, coercive persuasion, hypnosis and other topics at the core of BLUEBIRD and ARTICHOKE, and both received funding from numerous military sources and the CIA. Both men are therefore central to the history of psychiatric participation in mind control experimentation.

12

DR. EWEN CAMERON

The MKULTRA contractor about whom the most has been written is Dr. Ewen Cameron[65, 105, 184, 212, 278, 301, 313]. Dr. Cameron was the contractor for Subproject 68. It says in the Subproject 68 documents that Dr. Cameron was unwitting of CIA involvement, but this claim is implausible for a number of reasons. For one thing, the files often do not contain a complete account of the content or purpose of the Subproject.

A MEMORANDUM from Richard Helms, Acting Deputy Director (Plans) to Allen Dulles, Director of the CIA dated 3 April 1953 and entitled "Two Extremely Sensitive Research Programs" (MKULTRA and MKDELTA) includes the statement that, "Even internally in CIA, as few individuals as possible should be aware of our interest in these fields and of the identity of those who are working for us. At present this results in ridiculous contracts, often with cut-outs, which do not spell out the scope or intent of the work and which contain terms which the cut-out cannot incorporate in his contract with the researcher without revealing Government interest. Complete Government audits of such contracts are impossible for the same reason."

Born in Bridge of Allan, Scotland on December 24, 1901, Cameron immigrated to Canada in 1929 to take a job as a psychiatrist at Brandon Mental Hospital in Brandon, Manitoba. He was recruited by Dr. Thomas Pincock; one of the buildings in the Department of Psychiatry at the University of Manitoba in Winnipeg in the 1980's was the Pincock Building. Dr. George Sisler and Dr. John Matas, both of whom referred patients to Dr. Cameron when he was at the Allan Memorial Institute in Montreal, taught at the University of Manitoba into the 1980's, as did Dr. Gordon Lambert, who treated one of Dr. Cameron's mind control victims on her return to Winnipeg.

Despite these historical connections, I heard no conversation about Dr. Ewen Cameron or CIA mind control while a resident and then a staff psychiatrist in the Department of Psychiatry in Winnipeg from 1981 to 1991, despite the fact that plaintiffs, including Val Orlikow from Winnipeg, settled a suit with the CIA in 1988. Mrs. Orlikow's husband, David Orlikow, had been a prominent Member of Parliament from Winnipeg for many years. There was silence in psychiatry about CIA mind control, but no conspiracy of silence. No one was told to be quiet. From the perspective of academic psychiatry, mind control experimentation didn't exist, so there was no need to cover it up.

Throughout the twentieth century, academic psychiatry provided no public commentary, ethical guidance, peer review, or moral oversight of any kind concerning mind control experimentation, despite the fact that the leading psychiatrists and medical schools were well funded by the CIA and military for mind control research. Mental patients, cancer patients, prisoners and unwitting citizens were experimented on by mind control doctors at Yale, Harvard, McGill, Stanford, UCLA and the other major universities.

These human guinea pigs were never told that they were subjects in military and CIA mind control experiments, and they never gave informed consent. They received no systematic follow-up to document the harm done to them. The welfare of the "human subjects" was not a relevant variable in the academic equation. What counted for the psychiatrists, I think, was money, power, perks, academic advancement and the thrill of being a spy doctor.

Despite the code of silence, and despite later claims by the Canadian Psychiatric Association that Dr. Cameron was unaware he was working for the CIA (see Appendix H), unwitting investigator status for Cameron is implausible for several reasons. He was far too politically connected to be unwitting. At various times, Dr. Cameron was President of the Quebec, Canadian, American and World Psychiatric Associations, the Society of Biological Psychiatry and the American Geriatrics Society. Dr. Cameron was one of four co-founders of the World Psychiatric Association; another was Dr. William Sargant[273], the foremost British authority on brainwashing. Many Board Members and Presidents of the Society of Biological Psychiatry were LSD researchers, funded by the military or otherwise in the mind control network.

A letter from the CIA to Senator Pete Wilson dated 11 December 1985 states that the CIA contacted Dr. Cameron directly. On page 4, the correspondent says:

> First, the CIA did not instigate this research, create the protocol, or supervise the work. Rather, CIA contacted a prominent and highly respected Canadian psychiatrist, Dr. Ewen Cameron, who was conducting research into treatment of mental illness with drugs such as LSD, and the CIA provided minimal and partial funding for a short time period. In return, the CIA received periodic reports on his research into behavioral modification through a process which he termed "psychic driving."

Dr. Cameron was eulogized in obituaries in the *Canadian Psychiatric Association Journal*[15], the *Canadian Medical Association Journal*[61], the *American Journal of Psychiatry*[93], and *Recent Advances in Biological Psychiatry*[129], the latter written by Hudson Hoaglund, Ph.D., who was personally referred to J. Edgar Hoover by G.H. Estabrooks. Dr. Cameron received many awards including the Adolph Meyer Award, the Samuel Rubin Award and the Montreal Mental Hygeine Institute Award, given to "a scientist who has made an outstanding contribution to the mental health of the Canadian people."

In an article entitled "McGill University Department of Psychiatry 50th Anniversary," Pinard and Young[242] echo the sentiments of the eulogist:

> Since the department's inception in 1943, research has been a preponderant part of its mission; this was stated in the very first reports to the university by the department's founder, Ewen Cameron...

> The department's record has not been one of unblemished success. Cameron's drive led to the foundation and growth of the department, but also lead him to perform much publicized experiments of doubtful ethical or scientific value in which patients received multiple courses of ECT or doses of LSD.

In his obituary in the Canadian Psychiatric Association Journal[61] Cameron is eulogized as follows:

> As a diligent seeker after new knowledge, a gifted author, a renowned administrator and inspiring teacher he brought,

*not only to his professional colleagues but also to the community
at large, a wider and deeper understanding of the importance and
significance of the emotional life of man.*

Dr. Cameron began conducting unethical, unscientific and inhumane
brainwashing experiments at Brandon Mental Hospital in the 1930's.
He continued this work into the 1960's. In one paper[50] Dr. Cameron
describes treating schizophrenics with red light produced by filtering
light from fifteen 200-watt lamps through an inch of running water and
a layer of sodium salt of ditolyldisazo-bis-napthylanine s sulphuric acid
impregnated into cellophane.

The color red was chosen because it is the color of blood. In these
experiments, schizophrenic patients were forced to lie naked in red
light for eight hours a day for periods as long as eight months. Another
experiment involved overheating patients in an electric cage until their
body temperatures reached 102 degrees F.

After leaving Brandon Mental Hospital in 1936, Cameron took a job at
Worcester State Hospital in Massachusetts. The Worcester Foundation
for Experimental Biology received CIA money through MKULTRA
Subproject 8, and was the professional home of Dr. Cameron's eulogist,
Hudson Hoaglund[129]. At Worcester State Hospital, Dr. Cameron massively
over-utilized insulin coma therapy by putting patients in coma for 2 to 5
hours per day for up to 50 days in a row.

In a paper published in the *American Journal of Psychiatry* entitled
"Psychic Driving," Dr. Cameron[51] describes his brainwashing techniques
and says, "Analogous to this is the breakdown of the individual under
continuous interrogation."

Psychic driving was a procedure carried out in two stages; in the first stage,
patients were *depatterned*, which meant they were reduced to a vegetable
state through a combination of massive amounts of electroconvulsive
shock, drug-induced sleep and sensory isolation and deprivation. When
fully depatterned, patients were incontinent of urine and feces, unable
to feed themselves, and unable to state their name, age, location, or the
current date (see Chapter 16).

In the second stage, *psychic driving* was introduced. This consisted
of hundreds of hours of tape loops being played to the patient through
earphones, special helmets or speakers in the sensory isolation room. The

tape loops repeated statements of supposed psychological significance. If such procedures were carried out under third world dictators, they would be denounced as human rights violations by American and Canadian psychiatry, and would be called *brainwashing*.

There is a further reason to conclude that Ewen Cameron had a security clearance and was witting of CIA funding of his research; Dr. Cameron definitely had a security clearance with the U.S. government. In 1945 he was part of an American team that did psychiatric assessments of German War criminals including Rudolph Hess, who was examined at the request of the Military Tribunal in Nuremberg. Dr. Cameron must have heard about the mescaline research done in the death camps by Nazi psychiatrists. He himself instituted similar work at McGill when he began experimenting with LSD.

An example of a German psychiatrist recruited to the Allan Memorial Institute is Dr. Werner Kohlmeyer, who was born in Hanover on May 21, 1921. Dr. Kohlmeyer received his M.D. from the University of Gottingen in 1945, then did a year of internship in 1946 and two years of psychiatry residency in Hamburg in 1947-48. He did post-graduate training at the Allan Memorial Institute from 1951 to 1954[156]. Dr. Kohlmeyer became an Instructor in Psychiatry at Johns Hopkins School of Medicine in 1958 and an Assistant Professor in 1970. He was still resident in Baltimore as of 1986.

There is no evidence that Dr. Kohlmeyer was directly recruited by the CIA or military, however research he did at the Allan Memorial Institute was funded by The Medical Research and Development Division, Office of the Surgeon General, Department of the U.S. Army under Contract No. DA-49-007-MD-70 (Malmo, Smith, and Kohlmeyer, 1955). The outline of Dr. Kohlmeyer's professional career and recruitment to the Allan Memorial Institute is included to illustrate the flow of psychiatric personnel from Germany to McGill to Johns Hopkins[37]. German mind control doctors could have been brought over under PROJECT PAPERCLIP and provided cover under an immigration profile like that of Dr. Kohlmeyer. Dr. Cameron is a leading candidate for involvement in the recruitment and placement of PAPERCLIP psychiatrists, in part because he himself trained at Johns Hopkins for a period[129].

Rather than being the object of suspicion and investigation in the 1950's, Dr. Cameron was well regarded in the Canadian media. Favorable articles about him were entitled "Canadian Psychiatrists Develop Beneficial

Brainwashing"[195]; "New 'Personalities' Made to Order"[47] and "Two-Month Sleep, Shock New Schizophrenic Cure"[49]. Similarly, as recently as June 6, 1987, the official position of the Canadian Psychiatric Association on Dr. Cameron's brainwashing experiments was far from negative (see Appendix H):

> *... the fact that Dr. Cameron's research would not be accepted by today's standards of ethical and scientific inquiry, cannot be used as a retrospective critique of his work. What has to be recognized clearly is that in the intervening 20 to 30 years there has been a continuing progression of scientific and ethical research standards that included much more sophisticated peer review and ethical approval review now in place as part of standard practice. This represents the evolution of concern and control for all medical research using human subjects deriving in part out of concerns experienced in several fields of medicine. Such experiments would not be permitted in today's research climate.*

The position on Dr. Cameron taken by the Canadian Psychiatric Association is mistaken for several reasons. Dr. Cameron received a grant from Canada's Department of Health and Welfare for $57,750.00 for the years 1961 to 1964 for "A Study of Factors Which Promote or Retard Personality Change in Individuals Exposed to Prolonged Repetition of Verbal Signals." The Helsinki Declaration governing ethical rules for medical research was adopted in 1964; Dr. Cameron's brainwashing experiments clearly violated the principles of informed consent and protection of the patient from undue harm contained in the Helsinki Declaration.

Dr. Cameron's experiments also violated the informed consent provisions of the Nuremberg Code, which arose out of the war crime trials of the Nazi doctors, in which Dr. Cameron participated as a member of the American psychiatric team. He thus had direct knowledge of the medical atrocities the Nuremberg code was designed to prevent. The Canadian Psychiatric Association's position that Dr. Cameron's research would "not be permitted in today's research climate" is correct, but ignores the fact that the rules of ethical conduct in medical research have not changed since Nuremberg.

The fact that medical schools were routinely lax in ensuring that prevailing ethical codes were adhered to in the 1950's and 1960's is a condemnation of the medical schools, not a vindication of Dr. Cameron. The Canadian Psychiatric Association's argument concerning different ethical standards in the 1950's and 1960's is reminiscent of the U.S. Army's apologist strategy concerning brain electrode implant experiments at Tulane (see Chapter 8). I consider the Canadian Psychiatric Association's official position on the mind control experiments conducted by Dr. Ewen Cameron to be a violation of the Hippocratic Oath. Lies and silence concerning psychiatric mind control experimentation are a betrayal of the physician's ethical duty.

The fact that Dr. Cameron's unethical, inhumane, and grossly damaging experiments were published in the psychiatric literature is a condemnation of the editorial standards of the journals, not a vindication of Dr. Cameron. The only argument protective of the psychiatric journals is the fact that Dr. Cameron whitewashed the experiments for publication. Dr. Cameron's brainwashing experiments stopped in 1964, whereas the Tuskeegee Syphilis Study continued until 1972. The continuation of the Tuskeegee Syphilis Study under the auspices of the Center for Disease Control until 1972 does not provide vindication for Dr. Cameron, rather it provides further grounds for criticism of organized medicine.

The U.S. Government has officially apologized to and financially compensated the victims of the radiation experiments and the Tuskeegee Syphilis Study, and the Canadian Government has established a fund that compensates victims of unethical experiments by Dr. Cameron at the Allan Memorial Institute; compensation of $100,000.00 can be activated by documented victims by calling a toll-free number provided by the Canadian government. Given the positions taken by two federal governments on such medical experiments, the position of the Canadian Psychiatric Association on Dr. Ewen Cameron requires revision.

Dr. Cameron was not the only researcher at McGill funded by the CIA and the military. Another psychiatrist at McGill, Dr. Raymond Prince[248] was funded through MKULTRA Subproject 121. Dr. Prince was an unwitting investigator and is the only psychiatrist to have written about CIA mind control in the peer-reviewed medical literature. He is the only MKULTRA contractor to have publicly identified himself to date. No other MKULTRA contractor has engaged in any public discussion of psychiatric participation in CIA and military mind control.

Dr. Prince's MKULTRA work was published in a book edited by Ari Kiev[150, 246]. Kiev was a participant on the Hungarian refugee studies[127] funded through MKULTRA Subprojects 69 and 89. From 1962 to 1964, Dr. Kiev was a staff psychiatrist at Wiford Hall, USAF Hospital, Lackland

Air Force Base, San Antonio. In the book in which Dr. Prince's chapter on the Yoruba appears, Dr. Kiev himself references MKULTRA contractors Carl Rogers, Harold Wolff and Lawrence Hinkle, and British brainwashing expert William Sargant, who co-founded the World Psychiatric Association with MKULTRA contractor, Ewen Cameron. He also references Human Ecology Foundation Director, John Whitehorn (see Chapter 13).

Dr. Hassan Azima was a young McGill psychiatrist who was being groomed as a military mind control contractor prior to his death from cancer in his early forties. A colleague, Dr. Sarwer-Foner[274] gave the Hassan Azima Memorial Lecture at a meeting of the Society of Biological Psychiatry; Dr. Cameron was a Past President of the Society.

Dr. Azima[17, 18] worked at the Allan Memorial Institute, where he gave psilocybin to patients; psilocybin is the active ingredient of "magic mushrooms." He also attended LSD symposia and performed sensory isolation experiments[19] that caused damage to patients. Two patients with "obsessional neuroses manifested acute psychotic episodes. They were treated with electric shock, which resulted in improvement in both paranoid and obsessional features." Azima and Cramer[19] write:

> *Contrary to the above case, a hebephrenic-catatonic girl who remained in isolation for six days showed no perceptual alteration. Behaviorally, she manifested overt hostility, became quite talkative and self-assertive. Her F.D. [figure drawings] revealed gradual, but definite emergence of aggressive tendencies. She also experienced several spontaneous orgasms, and verbalized memories of her "sexual adventures."*

Another patient in the series is described as follows:

> *Another case of obsession neurosis, suffering severe motor compulsions, who had not responded to any form of treatment, was put in isolation with the explicit aim of provoking a psychotic disorganization. He remained five days in isolation, began to manifest signs of depersonalization on the second day, and showed several acute psychotic episodes, lasting about three hours on the fourth and fifth days. The disorganization manifested itself, in part, as a marked disinhibition. He experienced many spontaneous orgasms, and manifested overt erotic behavior toward the nurses. His eating habits deteriorated, and his behavior was like that of a very hungry*

*child during the feeding periods. In the post-isolation period
he showed some reorganization and lost some of his motor
compulsions. But because of the appearance of some paranoid
tendencies, he was put on electric shock therapy, which resulted
in considerable improvement and subsequent discharge.*

Dr. Azima[21] published a paper with Dr. Eric Wittkower, who worked
at the *Transcultural Psychiatry Institute* at McGill, where Dr. Prince
was employed. Dr. Wittkower founded and edited *The Transcultural
Psychiatric Research Review*. The *Review* was funded by CIA cutout the
Society for the Investigation of Human Ecology, which lists a payment
to Dr. Wittkower of $7,500.00 in its 1961 Annual Report. The Board
of Advisors for the *Review* included Dr. Ewen Cameron and Margaret Mead,
who received CIA money for her anthropology research, and who was married
to Gregory Bateson. Bateson took LSD supplied to him by a psychiatrist (see
Chapter 7), and both Bateson and Mead were members of the Cybernetics
Group, which was funded by CIA cutout, The Josiah Macy, Jr. Foundation.

Margaret Mead was funded by the OSS during World War II, as was
Gregory Bateson[134]. Bateson spent two years in Ceylon, India, Burma
and China as an OSS psychological warfare expert, and he also taught at
Columbia University under OSS and Navy auspices beginning in 1942.
Mead set up an OSS training unit with Kurt Lewin and later recruited
Rhoda Metraux to the OSS; Metraux became a close colleague and friend
of Mead's and lived with her for a period. Rhoda Metraux was a co-
author of MKULTRA lead psychologist, John Gittinger and MKULTRA
contractor Harold Wolff[128].

Margaret Mead's sister, Priscilla, was married to Leo Rusten, who worked
as a liaison with Hollywood for the Office of War Information, and later
founded the social science division of the RAND Corporation. Mead's
Research in Contemporary Cultures study was funded by RAND in 1948-
49, and the RAND Corporation later became an MKULTRA contractor
itself (Subproject 79).

After the war, Mead received a $1,000,000.00 grant from the Office of
Naval Research, which she used to assemble a team of 120 anthropologists.
In addition, she maintained a personal relationship with MKSEARCH
contractor Dr. James Hamilton from World War II until her last visit to him in
1978. These numerous interconnections between Mead, Bateson, MKULTRA,
MKSEARCH, the OSS and the Navy illustrated how the mind control network
involved the field of anthropology, as well as psychology and psychiatry.

Dr. Azima thanked Dr. Cameron and Dr. Cleghorn for their support in another paper[20]. Dr. Cleghorn[61] wrote an obituary on Dr. Cameron, and notes of his appear in Linda MacDonald's medical record along with notes by Dr. Cameron (see Chapter 16 and Appendix H).

Another McGill psychiatrist, Dr. James Tyhurst worked at the Allan Memorial Institute and received funding from Canada's Defense Research Board for studies of individual reactions to community disasters[304]. Disaster studies were also the subject of investigation in MKULTRA Subproject 126, which was approved by the CIA in 1960. Dr. Tyhurst attended a meeting with CIA personnel in 1951 in Montreal devoted to oversight of BLUEBIRD and ARTICHOKE[105]. He also worked at Hollywood Hospital in Vancouver, where hundreds of patients were treated with LSD[174].

In a paper entitled "An Evaluation of the Clinical Significance of Reserpine," Tyhurst and Richman[305] noted that:

> *In a 5-month period, while 5 out of 6 reserpine-treated patients developed complications in insulin coma, only 5 out of 36 non-reserpine patients developed complications. The complications seen in reserpine-treated patients included 2 prolonged comas, 1 cyanosis, 1 increased sensitivity to insulin, and 1 death with respiratory arrest.*

Dr. Donald Hebb, Head of the Department of Psychology at McGill during the 1950's, received funding from Canada's Defense Research Board for experiments on sensory isolation[105]. The network of doctors with CIA and military funding at McGill included Dr. Cameron, Dr. Hebb, Dr. Tyhurst, Dr. Wittkower and Dr. Prince, and in addition Dr. Azima was firmly established in the mind control network and using many of the same experimental procedures. LSD research was also done at McGill and Montreal General Hospital by Dr. J.H. Quastel[16]. Any claim that Dr. Cameron's CIA funding was an anomaly or isolated incident is therefore incorrect.

Medical experimentation by the Department of Psychiatry at McGill resulted in death, psychosis, vegetable states, organic brain damage, and permanent loss of memory among other damages. It resulted in the creation of amnesia, identity disturbance and depersonalization among other dissociative symptoms. Dr. Ewen Cameron was the main figure in these activities.

13
JOHNS HOPKINS UNIVERSITY

The Current Chairman of the Department of Psychiatry at Johns Hopkins is Dr. Paul McHugh, who was born in Lawrence, Massachusetts on May 21, 1931. He received his M.D. from Harvard Medical School in 1956 (research at Harvard was funded through MKULTRA Subprojects 84 and 92). He worked at Walter Reed Army Institute of Research in Washington from 1961 to 1964, where he did brain electrode implant research on monkeys with funding from the U.S. Army Medical Research and Development Command[187]. Dr. McHugh was an Assistant Professor of Psychiatry and Neurology at Cornell from 1964 to 1968; the 1961 Annual Report of CIA cutout the Human Ecology Foundation lists MKULTRA contractor Dr. Harold Wolff as Chairman of its Board of Directors. Dr. Wolff was a neurologist at Cornell.

Dr. McHugh became the Henry Phipps Professor of Psychiatry and Director of the Department of Psychiatry and Behavioral Sciences, the Johns Hopkins School of Medicine in 1975, a position he holds up to the present. The first two academic conferences held by the False Memory Syndrome Foundation (FMSF) took place in Baltimore and were co-sponsored by the Department of Psychiatry at Johns Hopkins. Dr. McHugh was a course director at the second meeting.

Faculty for the second FMSF conference on March 21, 1997 included Godfrey D. Pearlson, M.D., Professor of Psychiatry and Mental Hygeine, Director, Division of Neuroimaging, Johns Hopkins School of Medicine. His talk was entitled, "Brain Imaging Studies on False Memory and Trauma: A Critical Review." Johns Hopkins is currently participating in the Human Brain Project, which receives funding from the Office of Naval Research, and has contracts with the Army Research Laboratory for microelectronics development.

The 1961 Annual Report of the Human Ecology Foundation lists John C. Whitehorn, Professor and Director, Department of Psychiatry, Johns Hopkins University as a Director. John Clare Whitehorn was born on December 6, 1894 in Spencer, Nebraska. He was Henry Phipps Professor of Psychiatry and Psychiatrist-in-Chief at Johns Hopkins from 1941 to 1960. Dr. Whitehorn corresponded extensively with the Scottish Rite Research Committee and received research grants from them, as did MKULTRA and MKSEARCH contractor, Dr. Carl Pfeiffer.

Correspondence with Dr. Whitehorn, obtained from the Alan Mason Chesney Medical Archives at Johns Hopkins, includes an April 2, 1957 letter from William Malamud, M.D. Dr. Malamud was a co-author of Dr. Overholser[175], whose extensive mind control connections are described in Chapter 14.

The Supreme Council, 33 Degree Scottish Rite, Northern Masonic Jurisdiction, U.S.A. sponsored a conference on research in schizophrenia at Boston University School of Medicine on October 7, 1950, as described on Dr. Malamud's stationery. Opening remarks were by Commander Melvin M. Johnson. Speakers included Dr. Whitehorn, Dr. Franz Kallman[232], and Dr. Hudson Hoaglund, who was recommended to J. Edgar Hoover by G.H. Estabrooks (see Chapter 15). Estabrooks was himself a 32nd degree Mason. Although the Masons are not implicated as an organization in CIA and military mind control, connections in the network of doctors were maintained in part through high rank in the Masons.

The Josiah Macy, Jr. Foundation funded a conference on May 14 and 15, 1942 attended by: Dr. Whitehorn; Gregory Bateson (who first received LSD from a psychiatrist; see Chapter 7); Dr. Milton Erickson (who spoke at a conference organized by G.H. Estabrooks; see Chapter 15); Dr. Frank Fremont-Smith (Medical Director of the Josiah Macy, Jr. Foundation; see Chapter 7); and Dr. Harold Wolff (MKULTRA contractor and Director of the Human Ecology Foundation). On October 26, 1945, Dr. Whitehorn wrote to Dr. Fremont-Smith at the Josiah Macy, Jr. Foundation.

Also involved in this academic circle were anthropologists Clyde Kluckholm and Margaret Mead (wife of Gregory Bateson); the group continued meeting after the war with funding from the Josiah Macy, Jr. Foundation. According to Heims[125], the sociologist Talcott Parsons was also part of this academic group. Dr. Parsons recruited Russian-born Nazi collaborators to work at the Russian Research Center at Harvard University, which was supported by the Carnegie and Rockefeller foundations. These scholars were denied U.S. entry visas according to Heims, and therefore must have been brought into the U.S. through PROJECT PAPERCLIP or another similar program. There was an arrangement between Harvard University and the FBI to turn information from the Russian Research Center over to the FBI, but Harvard archives on these activities are closed to researchers, so the extent of the collaboration is uncertain. Dr. Parsons also worked for Army Intelligence and the State Department.

Dr. Whitehorn died in 1973. During his life, he served as a consultant to the War Department, the Naval Hospital in Bethesda, the CIA through the Human Ecology Foundation, and the Veterans Administration Hospital in Perry Point. He gave the Presidential Address to the American Psychiatric Association in 1951 and was an Associate Editor of *The American Journal of Psychiatry*.

The next Chairman of Psychiatry at Johns Hopkins was Seymour S. Kety, who held the position from 1961 to 1962. Dr. Kety and Dr. Franz Kallman attended the October 7, 1950 Scottish Rite Conference on Schizophrenia. Dr. Kallman's genetic theories of schizophrenia were intolerable even to the Nazis because they implied that many Aryan Nazis were carrying a recessive gene for schizophrenia; Kallman emigrated from Germany to the U.S. in 1933, where he recommended eugenics programs to the U.S. and state governments[145, 145, 232].

Besides being a researcher on the genetics of schizophrenia, Dr. Kety did experiments with LSD[293, 294]. On November 8 and 9, 1958, he participated in a Scottish Rite Conference at the Waldorf Astoria Hotel in New York; he chaired a morning session on November 8. Presenters included: Dr. Hudson Hoagland of the Worcester Foundation for Experimental Biology (MKULTRA Subproject 8 on LSD, 1953), who was personally recommended to J. Edgar Hoover by G.H. Estabrooks; Dr. Jacques Gottlieb, LSD and phencyclidine researcher (see Chapter 7); Dr. Franz Kallman; and Dr. John Whitehorn.

Dr. Kety was Chairman of NASA's bioscience advisory committee, and was a member of the Scottish Rite Schizophrenia Research Committee. He did LSD research with Dr. Louis Sokoloff while at the National Institute of Mental Health[16], and was funded by the Supreme Council, Scottish Rite, Northern Masonic Jurisdiction for work on "barbiturate semi-narcosis, insulin coma and electric shock"[149]. Dr. Kety also did work for the U.S. Naval Air Development Center[159].

From 1963 to 1973, the Chairman of the Department of Psychiatry at Johns Hopkins was Dr. Joel Elkes. Dr. Elkes did brain electrode experiments on conscious animals; one of his papers is entitled "A technique for recording the electrical activity of the brain in the conscious animal"[40].

Prior to 1963, Dr. Elkes worked at St. Elizabeth's Hospital, where the poet Ezra Pound was held as a political prisoner on psychiatric grounds by Dr. Overholser (see Chapter 14). He published hallucinogen research in a publication of CIA cutout the Josiah Macy, Jr. Foundation[80] and participated in chemical weapons research in England during World War II. On April 17 to 19, 1970, Dr. Kety spoke at a conference in Baltimore with Dr. Albert Hoffman, who discovered LSD at Sandoz Laboratories in Switzerland in 1943. In a 1970 newspaper article, Dr. Elkes[152] describes first taking LSD himself in the late 1940's.

The Department of Psychiatry at Johns Hopkins School of Medicine may experience *blowback* because of its involvement in CIA and military mind control. For instance, Department of Psychiatry Chairman, Dr. Paul McHugh[188, 189] claims that multiple personality never occurs as a natural disorder and is always caused by the therapist. Dr. McHugh[189] states that diagnosis and treatment of multiple personality is "a major folly, a folly astonishing in its wild presumptions" that has "misaligned psychotherapy," and been "a disaster for American psychiatry." Writers on multiple personality, he says, have "deranged the discourse of psychiatry and cultivated a Sherlock Holmes fantasy among many psychotherapists."

The book to which Dr. McHugh has contributed the Foreword, and in which he makes these statements, is by False Memory Syndrome Foundation Advisory Board Member, Dr. August Piper[243]. The title, *Hoax and Reality. The Bizarre World of Multiple Personality Disorder*, is typical of the attack on multiple personality spearheaded by members of the Scientific and Professional Advisory Board of the False Memory Syndrome Foundation.

FMSF Advisory Board Members Dr. Martin Orne and Dr. Louis Jolyon West are CIA and military mind control contractors with TOP SECRET CIA clearance. Both received MKULTRA contracts to study the dissociative disorders, implantation of false memories, and techniques for creation of Manchurian Candidates. The dissociative disorders, false memories and therapist-created multiple personality are the focus of the FMSF campaign.

Dr. McHugh and other FMSF Advisory Board members scoff at clinical multiple personality disorder. They claim that virtually all cases of multiple personality are iatrogenic, or created by the therapist. Dr. McHugh is firmly entrenched in the network of mind control doctors that created Manchurian Candidates. He is a productive academic, and Chairman of a major academic Department of Psychiatry, not a fool, yet he falls short of the most elementary scholarly standards in his attack on multiple personality disorder. Why? What is really going on here?

Perhaps Dr. McHugh is speaking from his experience, or the experience of his friends, colleagues, and Department of Psychiatry, in Cold War mind control experimentation. If clinical multiple personality is buried and forgotten, then the Manchurian Candidate Programs will be safe from public scrutiny. I would like to know whether Dr. McHugh himself, or other members of his Department of Psychiatry at Johns Hopkins University School of Medicine, are CIA or military mind control contractors.

14

OTHER DOCTORS IN THE NETWORK

Other doctors in the mind control network include Neil Burch, M.D. Dr. Burch was born on April 3, 1924. He died on December 17, 1987. He was the Director of the Research Division of the Texas Research Institute of Mental Sciences (TRIMS) in Houston. His coauthor on a number of publications was Bernard Saltzberg, Ph.D.[264, 268, 269, 270]. Dr. Saltzberg was in turn a coauthor of Tulane brain electrode specialist and CIA contractor, Dr. Robert Heath[265-267].

A paper by Saltzberg, Burton, Burch et al.[269] was published in *Aviation, Space, and Environmental Medicine*; four of the authors are said to be from the Naval Biodynamics Laboratory, and funding is said to be through Office of Naval Research Contract #N00014-76-C-0911. TRIMS documents describe grant applications being prepared for this project in 1976 for $61,050.00.

According to an article in the October 1, 1994 *Houston Chronicle*[198], Dr. Burch and Dr. William T. Lhamon received $300,000.00 in Air Force contracts for hallucinogen research between April, 1956 and April, 1961. Dr. Burch became a full-time Associate Professor of Psychiatry at Baylor College of Medicine in 1959. Prior to that he spent five years in the Air Force as a psychiatrist, according to a letter he wrote to the Chairman of the Texas Department of Mental Health and Mental Retardation (TDMHMR) on March 13, 1978. TDMHMR ran and was responsible for TRIMS.

Research appropriations for TRIMS were $1,100,000.00 in 1972 and $2,261,635.00 in 1983. Dr. Burch worked for TRIMS up till his death. The total research grants and contracts received by TRIMS from 1968 to 1983 was $16,358,810.00. This included grants to Dr. Burch from the Office of Naval Research (1967, $34,000.00), NASA (1968, $5,619.00; 1970, $152,079.00), and the CIA (1968, $7,886.00; 1968, $5,619.00; 1969, $68,315.00; and 1971, $39,757.00).

The CIA money was for development of an improved Galvanic Skin Response System (1968); On-Line Psychophysiological Analysis (1969); and Psychophysiological Correlates of Human Information (1971). These CIA grants are designated by the grant numbers XG-3061-68R, XG-3102 and XG-3245. These contracts came after the termination of MKULTRA and do not correspond to any of the seven MKSEARCH contracts. There must therefore be another still-classified CIA mind control program that ran at least into the early 1970's. The relevance of Dr. Burch's research on the galvanic skin response (GSR) is that the GSR is a component of the lie detector test.

Other military contractors at TRIMS included Dr. Saltzberg, who received a grant for $6,480.00 from the Department of the Navy in 1976 (Contract N06014-76-C-0911) for "Analysis of New Tapes and Develop Analytical Procedures Toward the Objective of Finalizing a Practical and Effective Protocol for Collection of Field Data."

The Office of Naval Research gave Dr. Saltzberg $213,252.00 from May 1, 1980 to June 30, 1984 to study "Analysis of Electrophysiological Signals Recorded From Rhesus Monkeys Subjected to Biodynamic Stress." This project is closely related to similar research conducted at other universities under MKULTRA Subprojects 45, 61, 74, 86, 106, 129, and 138. Another overlapping grant to Dr. Saltzberg from the Department of the Navy for $42,250.00 ran from December 1, 1983 to November 30, 1984.

Dr. Robert Smith at TRIMS received funding from the Scottish Rite Foundation to give PCP (phencyclidine or "angel dust") to research subjects under a 1977 grant for $39,108.00 to study "Acute vs. Chronic Effects of Phencyclidine: A Schizophreniform Pychotomimetic." The Scottish Rite Foundation also provided Dr. C. Smith $20,076.00 in 1979 to study "Sensory Integration in Schizophrenia;" this is presumably the same Dr. Smith, however it may be a separate individual from Dr. Robert Smith.

In 1979, NASA provided Dr. Fenimore at TRIMS $10,000.00 to develop a "Scopolamine Radioimmunoassay." Scopolamine is an anti-nauseant that was also used as a mind control drug by the U.S. Army (see Appendix I).

One of the ongoing research projects at TRIMS was the study of brain electrical activity in violent criminals, hence the contact between Dr. Burch and Dr. Louis Jolyon West[173]. Although TRIMS did not perform brain electrode implant experiments on prisoners or other subjects, a letter to Joseph Schoolar, Ph.D., M.D., Director of TRIMS, from W.J. Estelle,

Jr., Director, Texas Department of Corrections dated April 9, 1979 states that, "You may be assured of TDC's support of this research."

CIA mind control research at prisons was funded through MKULTRA. One of the most heavily funded MKULTRA contractors was Dr. Carl Pfeiffer, who acknowledges funding from CIA cutout, the Geschickter Fund for Medical Research in numerous papers[77, 101, 108, 109, 207, 236, 240, 239, 237, 241].

Research conducted at prisons by Dr. Pfeiffer includes a paper entitled "Quantitative electroencephalographic analysis of naturally occurring (schizophrenic) and drug-induced psychotic states in human males"[109]. Work for this paper was funded through MKULTRA Subproject 47. Subjects included: 21 inmates from the New Jersey Reformatory at Bordentown[38] ranging in age from 21 to 30 years; 9 volunteers from the laboratory staff ranging in age from 19 to 48 years; and 25 schizophrenic patients from the Clinical Investigative Unit of the Bureau of Research, New Jersey Neuropsychiatric Institute. Fifteen inmates and ten schizophrenic subjects received LSD but the laboratory staff received only placebo.

Subjects in Pfeiffer et al.[240] included 13 inmates from the New Jersey Reformatory at Bordentown who received amphetamines. Subjects in Murphree et al.[207] included inmates from the New Jersey Reformatory at Bordentown ranging in age from 21 to 29 years, with an average age of 23.6 years. Subjects in this study were given intravenous barbiturates.

Subjects in Demarr et al.[77] included 16 inmates at the U.S. Federal Penitentiary in Atlanta who received LSD. The ethics of this and other MKULTRA drug studies conducted in prisons are unacceptable because of the high percentage of drug addicts in prison populations, because meaningful informed consent is difficult to obtain in such circumstances, and because subjects were not informed that the research was funded by the CIA, despite the TOP SECRET clearance status of the principal investigators.

While he was Chairman of the Department of Pharmacology at Emory University, Dr. Pfeiffer gave LSD to inmates of the U.S. Federal Penitentiary in Atlanta under MKULTRA Subproject 47. He himself took a dose of LSD and had his reactions filmed by WSB-TV in Atlanta in 1955[67]. A portion of this film was broadcast on WSB's *Newsroom* program.

Born in Peoria, Illinois on May 19, 1908, Pfeiffer was named to the Board of Directors of the Oak Ridge Institute of Nuclear Studies in 1956, a site of radiation experiments reviewed in Chapter 3. He and

John R. Smythies of the Worcester Foundation for Experimental Biology (MKULTRA Subproject 8) co-edited an issue of the *International Review of Neurobiology*[238] which included chapters by: H.J. Eysenck (contractor on MKULTRA Subproject 111); Abram Hoffer[132], who did LSD research with Humphry Osmond[226, 227] in Weyburn, Saskatchewan before Osmond relocated to the New Jersey Neuropsychiatric Institute; and Dr. Robert Heath, CIA contractor at Tulane.

In one study funded by the Geschickter Fund, entitled "Hallucinatory effects in man of acetylcholine inhibitors"[241] prisoners at the U.S. Federal Penitentiary in Atlanta were given 150 micrograms of the experimental drug MER-16. The authors noted that:

> *Abood finds that oral administration of 10 to 20 mg. of JB-318, the tertiary amine analogue of Piptal, or JB-336, the n-methyl derivative of JB-318, produces a model psychosis characterized by visual and auditory hallucinations. We have not been able to give doses larger than 9 mg. because of the extreme mental effects.*
>
> *A similar possible acetylcholine antagonist, MER-16, produces extreme LSD-like effects when 150 mg. is given orally. Hallucinations last for three days and are characterized by repeated waves of depersonalization, visual hallucinations, and feelings of unreality.*

The authors also noted that MER-16 is a more effective hallucinogen than scopolamine, the drug studied by Dr. Fenimore at TRIMS.

Because Dr. Pfeiffer died on November 20, 1988, it is possible to obtain a version of the MKULTRA Subproject file in which Dr. Pfeiffer's name and signature, Emory University, the Atlanta Federal Penitentiary, the New Jersey Neuropsychiatric Institute and the New Jersey Reformatory at Bordentown have not been redacted. A memo from the file dated 24 March 1955 states:

> *Purpose: Pharmacological and clinical testing in animals and volunteers of chemicals and biochemicals which alter behavior. Provide consultation on special problems of TSD interest.*
>
> *Status: Study completed on threshold doses of LSD-25, a method of exploring antagonism of this drug by other agents. Work has been initiated to evaluate compound producing amnesia and*

having alcohol like effect on behavior will be started. Evaluation of effects of combinations of drugs of interest to TSD is ¼ complete.

Although one sentence in the memo is ungrammatical, its meaning is clear. The goal of MKULTRA Subproject 47 was to produce not a model psychosis, but a model dissociative state characterized by depersonalization and amnesia.

In a memo from the CIA to Senator Pete Wilson dated 11 December 1985, the unidentifiable CIA correspondent states:

It should also be noted that this matter has been considered at the highest levels of Justice and the Central Intelligence Agency and it is the considered judgment of the responsible officials that the United States has no legal responsibility for any of the alleged harms or injuries that may have been suffered by Mr. Weinstein [victim of mind control experiments by Dr. Ewen Cameron, see the book by his son313] or the other plaintiffs, and that neither Mr. Weinstein nor the other plaintiffs can demonstrate any causal relationship between the minimal CIA funding and their alleged injuries. This position is further supported by the fact that one similar case, arising from LSD testing financed by the CIA and conducted by the U.S. Public Health Service at Atlanta Federal Penitentiary, was fully litigated; in that case, judgment and costs were entered in favor of the United States.

Another site of LSD experiments on prisoners was the Oak Ridge Division, Penetang Psychiatric Hospital, Penetanguishene, Ontario, Canada. The principal investigator was Dr. Elliott T. Barker[27-30]. In a paper entitled "Defence Disrupting Therapy," Barker, Mason and Wilson[30] describe their patients as a group of inmates found unfit to stand trial or not guilty by reason of insanity. The crimes they had committed included murder, arson, and assault.

Dr. Barker is currently the President of the Canadian Society for the Prevention of Cruelty to Children. On the Society's web page (www.bconnex.net/~cspcc/crimeprevention/snug.html) there is a statement about child abuse by Michael Mason, Founding Member of the Society, dated April, 1975. This is presumably the same individual as M.H. Mason, Dr. Barker's coauthor[30]. In a footnote to that paper, Mason is identified as "Patient, Oak Ridge Division, Penetang Psychiatric Hospital."

Another of Dr. Barker's papers[27] is entitled "LSD In A Coercive Milieu Therapy Program." The LSD was given in a dosage of 500 micrograms as an intramuscular injection, a heavy hallucinatory dosage. Other drugs given to the inmates by Dr. Barker include scopolamine, barbiturates, and amphetamines, often in combination with each other. A third paper of Dr. Barker's was entitled "The Total Encounter Capsule"[29].

The authors of that paper describe keeping groups of prisoners naked in a small sensory isolation chamber called The Capsule for days at a time. While in The Capsule together for these prolonged periods, the prisoners were given LSD. Some were as young as fifteen years old.

Dr. Barker's proposition that arsonists, rapists and murderers as young as fifteen years of age, some with only third grade educations, can be treated effectively by combinations of addictive drugs and sensory deprivation which render them delirious and psychotic, is remarkable. An alternative explanation for the observation that, "The treatment method has now gained such high status among patients that requests for it exceed our capacity to give the drugs," is the hypothesis that the patients enjoyed getting stoned.

There is no evidence that Dr. Barker's LSD, amphetamine, scopolamine, barbiturate and sensory deprivation experiments were funded by the CIA or the military. Like the results of the Tuskeegee Syphilis Study, they were described in the peer-reviewed professional literature without stimulating letters to the editors of the journals. Two reciprocally interacting facts are evident: 1) it was not difficult for the CIA and military to identify willing mind control contractors because the medical profession was highly permissive of such experimentation, and 2) ethical and experimental norms established in secretly funded mind control research spilled over into conventional medicine and psychiatry.

Another line of mind control research began with Dr. John Lilly, whose work with dolphins was depicted in the movie *The Day of the Dolphin*. Dr. Lilly[169] described experiments in which he gave LSD to dolphins in a CIA-sponsored LSD symposium. Dr. Lilly was also the inventor of the flotation tank depicted in the movie *Altered States*. Lilly[168] described research he had done with flotation tanks at the Mid-Atlantic Regional Research Conference on March 9, 1956. One of the discussants of the paper was Dr. Winfred Overholser, who did work on mind control drugs for the OSS during World War II[184]. Other discussants of the paper were from Walter Reed Army Medical Center and MKULTRA institutions including Georgetown University, Harvard University, and the University of Minnesota. One was from Tulane, where Dr. Robert Heath did contract work for the CIA.

Dr. Lilly described sensory isolation research done at McGill by Dr. Donald Hebb (funded by Canada's Defense Research Board) and said of Hebb's subjects, "The development of hallucinations in the visual sphere followed the stages seen with mescaline intoxication." Commenting on sensory deprivation experiments done at the Allan Memorial Institute by Dr. Hassan Azima, discussant Dr. Herbert Zimmer says, "Of the 15 cases, eight showed a depersonalized state with varying degrees of visual, auditory and gustatory hallucinosis."

In Dr. Lilly's flotation tank, which contained a 10% magnesium sulphate solution at 84.5 degrees F., subjects were naked except for a mask which covered the entire head but allowed for breathing. Subjects floated suspended in the solution with their heads just out of the water, with no light or sound other than their own breathing and sound from the pipes circulating water through the tank. Dr. Lilly's flotation tank was a solitary, aqueous precursor of Dr. Barker's Capsule.

Discussant Dr. Ogden R. Lindsley, who did operant conditioning experiments on children age seven to twelve[22], told the following story in response to Dr. Lilly's (1956) presentation:

> *During the war I had the good fortune to fly in a heavy bomber for the U.S. Army Air Force and the misfortune of being shot out of it and put in isolation by the German Gestapo for about fourteen and a half days. Their method was to put you in a little room, not long enough to lie down in, with no furnishings, no window, and no light. They came once every twelve hours or so and brought water and black bread. I don't want to go into any emotional experiences in the room, because they were all very similar to those which Dr. Lilly has reported. Sometimes while there it would seem as though four days had gone by without any water, and then again it would seem that they came fifteen minutes after they had last appeared.*

An article in *The Dallas Morning News*, January 29, 1997, p 9A describes how the *Baltimore Sun* obtained a 1983 CIA manual through the Freedom of Information Act. The manual was used to teach non coercive interrogation techniques to foreign agents, including ones from

Central America. The manual taught techniques studied in BLUEBIRD, ARTICHOKE and MKULTRA; the same brainwashing techniques were used on Dr. Ogden Lindsley by the Gestapo, on Patty Hearst by the Symbionese Liberation Army (see Chapter 19), and on patients at Penetang Psychiatric Hospital by Dr. Elliott Barker. The CIA manual taught techniques for the induction of "intense fear, deep exhaustion, solitary confinement, unbearable anxiety and other forms of psychological duress," and was used until at least 1983. These are some of the building blocks for making Manchurian Candidates.

As part of his work in sensory isolation, Dr. Lilly[170] wrote a book entitled *Programming and Metaprogramming in the Human Biocomputer* in which he discusses LSD, interspecies communication, and the flotation tank. The book is also an early work in artificial intelligence, much of it written in engineering language. In it, Dr. Lilly provides a model of the mind as an interconnected system of parallel processing units.

This line of research has been pursued by cognitive psychologists funded by the Office of Naval Research, especially at the Massachusetts Institute of Technology (MIT), which was an MKULTRA and MKNAOMI institution. Andrew G. Knapp and James A. Anderson[151] published a paper entitled "Theory of Categorization Based on Distributed Memory Storage" in which they acknowledge support through Office of Naval Research Contract N00014-81-K-0136. Dr. William Adey of UCLA (see Chapter 10) was active in MIT's Neurosciences Research Program and received funding from the Office of Naval Research.

In his book *Society of Mind*, MIT psychologist Marvin Minsky[192] states that his work was funded by the Office of Naval Research over a period beginning with his graduate studies. The central thesis of Minsky's book is that the mind is a society of subsystems, that is, a distributed parallel network. Dr. Daniel Schachter[276] of Harvard published a book entitled *Searching for Memory. The Brain, the Mind, and the Past* which discusses the fact that memory is composed of subsystems; in the book, he acknowledges funding from the Air Force Office of Scientific Research. This research is directly relevant to understanding the structure of a Manchurian Candidate's mind, which is a society of subsystems or, in different language, an interconnected system of parallel processing units.

On December 11, 1996 in a posting on the internet list WITCHNT@MITVMA.MIT.EDU, Dr. Peter Freyd, husband of the Executive Director of the False Memory Syndrome Foundation, wrote:

Since we all want to be open about any money we might have received from military-related sources, let me confess.

I, too, must go on record. Starting in 1988, I've been getting a lot of money from the U.S. Office of Naval Research.

In 1968 I received a lot of money from the Kingdom of Iran. There were some who thought the Kingdom was a CIA front. Actually, the evidence is that the money was flowing in the other direction: the CIA might have been something of a Savak front.

Academics have been receiving research funding from military intelligence agencies into the twenty-first century. Much of the research is no doubt ethical and humane. Unfortunately, however, everyone in academia, and especially everyone in psychiatry and psychology with military funding is now under suspicion. This is the inevitable outcome of decades of deception, implausible denial, and looking the other way.

Another funding agency woven into the mind control network is the Scottish Rite Foundation. In a 1958 paper[175] Dr. William Malamud is identified as the Medical Research Director and Dr. Winfred Overholser as the Chairman of the Scottish Rite Research Committee. Another 1958 paper[231] states that second author, Dr. Sidney L. Werkman, received his M.D. from Cornell in 1952, where he worked under Dr. Harold Wolff, MKULTRA contractor and Director of CIA cutout The Human Ecology Foundation. Dr. Overholser worked with Dr. Joel Elkes when Dr. Elkes was Director of Research at Saint Elizabeth's Hospital, and prior to Dr. Elkes becoming Chairman of the Department of Psychiatry at Johns Hopkins[230].

Dr. Winfred Overholser, Sr.[229] gave his Presidential address to the American Psychiatric Association in Washington, D.C., in May, 1948. In a biographical sketch[196] Dr. Overholser is described as having been born in Worcester, Massachusetts on April 21, 1892. He received his M.D. in 1916, and saw military service in World War I. In a diary written in a field hospital in France, Dr. Overholser stated, "We are using suggestion and hypnosis when it is possible."

Dr. Overholser became the superintendent of St. Elizabeth's Hospital in Washington in 1937; over 5000 naval officers and enlisted men were treated as patients there during World War II. Psychiatric training was provided to 125 naval medical officers, nearly 100 nurses and about 800 hospital corpsmen during the War. Dr. Overholser is described in the biographical sketch as a 32nd degree Mason.

Dr. Winfred Overholser, Jr. was born on April 29, 1930. He received his M.D. from New York Medical College in 1955, and did his psychiatry residency at New York State Psychiatric Institute from 1956 to 1959; it was at the Institute that Dr. Paul Hoch killed Harold Blauer with an injection of U.S. Army mescaline in 1953.

Dr. Hudson Hoagland[129] of the Worcester Foundation for Experimental Biology (MKULTRA Subproject 8) wrote an obituary for Dr. Ewen Cameron (MKULTRA Subproject 68), was recommended to J. Edgar Hoover by G.H. Estabrooks, a 32nd degree Mason, and received money for LSD research from the Scottish Rite Committee, as did MKULTRA and MKSEARCH contractor, Dr. Carl Pfeiffer. A coauthor of Dr. Hoaglund's[252], Dr. Robert Hyde received TOP SECRET clearance as the contractor on MKULTRA Subprojects 8, 63, and 66.

Another coauthor of Dr. Hoaglund's, Dr. William Malamud[175,176] did lobotomy research when he was at the Worcester State Hospital[263]. These connections illustrate how the network of mind control doctors was structured. There was no central conspiracy; rather the network was maintained by diverse connections between individuals, institutions and agencies.

In a chapter in a book on brainwashing, Chodoff and Mercer[58] write:

> *As for the issue of the deliberate, systematic misuse of psychiatry to suppress political and religious dissent, no strong case can be made that this is a problem in the United States. The case usually considered most relevant is that of the poet Ezra Pound. Arrested at the end of World War II for his treasonous broadcasts in Italy, Pound was never tried but was found incapable of assisting in his defense by reason of mental illness. Later he was confined, under relatively comfortable conditions, at St. Elizabeth's Hospital in Washington, D.C. This judgment, largely the work of Dr. Winfred Overholser, superintendent of St. Elizabeth's Hospital, was made in spite of what seems to have been a lack of substantial clinical evidence of psychosis and the fact that Pound had written a lucid and detailed defense of himself to the U.S. Attorney General.*
>
> *The Pound case appears to constitute a political subversion of psychiatry. But it should be noted that the action was taken in the primary interest of the accused person rather than that*

*of the state, as is the case in the Soviet Union. Most important,
it was an isolated example, and very few similar ones have taken
place in the United States.*

Dr. Winfred Overholser, Sr. funded LSD research through the Scottish Rite Committee and was at the center of the mind control network beginning with his work for the OSS during World War II[184].

Only some papers from the extensive LSD literature acknowledge direct funding from the military. An example is a paper entitled, "Cognitive Test Performance Under LSD-25, Placebo and Isolation"[106] which acknowledges support through Air Force Contract No. AF33(616)-6013. The research was monitored by the Aero Medical Laboratory, Directorate of Research, Wright Patterson Air Force Base, Ohio.

Hallucinogen research would have flowed across the desk of Dr. Bruce Dill, who worked at the Aeromedical Laboratory research unit at Wright Field from 1941 to 1943. He was the Director of Medical Research at the U.S. Army Chemical Research and Development Laboratory, Edgeware Arsenal from 1947 to 1961. This is the time frame of both MKULTRA and MKNAOMI.

One of the most unexpected members of the mind control network was Carl Rogers, Ph.D. Dr. Rogers received TOP SECRET clearance for his work on MKULTRA Subproject 74. The paper based on Subproject 74, entitled "A Study of Psychotherapeutic Change in Schizophrenics and Normals: The Design and Instrumentation"[254] acknowledges funding from the Society for the Investigation of Human Ecology. The 1961 Annual Report of the Society lists Dr. Rogers as a Director.

The analysis of other doctors in the mind control network presented in this chapter is illustrative, and far from exhaustive. Contractors on CIA and military mind control research included leading psychiatrists and psychologists, Past Presidents and Awardees of the American Psychiatric Association, editors and associate editors of leading professional journals, Chairmen of academic Departments of Psychiatry, and their colleagues and coauthors. Many other doctors published similar research funded by other agencies such as the U.S. Public Health Service and the Scottish Rite Research Committee.

III. G.H. ESTABROOKS

G.H. Estabrooks requires a separate section of his own because he is the only mind control doctor who has publicly acknowledged the creation of Manchurian Candidates. The purpose of this chapter is to establish that Dr. Estabrooks was very well connected academically, and had professional relationships with documented CIA mind control contractors such as Dr. Martin Orne. Additionally, the documentation proves that Dr. Estabrooks conducted extensive training of military intelligence personnel and was a contractor of the War Department during World War II. G.H. Estabrooks was at the hub of the Manchurian Candidate programs. Because of the compartmented nature of the intelligence community, it is unlikely that there was only one centrally controlled Manchurian Candidate program.

15
G.H. ESTABROOKS

George Holben Estabrooks was born in St. John, New Brunwick, Canada on December 16, 1895. He moved to Colgate College in Hamilton, New York in 1927, and lived there till he died on December 30, 1973. Dr. Estabrooks did his B.A. at Acadia University in Wolfville, Nova Scotia in 1920 and his Ph.D. in psychology at Harvard in 1926. From 1921 to 1924 he was a Rhodes Scholar at Oxford and Exeter.

At age 19, Estabrooks became the youngest commissioned officer in the First Canadian Division. He was in the German gas attack at Ypres. While participating in a gas attack drill behind lines, he was exposed to mustard gas because of a tear in his mask. This almost killed him and eventually resulted in his being sent back to Canada. He developed tuberculosis and spent time in two TB sanitaria, one of them in Switzerland; there he met his future wife, the daughter of a Swiss watchmaker, whom he married in Rome twelve years later on July 20, 1933. She died in 1975, leaving behind their only daughter. Estabrooks led a stable, quiet personal life. Among other things, he was a 32nd degree Knight Templar Mason. His father, Leander Estabrooks, was a steamboat captain on the St. John River but was never known to drink or swear. Like his father, George Estabrooks was a teetotaller.

Dr. Estabrooks wrote many articles and books including *Man - The Mechanical Misfit*[83], *Hypnotism*[84], *Spiritism*[85] and *The Future of the Human Mind*[88]. He studied multiple personality very carefully. In his book *Spiritism*[85], Dr. Estabrooks describes experiments done to create multiple personality by a U.S. military psychiatrist, Dr. P.L. Harriman[111-113]. Dr. Harriman did not claim that any of his experimental multiple personality subjects were used in actual operations.

In his book *Hypnotism*, Dr Estabrooks[84] states that the creation of experimental multiple personality for operational use in military subjects, whom he refers to as super spies, is ethical because of the demands of war. He comments, in a chapter entitled "Hypnotism in Warfare" that:

> *The British are paying a terrible price for refusing to look reality in the face. We might easily do the same if we became over squeamish in our determination to protect ourselves ethically. We may rest assured that certain world powers will not hesitate one moment to use hypnotism directly they are convinced of its value. Then it will be incumbent on us to beat them at their own game, but under these circumstances the hand of the military must not be tied by any silly prejudices in the minds of the general public. War is the end of all law. When we speak of keeping within the rules of the game we are childish, because it is not a game and the rules never hold. In the last analysis any device is justifiable which enables us to protect ourselves from defeat.*

In a May 13, 1968 article in the *Providence Evening Bulletin[31]*, Estabrooks is described as a former consultant for the FBI and CIA, and is quoted as saying that, "the key to creating an effective spy or assassin rests in splitting a man's personality, or creating multipersonality, with the aid of hypnotism.... This is not science fiction. This has and is being done. I have done it."

In an obituary in the January 6, 1974 *Syracuse Herald American[56]*, the writer states:

> *But he knew the power of what he called "my curious little research hobby." Once I felt he was ready to tell me about his experiences in the war, how hypnotism might have been used in early "Manchurian Candidate" fashion, as a weapon of psychological warfare, but then he drew back to the style of conversation that stops just short of major revelation. You were left imagining all the cats struggling to be released from that bag of his.*

The "curious little research hobby" was the experimental creation of multiple personality for operational use by the military. The ARTICHOKE/BLUEBIRD documents contain a copy of Dr. Estabrooks' proposal to the CIA dated June 22, 1954. Although all names are whited out in the document, it is definitely written by Dr. Estabrooks for the following reasons: the writing style is characteristic; the vocabulary is characteristic; the content is characteristic; the time frame is correct; and the whited out name occupies the correct number of spaces to spell "Estabrooks."

Dr. Estabrooks' proposal and commentary from the CIA read as follows, with spelling, punctuation and grammatical errors uncorrected:

THE MILITARY APPLICATION OF HYPNOTISM

To: [Whited out]

From: [Whited out]

I choose two practical applications from many with which to illustrate my proposition:

1.   The safeguarding of the messages entrusted to couriers. In deep hypnosis the subject, military or civilian, can be given a message to be delivered to say Colonel X in Berlin. The subject may then be sent to Berlin on any perfectly routine assignment. The message will be perfectly safe and will be delivered to the proper person because

a.   the subject will have no memory whatsoever in the waking state as to the nature and contents of the message.

b.   it can be arranged that the subject will have no knowledge of ever having been hypnotized.

c.   It can be arranged that no one beside Colonel X in Berlin can hypnotize the subject and recover the message.

This hypnotic messenger, if I may use the phrase has in my opinion at least two very definite advantages over the ordinary courier. First he will never under any circumstance by a slip of the tongue divulge the true nature of his mission for the very simple reason that he has no conscious knowledge of what that mission may be. He is merely going on a routine replacement in say the Adjutant General's Office. This will be his story and the story which he believes.

Secondly, if by any chance, he is picked up through leakage if information from any other sources the message is safe. No amount of third degree tactics can pry it loose, for he simply does not have it in his conscious mind. Even if the enemy suspects the use of hypnotism the message is still safe for no one can hypnotize him except this Colonel X in Berlin.

May I point out that this technique is one which can be demonstrated under experimental conditions where you wish and when you wish allowing a certain amount of time to train the subjects in question.

2. A specific counterintelligence technique to be used against enemy agents. This particular use of hypnotism would be more complicated and more difficult than the rather simple case which I outlined in the preceding paragraphs, but is, I assure you, quite practical. I will take a number of men and will establish in them through the use of hypnotism the condition of split personality. Consciously they will be ardent Communists, phanatical adherence to the party line, ready and eager to submit to any discipline which the party may prescribe. Unconsciously they will be loyal Americans just as grimley determined to thwart the Communists at every turn in the road.

These men will again have no knowledge of anything that occurs in the hypnotic state - will have no knowledge of ever having been hypnotized and can only be hypnotized by such persons as the original operator may choose. Consciously they will associate with the Communists and learn all the plans of the organization. Once every month or at such time is advisable they will be contacted by a member of our intelligence department, hypnotized, and as loyal Americans will tell what they know. This sounds unbelievable, but I assure, you, it will work.

Once again the advantages. Your hypothetical counter spy will be placed in a very difficult situation - amounting at best to social ostracism, at worst criminal prosecution. He will not disclose his true role for the very simple reason that he can not. Consciously he is a Communist and will not in a moment of weakness admit to his relatives or to his friends that he is anything but a Communist. Again, if through some leakage, he is suspected of being an informer his true role is safely guarded, locked in the unconscious and impervious to all assaults from the outside.

[Whited out] I consider myself an authority on the theoretical applications of hypnotism to warfare and would point out that it is a highly specialized subject. The average psychologist or even

psychiatrist is as much at a loss here as would be the average chemist or physicist if called to supervise a very specialized project for which he had no particular training. I claim that I can demonstrate all my particular contentions to the satisfaction of the government agencies and request the opportunity to do so.

In closing, may I make one very significant point. The Russian literature is hard to get and carefully avoids any mention of the topic in question. Those Russian articles which I have been able to get leave no doubt about the fact that the Russian is just as conversive about the field of hypnotism as we are.

Respectfully submitted,
[Whited out]

15 July 1954

TO: Chief, Security Research Staff
FROM: Chief, Technical Branch
SUBJECT: [Whited out]

1. I have examined [whited out] proposals and I feel that I should make the following comments:

a) *The idea of a courier that has been hypnotized is not new and I am absolutely certain [whited out] did not invent this idea. We ourselves have carried out much more complex problems than this and in a general sense I will agree that it is feasible. However, there is no proof whatsoever that the hypnosis cannot be broken by another competent hypnotist [whited out] feels this is possible) and the entire test has not yet been subjected to actual field conditions (long travel, time, etc.).*

b) *As far as third-degree tactics are concerned, we do not know as yet what happens to an hypnotized individual under the third-degree or plied with chemicals of various types. Whether or not he will disclose hypnotic materials or indicate he possesses same has not been determined. Again this is a test that we hope to carry out in the future, as you know.*

c) *[whited out] proposal that a subject "will have no knowledge of ever having been hypnotized" is debatable. In regard to this, we are not yet certain but possibly through the use of subtle chemicals and/or a very careful cover, it might be done. It is conceivable it could be accomplished if the subject were not unduly suspicious, extremely naïve or very stupid but again this point is questionable.*

d) *[whited out] proposal about using hypnotized individuals as counteragents is also not new and we, of course, have discussed this many times. Whether or not it can in fact be demonstrated we are not sure and it is hoped that the field tests we are working on may help us along these lines.*

e) *[whited out] proposals are, of course, lacking in details and I am quite certain he has never carried any of these things out except in laboratory type experiments. We, of course, have been able to produce these results but again only in laboratory experiments and I assure you we would not be as emphatic about the success of these things as [whited out]*

f) *I think it very important that if [whited out] does come to Washington you and I should have the opportunity to discuss at length and in detail his ideas.*

g) *If you will recall, [whited out] among others long ago proposed the courier idea and in some ways [whited out] believes that given sufficient time and the opportunity for "correct training", he could condition individuals for these purposes if certain conditions were met. [whited out] you also recall is not greatly impressed by [whited out]*

[whited out]

In a 1971 article in *Science Digest*, Dr. Estabrooks[87] claimed to have created hypnotic couriers and counterintelligence agents for operational use during World War II:

One of the most fascinating but dangerous applications of hypnosis is its use in military intelligence. This is a field with which I am familiar through formulating guide lines for the techniques used by the United States in two world wars.

Communication in war is always a headache. Codes can be broken. A professional spy may or may not stay bought. Your own man may have unquestionable loyalty but his judgment is always open to question.

The "hypnotic courier," on the other hand, provides a unique solution. I was involved in preparing many subjects for this work during World War II. One successful case involved an Army Service Corps Captain whom we'll call George Smith. Captain Smith had undergone months of training. He was an excellent subject but did not realize it. I had removed from him, by post hypnotic suggestion, all recollection of ever having been hypnotized.

First I had the Service Corps call the captain to Washington and tell him they needed a report on the mechanical equipment of Division X headquartered in Tokyo. Smith was ordered to leave by jet next morning, pick up the report and return at once. These orders were given him in the waking state. Consciously, that was all he knew, and it was the story he gave his wife and friends.

Then I put him under deep hypnosis, and gave him - orally - a vital message to be delivered directly on his arrival in Japan to a certain colonel - let's say his name was Brown - of military intelligence. Outside of myself, Colonel Brown was the only person who could hypnotize Captain Smith. This is "locking." I performed it by saying to the hypnotized Captain: "Until further orders from me, only Colonel Brown and I can hypnotize you. We will use the signal phrase 'the moon is clear.' Whenever you hear this phrase from Brown or myself you will pass instantly into deep hypnosis." When Captain Smith re-awakened, he had no conscious memory of what happened in trance. All that he was aware of was that he must head for Tokyo to pick up the division report.

On arrival there, Smith reported to Brown, who hypnotized him with the signal phrase. Under hypnosis, Smith delivered my message and received one to bring back. Awakened, he was given the division report and returned home by jet. There I hypnotized him once more with the signal phrase, and he spieled off Brown's answer that had been dutifully tucked away in his unconscious mind.

The system is virtually foolproof. As exemplified by the case, the information literally was "locked" in Smith's unconscious for retrieval by the only two people who knew the combination. The subject had no conscious memory of what happened, so couldn't spill the beans. No one else could hypnotize him even if they might know the signal phrase.

Not all applications of hypnotism to military intelligence are as tidy as that. Perhaps you have read The Three Faces of Eve. The book was based on a case reported in 1905 by Dr. Morton Prince of Massachusetts General Hospital and Harvard. He started everyone in the field by announcing that he had cured a woman named Beauchamp of a split personality problem. Using post-hypnotic suggestion to submerge an incompatible, childlike facet of the patient, he'd been able to make two other sides of Mrs. Beauchamp compatible, and lump them together in a single cohesive personality. Clinical hypnotists throughout the world jumped on the multiple personality bandwagon as a fascinating frontier. By the 1920's not only had they learned to apply posthypnotic suggestion to deal with this weird problem, but also had learned how to split certain complex individuals into multiple personalities like Jeckyl-Hydes.

The potential for military intelligence has been nightmarish. During World War II, I worked this technique with a vulnerable Marine lieutenant I'll call Jones. Under the watchful eye of Marine intelligence I split his personality into Jones A and Jones B. Jones A, once a "normal" working Marine, became entirely different. He talked communist doctrine and meant it. He was welcomed enthusiastically by communist cells, and was deliberately given a dishonorable discharge by the Corps (which was in on the plot) and became a card-carrying party member.

The joker was Jones B, the second personality, formerly apparent in the conscious Marine. Under hypnosis, this Jones had been carefully coached by suggestion. Jones B was the deeper personality, knew all the thoughts of Jones A, was a loyal American and was "imprinted" to say nothing during conscious phases.

All I had to do was hypnotize the whole man, get in touch with Jones B, the loyal American, and I had a pipeline straight into the Communist camp. It worked beautifully for months with this subject, but the technique backfired. While there was no way for an enemy to expose Jones' dual personality, they suspected it and played the same trick on us later.

The use of "waking hypnosis" in counter intelligence during World War II occasionally became so involved that it taxed even my credibility. Among the most complicated ploys used was the practice of sending a perfectly normal, wide awake agent into enemy camp, after he'd been carefully coached in waking hypnosis to act the part of a potential hypnotism subject. Trained in auto-suggestion, or self-hypnosis, such a subject can pass every test used to spot a hypnotized person. Using it, he can control the rate of his heartbeat, anesthetize himself to a degree against pain of electric shock or other torture.

In the case of an officer we'll call Cox, this carefully prepared counter spy was given a title to indicate he had access to top priority information. He was planted in an international café in a border country where it was certain there would be enemy agents. He talked too much, drank a lot, made friends with local girls, and pretended a childish interest in hypnotism. The hope was that he would blunder into a situation in which enemy agents would kidnap and try to hypnotize him, in order to extract information from him.

Cox worked so well that they fell for the trick. He never allowed himself to be hypnotized during seances. While pretending to be a hypnotized subject of the foe, he was gathering and feeding back information.

Eventually Cox did get caught, when he was followed to an information "drop." And this international group plays rough. The enemy offered him a "ride" at gunpoint. There were four men in the vehicle. Cox watched for a chance and found it when the car skirted a ravine. He leaped for the wheel, twisted it, and over the ledge they went. Two of his guards were killed in the crash. In the ensuing scramble, he got hold of another man's gun, liquidated the remaining two, then hobbled across the border with nothing worse than a broken leg. So much for the darker side.

Dr. Estabrooks made one scholarly error in his article. *The Three Faces of Eve* was written by Thigpen and Cleckley[300]; Dr. Morton Prince's book about Miss Beauchamp was entitled *The Dissociation of a Personality*[247]. One might conclude from the *Science Digest* article, Dr. Estabrooks' proposal to the CIA, and the reaction to it by the Chief, Technical Branch, CIA, that Dr. Estabrooks' claims are exaggerated. It is clear that there was skepticism inside the CIA and in the minds of CIA consultants about the operational utility of the Manchurian Candidate.

If Dr. Estabrooks did in fact create and handle Manchurian Candidates during World War II, it is evident that the Chief, Technical Branch, CIA did not have access to this information as of July 15, 1954. Given the highly compartmented nature of intelligence agencies, it could be that Dr. Estabrooks actually did the work he describes in *Science Digest*. On the other hand, one must consider the possibility that he was exaggerating, not concerning the experimental creation of Manchurian Candidates, but about the degree to which they were used in actual operations.

There is nothing in Dr. Estabrooks' claims or procedures that is inconsistent with the BLUEBIRD and ARTICHOKE documents on Manchurian Candidates. Unfortunately, in this instance it is impossible to prove a negative, namely that Manchurian Candidates have never been used in field operations, because of the secrecy intrinsic to covert operations. All one can do is prove through documentation that events of interest did occur; lack of documentation proves nothing. In this regard, the denial of the operational reality of the Manchurian Candidate by Dr. John Gittinger, lead psychologist for MKULTRA, means nothing. Dr. Gittinger testified in *Project MKULTRA, the CIA's Program of Research in Behavioral Modification* (p. 62) that:

Senator SCHWEIKER. Mr. Gittinger, a moment ago you mentioned brainwashing techniques, as one area that you had, I guess, done some work in. How would you characterize the state of the art of brainwashing today? Who has the most expertise in this field, and who is or is not doing it in terms of other governments?

During the Korean War there was a lot of serious discussion about brainwashing techniques being used by the North Koreans, and I am interested in finding out what the state of the art is today, as you see it.

Mr. GITTINGER. Well, of course, there has been a great deal of work on this, and there is still a great deal of controversy. I can tell you that as far as I knew, by 1961, 1962, it was at least proven to my satisfaction that brainwashing, so called,

> *is some kind of an esoteric device where drugs
> or mind-altering kinds of conditions and so
> forth were used, did not exist even though "The
> Manchurian Candidate" as a movie really set
> us back a long time, because it made something
> impossible look plausible. Do you follow what
> I mean? But by 1962 and 1963, the general
> idea that we were able to come up with is that
> brainwashing was largely a process of isolating
> a human being, keeping him out of contact,
> putting him under long stress in relationship to
> interviewing and interrogation, and that they
> could produce any change that way without
> having to resort to any kind of esoteric means.*

Dr. Estabrooks' claims become more plausible if we consider other documented facts about his career and connections with intelligence agencies, within the field of hypnosis, and within the network of mind control doctors. Relevant documents are included in Appendix A.

Dr. Estabrooks was accepted as a contractor by the War Department on February 20, 1942. On July 13, 1939 he received correspondence from W.S. Anderson, Director of Naval Intelligence. On December 4, 1953 he addressed the Counter Intelligence Corps School at Fort Holabird; T.F. Hoffman of the Corps told Dr. Estabrooks in a letter dated November 18, 1953 that the Corps was studying *Hypnotism*[84], in which Estabrooks describes the hypnotic courier.

Dr. Estabrooks wrote countless letters to countless people. These are stored at Colgate College in Hamilton, New York. One, dated January 1, 1942 was to Colonel William Donovan, Coordinator of Information (COI); the COI was transformed into the OSS under Colonel Donovan's leadership. A statue of Colonel Donovan, who is regarded as the father of the CIA, stands in the CIA's headquarters in Langley, Virginia.

Other correspondence with intelligence agencies includes letters of: May 8, 1935 to the Chief Signal Officer, United States Army; November 13, 1935 from Headquarters U.S. Marine Corps; July 19, 1938 from R.S. Holmes, Director of Naval Intelligence; September 21, 1939 to Colonel R.V. Read at the British Embassy in Washington; October 7, 1940 to Superintendent E.W. Bavin of the Royal Canadian Mounted Police; January 26, 1942 from John V. Hinkel at Military Intelligence Division G-2; and August 29, 1942 from Paul Rath at Edgeware Arsenal.

Ernest Bavin, who received a letter from Dr. Estabrooks on October 7, 1940, was born in Cheltenham, England in 1988. He immigrated to Canada in 1908 and served in the 1st Battalion, Canadian Field Artillery, Canadian Expeditionary Force during World War I. He worked for various Canadian police forces before and after the War. From 1939 till his retirement in 1941, Mr. Bavin was in charge of the intelligence branch of the Royal Canadian Mounted Police.

From 1942 to 1944, Bavin worked in the Office of British Security Co-Ordination in New York as a liaison between the Canadian Directorate of Military Intelligence and the U.S. Army's Military Intelligence Division G-2 (with whom Estabrooks corresponded).

A May 8, 1945 letter to Mr. Bavin on British Security Co-Ordination stationery is signed by Bavin's boss, William S. Stephenson, Director. Stephenson is the intelligence officer known as *The Man Called Intrepid*[138,297,302]. William Stephenson worked closely with William Donovan, and was first introduced to J. Edgar Hoover by the boxer, Gene Tunney[302]. Tunney played a role in the recruitment of Candy Jones for Manchurian Candidate training in *The Control of Candy Jones*[23] (see Chapter 20). A June 4, 1945 letter from J. Edgar Hoover to Mr. Bavin thanks him for his close work with the FBI.

The Estabrooks archives contain voluminous correspondence back and forth between Dr. Estabrooks and J. Edgar Hoover beginning May 13, 1936 and continuing up to March 7, 1962. Hoover sent FBI personnel to Colgate College to meet with Estabrooks, sent him copies of his speeches, and acknowledged upcoming visits by Estabrooks to FBI headquarters. On June 25, 1937, Hoover acknowledged receipt of a, "current news clipping depicting experimental use of hypnotism by Dr. A. Herbert Kanter in the Ohio State Penitentiary at Columbus." Drug, interrogation and hypnosis experiments were conducted on Ohio prison inmates under MKULTRA Subproject 39. The archives also contain letters from Estabrooks to other FBI personnel.

In a letter of July 23, 1937, J. Edgar Hoover acknowledges a recommendation by Dr. Estabrooks that the FBI visit Dr. Hudson Hoaglund, Department of Biology, Clarke University, Worcester, Massachusetts. The Worcester Foundation for Experimental Biology was the site of MKULTRA Subproject 8, and Dr. Hoaglund[129] wrote an obituary for Dr. Ewen Cameron, contractor on MKULTRA Subproject 68. Dr. Hoaglund, who himself worked at the Worcester Foundation for Experimental Biology, was also a coauthor of a paper on LSD with Dr. Robert Hyde[252];

Dr. Hyde received TOP SECRET clearance for his work on MKULTRA Subprojects 8, 10, and 63. J. Edgar Hoover was aware of MKULTRA because he received correspondence from the Director of the CIA about it.

In an August 24, 1935 letter to Dr. Estabrooks from the Office of the Chief of Staff of the War Department, the correspondent notes communications received from Dr. Estabrooks by the Military Intelligence Division dating back to 1924. This is confirmed again in a letter from Military Intelligence Division G-2's Colonel Percy G. Black, dated February 2, 1945. Dr. Estabrooks also corresponded with other branches of the government including: the Office of Indian Affairs (undated); the Public Health Service (May 13, 1942); the Department of Health, Education and Welfare (August 11, 1959); and the Attorney General (September 2, 1959). He also wrote to Winston Churchill, to whom William Stephenson reported.

Dr. Estabrooks ran a symposium for the U.S. Army Intelligence School at Fort Holabird in Baltimore on April 5-7, 1963. A list of Registered Members of Symposium includes personnel from U.S. Army Intelligence, with ranks of Major and Lieutenant Colonel, and 29 M.D. physicians.

Dr. Estabrooks was also very well connected in academia. He corresponded with Aldous Huxley, and his brother, Sir Julian Huxley. Aldous Huxley[137] described a science fiction world of the future in which citizens were controlled with the drug *soma* in his book *Brave New World*. Gordon Wasson[310] wrote a book on the hallucinogenic mushroom *amanita muscaria* entitled *Soma. Divine Mushroom of Immortality*. Wasson was also the contractor on MKULTRA Subproject 58, which funded an expedition to Mexico to collect hallucinogenic mushrooms. In a symposium sponsored at Colgate College by Dr. Estabrooks on April 7, 1962, Aldous Huxley gave an evening talk at 8:00 P.M. entitled "Human Potentialities."

Dr. Estabrooks also wrote to Dr. Wilder Penfield, the McGill neurosurgeon and coauthor of MKULTRA Subproject 62 and MKSEARCH contractor, Dr. Maitland Baldwin[234].

Estabrooks invited MKULTRA Subproject 84 contractor, Dr. Martin Orne to speak at a symposium on hypnosis at Colgate College on April 1-2, 1960. The papers presented at this symposium were later published as *Hypnosis: Current Problems*, edited by Dr. Estabrooks[86]. The title of Dr. Orne's[216] chapter in this volume is "Antisocial Behavior and Hypnosis." In this chapter, Dr. Orne references Dr. Estabrooks' (1943) book *Hypnotism*, which describes the hypnotic courier or super-spy.

Dr. Orne's research for his chapter in *Hypnosis: Current Problems* was supported by contract AF49(638) 728 from the Air Force Office of Scientific Research. Dr. Orne's colleague and coathor, Ronald E. Shor, Ph.D.[284] is referred to as "Ron" in an August 22, 1961 letter from Dr. Estabrooks to Dr. Orne (see Appendix A). The research described in Dr. Shor's[283] chapter in the book was funded by the National Institute of Mental Health, a subdivision of the National Institute of Health (MKULTRA Subprojects 36, 45, 55, 62, 117, and 125), the Public Health Service (MKULTRA Subproject 36), Air Force contract AF49(638)-728 and CIA cutout, the Society for the Investigation of Human Ecology.

Among the colleagues thanked in Dr. Shor's chapter are three Members of the Scientific and Professional Advisory Board of the False Memory Syndrome Foundation, Dr. Martin Orne, Dr. Ulric Neisser, and Emily F. Carota (now Emily Carota Orne).   Not thanked in that particular publication is Board member Dr. David Dinges[222].

Other speakers at the 1960 hypnosis symposium included two of the other leading experts on hypnosis of the twentieth century, Dr. Ernest Hilgard and Dr. Milton Erickson. Dr. Erickson returned to Colgate College to talk at the Colgate University Symposium on Hypnosis on April 5-7, 1962. Dr. Hilgard is a member of the Scientific and Professional Advisory Board of the False Memory Syndrome Foundation. A coauthor of Dr. Orne's[94] who took over from him as Editor of the *International Journal of Clinical and Experimental Hypnosis*, Dr. Fred Frankel, is also on the Board of the False Memory Syndrome Foundation, but was not invited to the Colgate Symposium.

Other chapters in *Hypnosis: Current Problems* include one by Dr. Seymour Fisher, Chief, Special Studies Unit, Psychopharmacology Service Center, National Institute of Mental Health. It is implausible, because of his position, that Dr. Fisher was unwitting of CIA and military funding of mind control research.

Dr. Estabrooks did experiments on children. These were conducted at Rome State School in Rome, New York, with the approval of the Superintendent in a letter dated December 19, 1935. Estabrooks also did experiments on children at St. John's Orphan Asylum and the House of the Good Shepherd, run by the Utica Community Chest in Utica, New York. The Director of the Utica Community Chest, A.J. Derbyshire told Dr Estabrooks in a letter dated December 7, 1935 that he could supply fifty children age 9 to 12. This was to be facilitated by a Sister Callista.

Dr. Estabrooks corresponded with J. Edgar Hoover about using hypnosis to interrogate juvenile delinquents and applied to the Department of Health, Education and Welfare for a research grant. He also wrote to Hoover on June 8, 1936 about the possibility of combining drugs with hypnosis. In August 11, 1959 correspondence with Murray Aborn, Ph.D., Executive Secretary, Mental Health Study Section, Division of Research Grants, Department of Health, Education and Welfare, Estabrooks wrote:

> *By preference, I would hope to obtain the services, full-time, of a competent clinical psychologist, working with a psychiatric consultant, and a man well-versed in the use of hypnotism with children. This is a rather specialized field. There are two pediatricians in this area, both, of course, M.D.'s, who have had extensive practice in hypnosis, but they also have their regular practices. I doubt if this would be satisfactory. I am quite convinced I can obtain the clinical psychologist in question from, say, the Clinic at Johns Hopkins, from the George Washington Medical School, from the Harvard or Yale Medical Schools. He will, of course, occupy a crucial position, and should come very well recommended.*

Johns Hopkins, Harvard and Yale were all MKULTRA institutions. Given the military intelligence and academic connections of Dr. Estabrooks, and the fact that all his techniques and results were achieved in real-life simulations under BLUEBIRD and ARTICHOKE, it is probable that his claims to have created and handled Manchurian Candidates during World War II are accurate and factual. His experimentation on children raises the possibility that he or other investigators have attempted to create Manchurian Candidates in children. Such a possibility might seem far-fetched until one considers the LSD, biological and radiation experiments conducted on children, the effects on children of the Tuskeegee Syphilis Study, the fact that four MKULTRA Subprojects were on children, and the fact that hypnotic subjects described in the BLUEBIRD and ARTICHOKE documents include girls nineteen years of age.

Dr. Estabrooks is the only psychiatrist or psychologist to have claimed in public that he created Manchurian Candidates.

IV. Case Histories

In this section, case histories are presented. All cases involve the creation of altered states of consciousness and dissociative symptoms. Palle Hardrup, Patty Hearst and Candy Jones are Manchurian Candidates. Their cases illustrate in detail how Manchurian Candidates are created, using the methods of destructive cults[328], Chinese Communist interrogators, and BLUEBIRD and ARTICHOKE doctors.

Mary Ray, William Jordan and William Chaffin were subjects in military LSD experiments. They experienced dissociative symptoms, including amnesia in the two men's cases, but they were not Manchurian Candidates. Their cases illustrate the fact that many different elements of BLUEBIRD, ARTICHOKE, MKULTRA, MKDELTA, MKSEARCH, and MKNAOMI were designed to induce dissociative states and dissociative symptoms including amnesia. The techniques for creating Manchurian Candidates were studied as separate components of the overall process in many different experiments and projects.

Linda MacDonald has had complete amnesia for her life before age twenty-six ever since she was *depatterned* by MKULTRA contractor, Dr. Ewen Cameron. The utility of such amnesia from an intelligence perspective is obvious. Subjects for Cameron's experiments were civilian patients seeking treatment at one of the leading medical schools in North America, McGill University. Linda MacDonald's story brings the human costs of the experiments into focus.

Sirhan Sirhan and Mark David Chapman provide examples of the self-created Manchurian Candidate assassin. They illustrate the point that mind control methods can be applied through self-hypnotic and self-training procedures, a possibility discussed by MKULTRA contractor Alden Sears in his Subproject documents.

16

LINDA MACDONALD

Linda MacDonald was born in Vancouver on August 6, 1937. She was 56 when I interviewed her at her town house in Vancouver surrounded by books, music, a guitar and photographs of her children. She is an attractive, lively, interesting person. I didn't see the slightest hint of any kind of mental illness in seven hours of conversation. No one in her family has ever received psychiatric treatment, other than her, and she herself has not received any treatment since 1964. She has never had a drug or alcohol problem and has never been in trouble with the law. Linda MacDonald was a victim of Dr. Ewen Cameron's unethical, destructive mind control experiments.

In Linda's case, depatterning was achieved through 102 electroconvulsive therapy (ECT) treatments given to her between May 1 and September 12, 1963. Linda MacDonald and other depatterning subjects at the Allan Memorial Institute did not receive the usual amount of electricity to their brains per ECT treatment. Dr. Cameron[52, 53, 55] used a technique called the Page-Russell technique in which the button on the ECT machine is pushed six times per treatment, instead of the usual one.

Depatterning was combined with psychic driving in many patients[51, 54] but not in Linda MacDonald's case. In depatterning, tape loops were played repeatedly to patients so that they heard the same message in "250,000 to 500,000 repetitions over a period which averages 20 days"[54]. According to Dr. Cameron[51], "The effectiveness of the procedure has been studied under a variety of conditions, among them drug disinhibition, ordinary and prolonged sleep treatment, hypnosis under stimulant drugs and after prolonged psychological isolation."

Linda MacDonald's "treatment" at the Allan Memorial Institute involved intensive application of three of these brainwashing techniques; drug disinhibition, prolonged sleep treatment, and prolonged psychological isolation. These were combined with the electrical equivalent of 612 conventional ECT treatments. The amount of electricity introduced into Linda MacDonald's brain exceeded by 76.5 times the maximum amount recommended in the ECT Guidelines of the American Psychiatric Association, which state that a course of ECT should consist of 4 to 8 treatments.

Dr. Cameron's depatterning technique resulted in permanent and complete amnesia. To this day, Linda MacDonald is unable to remember anything from her birth to the time she entered the Allan Memorial Institute in 1963. Dr. Cameron created a type of dissociative disorder in Linda MacDonald. He demonstrated what was considered to be in doubt in the BLUEBIRD and ARTICHOKE documents; he proved that doctors skilled in the right procedures can erase a subject's memory.

The Linda MacDonald who was born in Vancouver in 1937 is not the Linda MacDonald I interviewed. The Linda I talked to is a new and separate identity that was created by Linda herself, after discharge from the Allen Memorial Institute. Linda referred to herself before age 26 as if she was talking about another person, whom she referred to several times as "Little Lindy." She said that was how it seemed to her, that her original self was another person, not her.

After destroying Linda MacDonald's identity and memory, Dr. Cameron allowed a new identity to evolve spontaneously outside the walls of his institution. The new identity wasn't used for anything by Dr. Cameron, it was simply an experimental by-product discarded by him without any follow-up. At the time of discharge, Dr. Cameron gave Linda's husband three instructions:

1. Don't give her back her past.
2. Keep her away from her family as much as possible.
3. Don't teach her anything until she takes some initiative.

As recorded by the nurses in her chart (see Appendix H), Linda was reduced to a vegetable state by the depatterning. She was completely disoriented, and didn't know her name, age or where she was. She didn't recognize her children. She couldn't read, drive, cook or use a toilet. Not only did she not know her husband, she didn't even know what a husband was.

For the first few months after discharge, Linda couldn't remember where her children were as soon as they went outside to play. She drew a map of the surrounding four blocks and put the children's names on it to keep track of their locations. While Linda was trying to relearn basic human functions and self-care, a nanny kept track of everything for her.

It took three to four years for Linda to recover her short-term memory fully. One of the highlights of her rehabilitation, which she did entirely on her own, was the time she announced excitedly, "Kids, look what I'm doing!" She had learned how to scramble an egg. It was not till the summer of 1964 that her husband, Tom, taught her C, G and D chords on the guitar; she had been a good guitar player before entering the Allan Memorial Institute.

When Linda was admitted to the Allan on March 28, 1963 her children were: a boy age 6, a boy age 5, a girl age 3, and twins age 1. She bore another son in 1966. Her oldest child was born in Toronto, the second in Quebec, her third in the United States, and the twins in Quebec. Despite all these moves and household responsibilities, compounded by the fact that her twins were born premature and spent a month in incubators, she functioned well up until March 28, 1963. There were a few things she was unable to do because of her depression, but not many; for instance, she was unable to sing in a choir.

Linda had never had any mental health problems requiring treatment until after the birth of her twins, when she developed a postpartum depression. She was treated by her family doctor, Dr. Rosenhec with Dexedrin (see a letter from Dr. Cameron to Dr. Rosenhec in Appendix H). This caused such severe insomnia that she was often up in the middle of the night vacuuming her house. It was Dr. Rosenhec who referred her to the Allan Memorial Institute.

Judging by things her relatives have told her, and by the medical record, it appears that Linda also had a dissociative disorder prior to March 28, 1963. She had gone into a strange state several times in which she didn't recognize people and couldn't talk (see Appendix H), and she heard a voice talking in her head. Other symptoms and the circumstances of her collapse into the strange state in August, 1961 can't be described because of confidentiality reasons.

Linda also had a cult background. Her mother belonged to a group called *Moral Rearmament*, also called *The Oxford Group*. The cult had its headquarters in Switzerland. Its doctrine was one of absolute purity, honesty, love and unselfishness. According to cult routine, the day was begun with a quiet time alone with God, then each member of the family shared with the others what had been done in words and thoughts on prior days. The children went to weekly meetings downtown. Full-time members lived communally in big houses that the children visited. According to Moral Rearmament, if a girl wore a bra, she was enticing a young man.

Information on the Oxford Group can be found on their web page at www.mra.org.uk.

On June 1, 1951 Dr. James Tyhurst attended a CIA meeting at the Ritz-Carlton Hotel in Montreal to discuss brainwashing. Also present were Dr. Donald Hebb, unidentified CIA personnel, and O. M. Solandt, Chairman of Canada's Defense Research Board, which funded research by both Dr. Hebb and Dr. Tyhurst at McGill. In the minutes of the meeting it says that[105]:

> *It was pointed out that there had been a number of previous times in the history of western culture when confession was a feature. These were the period of inquisition, of Salem witch trials, and of particular sub-groups such as the revivalist sects and the Oxford Group. It is possible that study of such phenomena might give clues to the central problem.*

The problem being discussed at the CIA meeting was how to change peoples' attitudes, beliefs, and identities. Experiments to achieve this goal were conducted under BLUEBIRD, ARTICHOKE, and MKULTRA and at McGill by Drs. Cameron, Hebb and Azima. Is it a coincidence that the CIA was interested in the mind control methods of the Oxford Group, to which Linda MacDonald belonged? Did her membership in the Oxford Group result in her being selected for depatterning? There is now no way to know.

Were other members of the Oxford Group or other small cults depatterned by Dr. Cameron? Did any of his depatterning patients have classified information of any kind? At least partial answers to these questions, which have never been asked before, may be sitting in the medical records department of the Allan Memorial Institute.

Linda's boyfriend, her future husband, didn't like the Oxford Group. Linda said he described her as "helly-holy-helly" during her teen years. He said she alternated back and forth in three-month cycles between moral restraint, and smoking and being sexually active. The summer

Linda became engaged, she went to the Moral Rearmament Canadian headquarters in Mackinaw. She was considering becoming a full-time member. She returned home to Ottawa with cult team leaders and told her mother she was planning on becoming a full-time member. Her mother blew up and dropped out of the Oxford Group, taking her daughter with her.

Later, when her boyfriend took her to Mackinaw for a romantic weekend, there was a lot of what Linda called "swooshy water" around. For unknown reasons, water triggered several pseudoseizures during the period Linda was recovering from her depatterning. Whether these seizures had anything to do with something that happened to her at the Moral Rearmament camp, is unknown.

There is no documentation that Dr. Cameron knew anything sinister or secret about the Oxford Group. However, there is a connection to politics, power, and weapons in Linda MacDonald's life. Her husband worked for the Canadian Armament Research Development Establishment (CARDE). His immediate boss at CARDE was a man who sold arms to Saddam Hussein. His boss was also tied into the Iran-Contra affair and was murdered in Europe a few years ago. It is unlikely that Linda MacDonald's memory was wiped out for political, intelligence, or military reasons based on her husband's employment at CARDE, unless he told her classified secrets and she was considered a bad security risk. However, the question arises whether any of Dr. Cameron's depatterning subjects were selected for intelligence reasons, in which case the function of other subjects would in part be to provide cover.

In her childhood and adolescence, Linda was a singer. She and her sister made a record at the Chateau Laurier, a famous old Ottawa hotel. Commenting on the tape, Linda said to me, "It's funny to listen to the other Linda - no way you would guess the voice on the tape is the same person."

Describing the other Linda's admission to the Allan Memorial Institute, Linda said, "She walked in with her guitar under her arm."

The Linda who was erased by Dr. Cameron was a very lively person. In 1955, her boyfriend moved to another city to go to university. She was left behind with her parents in Ottawa. Her parents liked Tom (a pseudonym) but didn't want the couple to get married yet. Linda's solution?

She borrowed $5.00 from her sister and caught a bus to Toronto, on the pretense of going to a football game. She and Tom were married in Toronto that night at 6:00 P.M. She caught the midnight bus back to Ottawa and sang in church as a soloist the next day. That Christmas her parents changed their minds and decided it would be all right for Tom and Linda to get married the next summer.

In response, Linda told her parents she was already married, which did not go over well. Her mother kicked her out of the house. Linda went to live in the attic of Tom's parents' house initially, because they were away in Florida. During her life before and after the Allan Memorial Institute, she has done many resourceful things.

Linda has a good relationship with her parents now, and has had for many years. During the period from March 28 to September 12, 1963 while she was at the Allan Memorial Institute, her parents were not allowed to visit her, except for one visit by her father in August. The only time Linda has ever seen her father cry was during a 1984 television interview, in which he described Linda's vegetable state during that August visit. Linda and Tom divorced in 1972, and she has never remarried.

Since 1972, Linda was always worked and supported herself. She has had a variety of interesting, responsible jobs including singing at a Hyatt Hotel, managing property, and working as a rehabilitation officer for the Canadian government.

Life changed for Linda when the Canadian Broadcasting Corporation program, *The Fifth Estate*, aired a segment on Val Orlikow and Dr. Cameron on January 17, 1984. On January 20, the Canadian government delivered its first formal protest about MKULTRA to the U.S. State Department. A Vancouver newspaper ran a full page story on Robert Loggie, a Vancouver man who had been experimented on by Dr. Cameron; Loggie was a plaintiff in the class action suit against the CIA for Dr. Cameron's MKULTRA experiments, which was settled out of court for $750,000.00, divided among the nine plaintiffs, in 1988.

Linda's mother phoned her about *The Fifth Estate* program. Linda's response was, "Mother, that has nothing to do with who I am now."

Despite her response to her mother, Linda shook a lot in reaction to the news, was scared, and didn't know what to do. Through a reporter she got in touch with Jim Turner, a Washington lawyer representing the nine Canadian plaintiffs in the suit against the CIA. He advised Linda that she could not be a party to the class action suit against the

CIA because she was "treated" by Dr. Cameron after his CIA funding had stopped. The Canadian government had picked up the funding by 1963 (see Canadian government grants to Dr. Cameron in Appendix H). Eventually, with much effort, she was referred to Canadian lawyer, Tom Berger, who got her $100,000.00 plus legal fees from the Canadian government. As part of her settlement, Linda agreed never to sue the Allan Memorial Institute.

The purpose of Dr. Cameron's depatterning was to create amnesia. Whether Linda MacDonald's amnesia should be classified as *dissociative amnesia* by the diagnostic rules of the American Psychiatric Association[12], or a form of organic amnesia depends on whether her memory is permanently erased, or intact but inaccessible. It is possible that intensive psychotherapy could result in the recovery of accurate memories. It would be difficult to demonstrate whether the recovered memories were indeed accurate, and if they were, whether she remembered them herself or reconstructed them from information provided by relatives since 1963.

When I interviewed her in 1993, the possibility of recovering the "erased" memories was a moot point because Linda had decided against any such attempt on the grounds that it would be too painful and stressful, with uncertain benefits. Today, she is considering trying to recover her stolen past through therapy. Whether that is possible, and whether it would be helpful, is unknown.

17
<u>Mary Ray</u>

Mary Ray was employed as a research assistant at the University of Minnesota from 1964 to 1966. She became an experimental subject when her boss, Dr. Amedeo Marrazzi, gave her an injection of 65 micrograms of LSD on January 15, 1966, as part of an experiment funded by the Air Force. She had a bad reaction to the LSD and was kept in the hospital overnight under the care of Dr. James Janecek, who sent a copy of his discharge summary to Dr. W.L. Pew. Dr. Janecek described Mary Ray as "acutely psychotic, hallucinating freely, complaining of tremendous fear of not coming out of this state, experiencing rapid passage of time and completely disoriented as to time, place and person."

Dr. Janecek's diagnosis was, "Acute brain syndrome associated with LSD" and he stated that, "This patient should not receive LSD again or any other hallucinogenic drug." In view of her symptoms and reaction, it is doubtful that the actual dosage of LSD was 65 micrograms. It is much more likely that the dosage was in the range of 400 micrograms referred to by Dr. Louis Jolyon West [2] (see Chapter 7).

There is no evidence from Dr. Janecek's C.V. or publications that he was ever involved in mind control research. His military service in Vietnam as Commanding Officer of the 175th Medical Detachment, with the rank of Major, was from June, 1967 to October, 1969, which is subsequent to his treating Mary Ray.

Mrs. Ray's description of her bad LSD trip in Senate testimony matches the medical record of Dr. Janecek closely (*Biomedical and Behavioral Research, 1975*, pp. 122):

Mrs. RAY.   *I went through a state of absolute terror, panic, I have a very hard time verbalizing because unless a person has been through this, it is very hard to explain. I started out after the injection with nausea and shaking and feeling cold and wanting to run away, but not knowing from what. As I got worse and worse, I realized something was very wrong. I felt they may have given me too much or maybe they accidentally went into a vein, and I told the student that I wanted to go to the emergency room.*

I was absolutely desperate, and he said he was sorry, but he could not take me there without some sort of authority. This was on a Saturday, and there just was nobody in the building. There was no one but the two of us who I knew of. He got on the telephone and tried dialing Marazzi who never seemed to be around. He was never around when I was around. He dialed all kinds of people and could not get through, so I tried to go out through the window. He was holding on to me. He hollered, and another student walked through, and the two of them took me to the emergency room. At this time it was about the worst. I was in a state of becoming the universe. I became objects. I was no longer a person. I was in a state of absolute terror.

The closest thing I can remember being like that was as a child, when I was given ether, the feeling before losing consciousness, and this time I could bring myself back enough to realize that I was a person out of this billowing black seething weirdness, this horror.

I looked down and I saw my arms which were two white rivers with black threads and they were my veins. I realized even though I was not really a person that I could end all this nightmare, this hell, by cutting my veins.

Then I concentrated on this problem for what seemed like centuries, because time did not exist. It was a strange time disorder. I tried desperately to kill myself, and at this point there was no question in my mind that if I had some sort of sharp instrument, and if I were alone, I would have killed myself.

And no one seemed to know how to handle the situation. No one seemed to know what to do. It seemed like kids playing scientists.

Senator KENNEDY. There was no adequate medical supervision during this period of time?

Mrs. RAY.   When I saw patients going in I never saw Dr. Marazzi around. There were just students.

Senator KENNEDY. Were you permitted to go to the emergency room
                   when you wanted to?

Mrs. RAY.   No, the student told me he just could not take me
                   there; he had to get some authorization first.

Senator KENNEDY. And you contemplated suicide?

Mrs. RAY.   It was not just contemplating; I was desperately
                   trying to find out how I could commit suicide.

Senator MATHIAS. Is that why you tried to get out the window,
                   that you were just trying to escape?

Mrs. RAY.   At that point I did not consider it suicide. I was
                   just trying to get away. I wanted to run away.

Senator MATHIAS. It was just getting out of there that was important.

Mrs. RAY.   Yes. I did not care that I was on the third floor.
                   I just had to be away. I was like an animal in a
                   cage. I did not want to be trapped. I was held
                   against my will, even though I guess I should not
                   have been.

Asked by Senator Kennedy about the long term side effects of the bad
LSD trip, Mrs. Ray testified:

Mrs. RAY.   Before this I was quite a relaxed person despite a
                   rather traumatic life, and right after that, starting
                   the date I got the LSD, I have been overwhelmed,
                   flooded with anxiety almost 24 hours a day. It
                   has never changed, and this is over 9 years ago.
                   That is the most important problem I have had,
                   flashbacks to more or less a degree, a feeling
                   of going back to that terrible world. I have had
                   nightmares, I have developed an intolerance to any
                   sort of stimulants. One cup of coffee after noon
                   will keep me awake all night, and things like that.

                   But at the time it influenced me quite a bit
                   because I had to quit school. I was hospitalized
                   when I had the LSD experience, but that was not
                   the end of it. I had to go through 6 ½ months
                   of psychiatric therapy. I was referred to a
                   psychiatrist the next week, and that was very
                   expensive for a student. To add insult to injury,
                   I received a hospital bill after I was admitted for
                   the treatment for me under the LSD, which I sent

to Dr. Marazzi. After that point I never seen or heard from him again.

Senator KENNEDY. *Do you want to try to get some kind of additional follow-up help or assistance?*

Mrs. RAY.   *Not from them.*

Senator KENNEDY. *You did not care if you ever saw them again?*

Mrs. RAY.   *I did not want to ever see him again.*

Dr. Amedeo Marrazzi was born in New York City on February 6, 1905. He died in Grosse Pointe, Michigan on January 11, 1980. His LSD research was funded by Air Force grant AF-AFOSR-764-65. Dr. Marrazzi published papers with both William L. Pew, M.D. and Richard Meisch, M.D.[186].

In a paper entitled "Quantified LSD Effect on Ego Strength"[186], an 18-year old girl identified as J.M. is described as "having entered a period of mutism lasting three days." The paper contains J.M.'s Minnesota Multiphasic Personality Inventory (MMPI) profiles for Pre LSD (8/30/65), Post LSD (9/14/65) and Recovery (9/22/65). The Pre-LSD MMPI is normal. The Post-LSD profile is highly abnormal with a huge elevation on the schizophrenia scale, but has returned to normal by 9/22/65. This is likely the same patient described by Mary Ray in her Senate testimony:

Senator KENNEDY. *How old were these test subjects?*

Mrs. RAY.   *I remember one girl of 17, although I saw her written up as 18, and I remember another girl of 19, and the 18-year old definitely did not want to be part of the experiment.*

Senator KENNEDY. *How did you know she did not?*

Mrs. RAY.   *I saw her as they were taking her in, and she said she won't go, she won't go, and they said, "Yes, you will," and she said, "Don't take me back to that hell.": which makes me think she had had a previous experiment.*

Senator KENNEDY. *What was she doing in there? You were all not forced or required to do this, were you?*

Mrs. RAY.   *She was a patient, and she was forced. They told her she had no choice. I remember this little episode very well. There was an aide on her arm restraining her, and an orderly on another, and she kept saying she did not want to go in, and*

> *they said - I do not know which it was who said*
> *that, but they said, "You have to go; you have*
> *no choice."*

Senator KENNEDY. *What did the doctor tell her?*

Mrs. RAY.   *There was no doctor there. But I went back then*
> *about 1 or 2 hours later, and at this point she*
> *was totally disintegrated. She was absolutely*
> *psychotic. Before this she was a very normal*
> *appearing person; she would gossip and joke.*
> *I even remember a joke she told me. She was*
> *attractive and talkative. But afterwards she*
> *was just a mess. She was taken back to the ward,*
> *and she was for like 4 days mute, and you could*
> *not get through to her in any way. I tried to test*
> *her, and I went into her room and she was just*
> *staring straight ahead. I went like this [waving*
> *hands], and it was nothing; she did not seem to*
> *see me. I took her to the testing room where there*
> *were four others, and she walked right through a*
> *chair as though it was not there. Any position*
> *I put her body in, she would stay in.*

Dr. Marrazzi worked as the Director of the Veterans Administration Research Laboratories in Neuropsychiatry in Pittsburgh from 1954 to 1964 before moving to the University of Minnesota. Prior to that he was Chief of the Toxicology Branch at the Chemical Corps Medical Laboratories, Army Chemical Center, Maryland (Edgeware Arsenal) from 1948 to 1951. From 1951 to 1956 he was Assistant Scientific Director of the Medical Directorate at the Chemical Warfare Laboratories. This puts him in the thick of the action for MKULTRA and MKNAOMI.

A letter from CIA Director Allen Dulles to the Secretary of Defense dated December 3, 1955 confirms that the CIA funded research by the Army, Navy and various universities. The letter specifically identifies the Army Chemical Corps and the Office of Naval Research. Six individuals are identified in the letter: Dr. Wilson Greene, Technical Director, Chemical Corps, Chemical and Radiological Laboratories, Army Chemical Center; Dr. Amedeo Marrazzi (his first name is spelled incorrectly in the letter), Medical Center, Army Chemical Center; Captain Clifford P. Phoebus, Chief, Biological Services Division, Office of Naval Research; Brigadier General Don D. Elickinger, ARDC, U.S. Air Force; and Lieutenant Colonel Alexander Bahlin, Office of the Assistant Secretary of Defense (Research and Development).

In his Presidential Address to the Society for Biological Psychiatry, entitled "An Experimentalist Looks at Psychiatry," Dr. Marrazzi[185] discusses the substance, taraxein extracted from the blood of schizophrenics by CIA contractor Dr. Robert Heath. He describes his own LSD research and includes a photograph of a "Skinner booth for humans" (see Appendix L). Dr. Marrazzi's LSD experiments were carried out in an Ames leaf room.

The Ames leaf room was created by Dr. A. Ames[13] on contract to the Office of Naval Research. It is a room in which the walls, floor and ceiling slope at strange angles. The subject sits just inside the room, which has one open end, such that his peripheral vision cannot detect anything outside the room. The surfaces of the room are entirely covered with leaves. The subject then puts on special goggles with anisokonic lenses that further distort all the angles of the walls, floor and ceiling. Added to this extreme perceptual distortion are the effects of the LSD given to the subject.

As depicted in the photograph in Marrazzi's[185] paper (see Appendix L), the subject is instructed to adjust a white bar at the far end of the Ames leaf room until it appears horizontal. This is done using two controls the subject can grasp with his hands. The purpose of the experiments, according to Dr. Marrazzi was to provide a measure of the subject's resistance or susceptibility to "cerebral disintegrative stress," which, translated, means resistance to brainwashing and intensive interrogation. Subjects were a group of healthy nurses containing "a sub-group that a psychiatrist had assessed as normal but labile and potentially more apt to succumb to stress."

The references for Dr. Marrazzi's[185] Presidential Address to the Society of Biological Psychiatry include papers by Dr. Robert Heath, CIA contractor and brain electrode specialist; Dr. Wilder Penfield, co-author of MKULTRA and MKSEARCH contractor, Dr. Maitland Baldwin; Office of Naval Research contractor, Dr. A. Ames; and Dr. Paul Hoch, who killed Harold Blauer with an injection of U. S. Army mescaline in 1953.

Officers of the Society of Biological Psychiatry in 1964-65 included MKULTRA contractor, Dr. Ewen Cameron; Dr. Lauretta Bender, who gave LSD and psilocybin to children; and Dr. Hudson Hoaglund of the Worcester Foundation for Experimental Biology (MKULTRA Subproject 8). The volume of *Recent Advances in Biological Psychiatry* in which Dr. Marrazzi's Presidential Address is published includes four other papers on LSD.

Other subjects of military LSD research also testified at the 1975 Senate Hearings, including William F. Chaffin and his wife. Chaffin participated in an Air Force mind control experiment in July, 1958. He learned that the substance he took was LSD only in 1975, after a story about LSD testing at Edgeware Arsenal was published. Mrs. Chaffin testified that she thought a miscarriage she suffered might have been due to the LSD causing a deformed fetus. The couple testified (*Biomedical and Behavioral Research, 1975*, pp. 127):

Senator KENNEDY. Mrs. Chaffin, do you have a gun in your house?

Mrs. Chaffin.   *Yes, sir, we do.*

Mr. CHAFFIN.   *Yes, sir, we do.*

Senator KENNEDY. Could you tell us, Mrs. Chaffin; I understand you had a rather frightening experience one time.

Mrs. CHAFFIN.   *Yes, sir. He did take the gun and start out with it and I asked him where he was going. It was about ten o'clock, after dark. I knew he had no reason to carry a gun. He said, "I don't know. I'll be back." He had been rather moody all day, and I just asked him why he was taking the gun. He said he was going to shoot himself, and that is when I told him that if he left the house with the gun, I would call the police and have them track him down. But he seemed to have no memory of it at all.*

Senator KENNEDY. Mr. Chaffin, as I understand, you have no memory of this incident, is that right?

Mr. CHAFFIN.   *Yes, sir, that is right. I have no memory of this specific instance at all.*

Senator KENNEDY. Or any incidents involving this?

Mr. CHAFFIN.   *I have had other instances of extreme depression, actually blank memories up to a certain point; as I say, extreme depression, virtually indescribable, as far as contemplating taking my own life.*

Senator KENNEDY. Did you ever have these prior to the time you took the drug?

Mr. CHAFFIN.   *No, sir. I can honestly say I had no such experiences as this.*

The amnesia William Chaffin describes is unlikely to be due to a single dose of LSD or to a major depressive disorder. It is likely that other drugs, such as scopolamine, were administered along with the LSD, or alternatively Mr. Chaffin may have experienced other brainwashing techniques for which he is amnesic. At any rate, the outcome of the experiments on Mr. Chaffin included recurrent amnesia for behavior that was out of character, and neither the behavior nor the amnesia occurred prior to the experimentation. These symptoms are elements of the Manchurian Candidate. I am not saying that William Chafin was a Manchurian Candidate himself – he was a subject in studies that were relevant to the Manchurian Candidate Program.

Bits and pieces of the procedure for creating Manchurian Candidates were studied one at a time and in numerous different combinations, spread out across many different intelligence agencies, and under many different overlapping cryptonyms.

Another LSD subject who testified to Senator Kennedy in 1975 was Colonel William R. Jordan. He was one of 34 men who received LSD at Fort Benning, Georgia in 1960. He described the effects of the drug as including "nausea, vertigo, and then facial disorientation and complete disintegration of everything around us.... We had periods of lucidity and almost total awareness that we were being experimented on, but yet following that there were enormous gaps, complete periods of blanks, where we did not know what was going on, and we were only told after the fact what we had done."

The long term side effects experienced by Colonel Jordan included "periods of transitory confusion, vertigo" and beginning in December, 1961, epileptic seizures. Medical investigation of the seizures was done at Valley Forge Hospital and Walter Reed Hospital. The Senate hearing documents include 38 pieces of correspondence generated while Colonel Jordan attempted to get a response from the U.S. Army concerning his seizures. In response to Colonel Jordan's initiative, the Army attempted to do the first follow-up on the subjects in 1972.

The results of these efforts are summarized in a memorandum by Kenneth R. Dirks, M.D., Brigadier General, MC, Assistant Surgeon General for Research and Development, dated July 15, 1975; of the 34 men, 19 were examined at Walter Reed Hospital, 7 declined examination, 7 did not respond or were still being sought, and one had been killed in Vietnam. Dr. Dirk estimated that about 1,500 Army subjects took part in LSD experiments at Edgeware Arsenal, Fort Benning, and other locations. Other estimates put the figure at 4000 subjects.

Mary Ray, William Chaffin, and William Jordan had acute reactions and long term side effects that suggest they were given higher doses of LSD than reported, or that the LSD was combined with other drugs such as scopolamine. The degree of amnesia, nausea and vertigo created by the LSD seems more typical of anticholinergic medications or other compounds.

Mary Ray is the only LSD subject for whom Senate testimony is corroborated by medical records. She is also the only subject whose mind control doctor is identified by name. The fact that Dr. Marrazzi administered LSD to subjects on contract to the Air Force is documented in his own publications, which makes Mrs. Ray's testimony uniquely corroborated. Thousands of other LSD subjects might have similar stories to tell, and those subjects represent only a small subset of the mind control drug experiments, since the Army alone lists over 130 mind control drugs it tested in the 1950's, 60's and 70's.

18

PALLE HARDRUP

Palle Hardrup, a Danish man, was 31 years old when he was found guilty of murder and bank robbery on July 17, 1954. The robbery and murder of two bank employees had taken place on March 29, 1951. Hardrup also robbed a bank on August 23, 1950, but no one was killed during that holdup. Palle Hardup was subjected to the classical methods of mind control studied in BLUEBIRD and ARTICHOKE, and is the best documented and studied example of a real Manchurian Candidate. His story proves that Manchurian Candidates can in fact be created, be programmed to commit crimes, and be amnesic for those crimes. The 1958 book describing the case, *Antisocial or Criminal Acts and Hypnosis: A Case Study* could be used as a training manual for Manchurian Candidate programs.

Using different vocabulary consistent with Danish terminology at the time, the jury found that Palle Hardrup had multiple personality, and concluded that the multiple personality had been created deliberately by his programmer and handler, Bjorn Neilsen. The verdict was appealed to the Supreme Court, which upheld it in a decision rendered on November 18, 1955. The case also went to the Special Court of Appeal, where the initial jury decision was upheld on June 29, 1957. Over 50 witnesses were called at the original trial, numerous experts testified, and the Danish Medico Legal Council reviewed the case.

In their report of February 17, 1954, the Medico Legal Council, also called the Board of Forensic Medicine, wrote that, "even though the actual symptoms of the mental disorder now seem to have disappeared Hardrup cannot be regarded as cured. The profound split in his personality, which has been established, will certainly only slowly be straightened out." This analysis was reconfirmed by the Medico Legal Council in its final report of May 3, 1957.

The jury found Hardrup guilty on all charges but not responsible for his actions on account of insanity. The man who transformed Palle Hardrup into an amnesic bank robber, Bjorn Neilsen, was found guilty of robbery, attempted robbery and manslaughter, even though he was not physically present at any of the crimes. The jury found that Neilsen had planned and instigated the crimes and had compelled Hardrup to carry them out through various forms of influence including hypnosis. Neilsen was sentenced to life imprisonment. Neilsen's verdict went through the Danish appeal process and was not changed. On February 2, 1956 Hardrup was transferred to the State Institution for Psychopathic Delinquents - what became of him in the end, and whether he is still alive, is unknown. He would now be 82 years old.

How did Neilsen turn Hardrup into a Manchurian Candidate? The explanation begins with Palle's childhood. Contrary to expectation, Hardrup's childhood was stable, normal and non-traumatic. His identical twin brother never got into any kind of legal trouble, his father worked regularly, there was no alcoholism or violence in the home, and Palle never had behavior problems, school problems or trouble with delinquency. He is described as having been a pleasant, truthful, idealistic adolescent. Dr. Reiter interviewed the family repeatedly and established that there was no family history of substance abuse, mental illness, seizures, suicide or criminal behavior. Both parents and sons agreed that the marriage of Palle's parents had been happy and harmonious.

The family was solid and middle-class. They owned a piano and both sons were musical. Palle's brother had many interests including gliding, mechanics, travel and popular science. Palle is said by Dr. Reiter to have been lively, practical, economical and to have had a good memory, powers of concentration and judgment. Both boys were physically healthy, and Palle never had any serious illnesses or head injuries.

This normal background is important because it proves that Neilsen did not exploit a pre-existing criminal personality in Palle Hardrup, or pre-existing mental illness. This finding is consistent with the fact that destructive cults recruit primarily psychiatrically normal individuals, using many of the classical techniques of mind control employed by Bjorn Neilsen[102, 289]. It also matches the normal pre-abduction psychiatric profile of Patty Hearst (see Chapter 19).

Palle Hardrup's sexual life was normal. He was heterosexual. He had satisfying sexual intercourse a number of times with different women prior to his marriage, but no pattern of unusual promiscuity. One of these women got pregnant by him and he voluntarily paid her child support although he never knew the child.

In 1939, Palle became an apprentice to a toolmaker and subsequent to that he worked as a journeyman. His life started to go wrong after the Germans occupied Denmark on April 9, 1940. Palle was seventeen at the time. An anticommunist and a Danish nationalist, he was unhappy with what he saw as Danish apathy and defeatism, which he saw as partly responsible for the German occupation. He joined a rifle corps and from there was recruited to the Nazi Party. How this recruitment took place and why Hardrup agreed to it is not made entirely clear by Dr. Reiter.

In September, 1944 Hardrup was called up by the Danish army to take part in the civil defense of Denmark. The recruiter rejected him on the grounds that he was serving in a Nazi volunteer brigade, the Schalburg Corps. The German police commandeered Hardrup as an interpreter, but he didn't like this work and tried to escape it by shooting himself in the leg with a pistol. He was released from duty by the Nazis and went home for several months to recuperate. Once healed, he returned to the Schalburg Corps but was not required to work as an interpreter.

On February 1, 1945 Hardrup joined the Nazi Hipokorps, an organization that had persecuted Danish Jews in 1943. At the end of the war he tried to leave Denmark with some German troops, but he was arrested by the Danish police on May 8, 1945. On September 9, 1946 Hardrup was sentenced to fourteen years in prison, less the sixteen months he had served. On October 27, 1949 his sentence was reduced to ten years by royal decree and he was released on probation at that time.

During the early part of his inprisonment, Palle Hardrup was depressed, disillusioned and directionless. He realized that the ideals which led him into the Nazi Party were mistaken. During this period Palle was examined twice by a psychiatrist, Dr. Max Schmidt, as part of a series of routine examinations of war criminals. Dr. Schmidt found no signs of mental illness (Hardrup was unhappy and despondent but not clinically depressed). Dr. Schmidt wrote in his report of the second examination, conducted on September 16, 1947 (pp. 75):

The subject is of normal intelligence. He seems somewhat boyish in his political idealism, but is not otherwise immature. He has earlier been under the influence of his Nazi comrades in the Copenhagen Rifle Club, and at the age of seventeen he joined the N.S.U. [Nazi Party]. He took part in the work of the party and became an enthusiast Nazi and anticommunist. His political crimes must be regarded as a result of these beliefs. It seems likely that he belongs to the idealistic type of subject.

The criminal prognosis must be regarded as good.

Dr. Schmidt concluded that Hardrup became a Nazi out of political idealism, not because of a criminal character. He thought that the risk of future criminal activity was low. Prison reports from 1946 and 1947 described Hardrup as, "Polite and well behaved. Young idealist. Works well," and, "Quiet, steady prisoner."

The picture of Hardrup at the time he first met Bjorn Neilsen is similar to a freshman college student being recruited by a destructive cult. Alone, away from home, idealistic, subject to influence by others, directionless and unhappy, he was vulnerable to control and manipulation. Although not fundamentally criminal, Hardrup did have an antisocial streak in him. He had joined the Nazi Party. He did not commit any human rights violations himself while in the Schalburg Corps and the Hipokorps, but the Nazis, for whom he worked, certainly did. The seeds of the future Manchurian Candidate bank robber and murderer were already there when Bjorn Neilsen began his mind control experimentation.

Neilsen was a repeat offender. In 1933 he was found guilty of theft, and in 1938 of attempted robbery. In January, 1947 Neilsen was sentenced to twelve years in prison for being a member of the Nazi Frikorps Danmark. While a member he supplied the Nazis with information about Danish resistance fighters. Under cover of the resistance movement he blackmailed two Danish businessmen. Like Hardrup, he was released from Hortens State Prison in 1949.

Hardrup and Neilsen got to know each other in the spring of 1947 while working in the same workshop. While in the workshop they discussed their mutual interests in the philosophy of religion, yoga, spiritualism, hypnosis and politics. Neilsen told Hardrup that he had participated in hypnosis experiments at the Society for Psychical Research - he suggested to Hardrup that they share the same cell so that they could conduct hypnotic experiments together. Hardrup asked and received permission to share a cell with Neilsen. For eighteen months he was continuously either alone in his cell with Neilsen, or working beside him in the workshop.

Neilsen began his mind control experiment immediately, working along by instinct. There is no evidence that he had prior training in mind control. Right away we see the degree of control and influence required to create a durable, operational Manchurian Candidate.

Palle Hardrup was an excellent hypnotic subject. Neilsen began an intensive program of hypnotic conditioning involving hours per day of trance exercises. These usually occurred in the evening. Often Hardrup would go to sleep without having come out of trance. Neilsen characterized these sessions as mainly yoga training. He gave Hardrup suggestions about emptying his mind, transcending, experiencing peace and relaxation, and establishing direct contact with a deity. He also instructed Hardrup to begin isolating himself from his fellow prisoners. Hardrup's world was narrowed down to a hypnotic focus on Neilsen.

After some time, Neilsen introduced the guardian spirit, "X." X was a guiding spirit who spoke through Neilsen - Neilsen was but the vehicle for the divine counsel of X. X told Hardrup that his misfortunes to date were all tests to strengthen him for future tasks, and to prepare him for his destiny. X took complete control of all subsequent yoga training.

Gradually, Neilsen conditioned Palle Hardrup so that it was no longer necessary to induce hypnosis. Hardrup experienced Neilsen as X incarnate speaking directly to him even without hypnosis. Whenever Neilsen spoke, it was X speaking. X taught Palle about Samadhi and how yogis attain that transcendent state through denial of their bodily needs. X was there to guide Hardrup to Samadhi and enlightenment.

As a test of Hardrup's progress, obedience, spiritual earnesty and allegiance to X, X began to assign him certain tasks. One was to have another worker removed from the workshop. Hardrup succeeded in doing so through his manipulation of the other worker. X also instructed Hardrup over and over never to speak to anyone about the secret relationship between Hardrup and X. Disobedience would mean that Palle would never attain Samadhi.

Although Hardrup was destined to transcend to a higher plane, X said, there was a reason he was born in Denmark at that time. Palle Hardrup was to create the Danish National Communist Party. Through this Party,

Hardrup would realize his destiny of uniting all of Scandanavia under one government. The Party would also set in place an organization to ferry all the leading intellectuals out of Denmark should the Russians invade. The divine nature of this mission was emphasized over and over again by X.

X instructed his pupil that all true yogis are vegetarians. As a result Hardrup stopped eating meat - Neilsen then got to eat both portions of meat delivered to their cell. As well, Hardrup sat in the lotus position for hours on end to practice denial of his body. To further separate from material needs, Hardrup gave Neilsen his watch on instruction from X.

Neilsen built on this program by citing vague references from books he checked out of the prison library, including the prophecies of Nostradamus. Everything that X said was a direct emanation from the divine kingdom. As another test, X had Hardrup agree that he would have sex with women once released from prison only on direct orders from X. Hardrup was also told to practice his "concentrations" as X called them, even when X was not around.

Sometime late in 1947 or early 1948, X began to talk to Palle about schemes to raise money. The money would be used to finance the activities of the Danish National Communist Party. One scheme was an engine that ran on water. Amazingly, the engine idea actually made front-page headlines in a Danish newspaper on February 17, 1948. The Minister of Justice had drawings of it that Pale had submitted.

When Palle's father heard about the engine he had a lawyer draw up a deed of partnership between Hardrup and Neilsen, to protect his son's interests should the invention actually work. X ordered Hardrup to sign the deed, which he did. Afterwards, X had him sign a second contract transferring all rights to Neilsen, and voiding the first contract. Following this, the tests that X devised began to become more sinister.

In order to sever all ties with the material world, Hardrup began a series of hypnotic exercises involving money. In preliminary exercises, Hardrup would imagine moving money from the table in their cell to a safe or a "poor old woman's money box." This was experienced by Hardrup as a transcendent act of love and kindness. The tasks soon escalated. Soon, under orders from X, Hardrup was imagining robbing banks and committing murders.

Any qualms or conflicts about robbery and murder were interpreted by X as the reactions of the physical body These Hardrup had to reject and transcend. He was reminded that if he failed to progress on the path to Samadhi, he might lose X and be consigned to despair and eternal damnation. One of the ways to stay on the path was for Hardrup never to allow himself to be hypnotized by anyone else, ever at anytime. Dr. Reiter called this procedure "locking," the same term G.H. Estabrooks used in his 1943 textbook *Hypnotism*, which Reiter references.

The bank robberies that Hardrup practiced in his hypnotic trances were rehearsed in minute detail, including the shooting of bank employees. Another hypnotic exercise involved Palle killing his mother, a true test of his renunciation of earthly ties.

Sometime in 1947, X introduced a contingency plan in case Neilsen and Hardrup were ever separated in the future. He inserted an access code, the letter "X." This would be transmitted to Hardrup in a letter disguised as "XH2O." This code would not alert authorities because of the prior work on the water engine. The purpose of the code was to reinforce Hardrup's loyalty to X and to trigger him to follow any other instructions.

Neilsen and Hardrup were then separated for a period of time due to Hardrup's transfer to another prison camp. After a month in prison Hardrup received a letter from Neilsen that concluded, "Many greetings X." This letter was produced at trial. Neilsen was shortly thereafter transferred to the same prison. The two men arranged to have beds beside each other in the same dormitory.

X began to instruct Hardrup on the necessity of setting up "fighting units" for the Danish National Communist Party. X told Hardrup that he needed to escape from prison to carry out this work. Hardrup was told that he should go to Germany for several weeks to escape the Danish authorities. Then he would return to Denmark, go underground, and carry out his mission. When Neilsen was eventually released, he would join Hardrup. X would provide further instructions at that time.

Hardrup now began to hear X's voice talking to him even when Neilsen wasn't physically present. He had internalized his guardian spirit, possibly to protect himself from losing X should he and Neilsen ever be separated again. Separation did occur because Neilsen was transferred back to his previous prison, from where he sent Hardrup a Christmas card containing the message that Hardrup "was to get going with 'XH2O'."

Palle became obsessed with escaping, and soon succeeded in doing so. As per instructions, he went to Hamburg. One evening he hallucinated meeting X by the roadside (Neilsen was still in prison), and received further encouragement from him. Again as per X's orders, Hardrup crossed back over the frontier after two weeks. He was immediately arrested and put back in prison.

Now followed a period in which Neilsen and Hardrup were separated for nine months. Prior to his eventual release on October 29, 1949, Palle received many letters from Neilsen signed, "Greetings from X." Neilsen had been released before him, and Hardrup immediately established contact again as soon as he was free. Neilsen began working on plans for them to set up a "Psychophysical Institute," which would require financing, and he resumed the intensive hypnotic training.

Palle's father had given him about $65.00 on his release, which he immediately turned over to X. Neilsen administered this money on behalf of X. Hardrup started work early in 1950 and turned over almost his entire earnings to X/Neilsen. This made Palle's father suspicious about Neilsen's influence, so X began to instruct Palle to sever connections with his family. X also instructed Hardrup to obtain a pistol, which he did.

On February 11, 1950 Palle Hardrup was introduced to a girl named Bente by Neilsen. X had decided that Hardrup should marry her, and told him that he should make a pass at Bente when he took her home from the cinema. Ever obedient, Hardrup took Bente to his home to have sex, but his brother was there so the plan was thwarted. The next day Palle could not remember Bente's first or last name. In less than two weeks they had had intercourse.

The couple soon became engaged, as X had instructed. Prior to the wedding, X devised another test of Palle's commitment. He instructed Palle to arrange for Neilsen to have intercourse with Bente. This actually took place. Ten days later, on April 4, 1950, Palle and Bente married. One of the reasons Palle gave for why Neilsen had to have intercourse with his fiancee, was that Neilsen's wife was having her period.

In June, 1950 Neilsen began training Hardrup for the first bank robbery in earnest. There was much emphasis on the need to finance the escape plan for Denmark's intelligentsia in the event of a Russian invasion. The robbery was rehearsed in minute detail countless times. The robbery was carried out on August 23, 1950 with a take of just under $2,000.00. All this money, plus much of Hardrup's ongoing income, was turned over to X.

Plans for the second robbery began in early 1951. Preparations included the same detailed enactment of the crime during hypnotic trance. Constant reminders by X reinforced the belief that Palle's transcendence of the reincarnation cycle depended on his successful performance. Shortly before the second robbery there was a hypnotic session amplified by chloroform.

On March 29, 1951 Hardrup was caught by police immediately after the failed second robbery, having killed two bank employees. Under the influence of Neilsen's locking mechanism (never to mention X, or Neilsen's connection with X; never to let himself be hypnotized by anyone else), Hardrup told police that he had acted alone. He said he was trying to raise money for the Danish National Communist Party.

Neilsen did not become a suspect because of any evidence or anything Hardrup said. Fellow prisoners from Hortens State Prison told police that they suspected Neilsen was involved. Neilsen was interrogated and held in custody, but he stuck to an elaborate story in which Bente was identified as the mastermind behind the crime, and Palle was described as a fanatic. Neilsen had carefully set up circumstantial evidence to support his explanation.

In the course of legal hearings in the spring of 1951, Hardrup began to talk about being controlled by his guardian spirit, X. He claimed to have met X in February, 1947, prior to his first meeting with Neilsen. Hardrup denied that he had committed the 1950 robbery but in October, 1951 Bente informed police that she thought her husband had committed the crime.

Hardrup denied that his wife was correct, then a few days later confessed, then the next day withdrew his confession. By Christmas, 1951 he had written a lengthy account of the hypnotic conditioning by Neilsen. He stated that he was now free enough of Neilsen's influence to maintain a stable story. In April, 1952 Hardrup began a court-ordered psychiatric examination by Dr. Paul Reiter. Reiter delivered a 370-page report in June, 1953.

Initially, Dr. Reiter found Palle Hardrup to be unhypnotizable, until he broke through the locking mechanisms. This required a combination of growing trust, discussion of the evidence, extrication of Hardrup from Neilsen's influence, and hypnosis. Once the locking was undone, Hardrup proved to be highly hypnotizable. Dr. Reiter easily induced amnesia for posthypnotic suggestions.

In November, 1952 Neilsen had a secret conversation with Hardrup while the two were in court. For two weeks afterwards Hardrup hallucinated X's voice and was anxious and agitated. This gradually settled down and went away.

Testimony at the trial included both wives, Mrs. Hardrup and Mrs. Neilsen, corroborating events of which they were aware (the two couples spent a lot of time together). The Hardrups had a daughter, and Bente stuck by her husband throughout.

The Palle Hardrup case is not an isolated example of the documented Manchurian Candidate. Dr. Reiter reviews other similar cases in his book, including ones that came to trial and resulted in conviction of the hypnotizer. One is the 1936 Heidelberg case documented in a book written in German by Dr. Ludwig Mayer (*Das Verbrechenin Hypnose*, J.F. Lehmann, Munich, Berlin, 1937). Mayer was the most prominent German hypnosis expert of his time.

The hypnotist in the Heidelberg case was sentenced to ten years in prison for crimes committed by a 24-year old woman. The woman was acquitted. The hypnotist had inserted a locking mechanism involving verbal codes that were required for her to enter trance.

In another case, A German schoolteacher in Thuringia came under the influence of a criminal hypnotizer in 1921. In this case the schoolteacher was found guilty of arson and insurance fraud, but the hypnotizer was not convicted. Re-interviewed in 1952, the schoolteacher was almost completely amnesic for the years 1921 to 1933 (he was released from prison in 1928). Under hypnosis he gave a complete account of how he was made into a multiple personality that exactly matched a 200-page transcript of the account he had given under hypnosis in 1926. Both the tape recording and the transcript from 1926 were in Dr. Reiter's possession when his book on Palle Hardrup was published in 1958.

Hypnosis was only a single element in a complex mind control experiment conducted by Bjorn Neilsen, as the jury understood. The debates by academic expert witnesses at the trial as to whether a person can be compelled to commit crimes with hypnosis alone were correctly viewed by the jury as irrelevant to the real-world business of creating a Manchurian Candidate. Hypnosis is only one tool among many required for creating a Manchurian Candidate.

The Palle Hardrup case provides compelling evidence that the creation of Manchurian Candidates claimed by G.H. Estabrooks, and described in BLUEBIRD and ARTICHOKE documents, is real. The methods used by the creators of Manchurian Candidates are those of classical thought reform, brainwashing, mind control, and coercive influence, all terms for the same process. The methods have been used by leaders of destructive cults, MKULTRA contractors, professors of psychology and psychiatry at McGill University, and probably the KGB and other intelligence agencies. The Manchurian Candidate is fact, not fiction.

19

PATTY HEARST

Patty Hearst was born in San Francisco on February 20, 1954. She has four sisters: Anne, one year younger; Vicki, two years younger; Gina, five years older; and Cathy, fifteen years older. Their father is William Randolph Hearst, owner of a media empire including *The San Francisco Chronicle* and Avon Books, which published *Patty Hearst. Her Own Story*[115]. The Hearst girls grew up more-or-less normal, with no serious trauma and no serious mental health problems.

On February 4, 1974 the Symbionese Liberation Army (SLA) broke into Patty Hearst's apartment in Berkeley, California, tied up her boyfriend, Steven Weed, and abducted her at gunpoint. She was gagged, bound, blindfolded and hit on the left cheek with a rifle butt before being taken out of her apartment. There were several bursts of gunfire before she was driven away. She was transported to the SLA's hideout and immediately placed in a closet, still blindfolded.

For about forty days, Patty Hearst was kept in solitary confinement in the closet with no contact with the outside world. Besides profound sensory deprivation, she was subjected to food and sleep deprivation, sexual molestation, frequent interrogations and mock FBI raids staged by the SLA. During these she thought she might be killed at any time. Once out of the closet she was subjected to further interrogation and threats. Her autobiography makes it clear that the SLA used the classical techniques of thought reform, coercive persuasion, mind control, or brainwashing.

The SLA was an underground revolutionary group led by Donald DeFreeze. There were seven members, three men and four women. Donald DeFreeze was an uneducated black petty criminal. He was a maximum security prisoner at Vacaville State prison at the same time the CIA was conducting mind control experiments there under MKSEARCH Subproject 3.

These experiments involved administration of the drug pemoline to Vacaville prisoners under the direction of Dr. James Hamilton, as confirmed in an October 18, 1978 letter from Frank C. Carlucci, the Deputy Director of the CIA to Congressman Leo Ryan (see Appendix J).

According to Mae Brussell[44], Donald DeFreeze was a subject in an experimental behavior modification program run at Vacaville State Prison by Colston Westbrook. Westbrook was a CIA psychological warfare expert, and advisor to the Korean CIA. From 1966 to 1969 he was a CIA advisor to the Vietnamese Special Police Branch. In Vietnam he worked under cover as an employee of Pacific Architects and Engineers[306].

According to Brussell, Westbrook returned to the U.S. in 1970 and got a job at the University of Berkeley. He entered Vacaville State Prison under cover of the Black Cultural Association, and there designed the seven-headed cobra logo of the SLA and gave DeFreeze his African name, Cinque.

Westbrook's[331] M.A. thesis from the University of California, Berkeley was entitled "The Dual Linguistic Heritage of Afro-Americans." It is about ebonics. His thesis committee consisted of Jesse Sawyer, Kenneth Johnson and Julian Boyd and his M.A. degree was conferred on June 15, 1974. The thesis is dedicated to, "My wife Eposi and our son Ngeke Colston Ngomba-Westbrook."

In his thesis acknowledgments, Westbrook describes working as a teaching assistant in linguistics at Berkeley. He says on page 84 that he was born on September 14, 1937 in Chambersburg, Pennsylvania, second son to Edward Cody Westbrook and Virginia Ruth Colston. He describes serving three years in the Army, and being assigned to Travis Air Force Base, California in 1960 after an assignment in Korea.

Westbrook states in his thesis that he did contract work in Vietnam for the U.S. Army and the Agency for International Development before returning to the University of Berkeley in September, 1970. On page 58 of his M.A. thesis, Westbrook writes under footnote 62:

> *During the writing of this thesis, the "Symbionese Liberation Army" kidnapped Patricia Hearst. Thinking that the alleged leader of the SLA would respond more directly to Black English, this writer read a three-page open letter to news media people which was presented as a "BIZARRE LETTER TO CINQUE" by an unofficial news publication of the University of California,*

Berkeley (See The Daily Californian, Tuesday, March 5, 1974).
Cinque acknowledged the letter in a subsequent tape by stating–
for the first time – his reborn name. That and other rejoinders
were evidently too subtle for many people to understand.

Brussell states that Westbrooks' control officer was William Hermann,
who was connected to the Stanford Research Institute and the Rand
Corporation, which were both MKULTRA institutions. Hermann
was also linked to the UCLA Center for the Study and Prevention of
Violence, headed by MKULTRA contractor, Dr. Louis Jolyon West. In her
autobiography, Patty Hearst[115] describes DeFreeze as being convinced that
Westbrook was an intelligence officer. She says (pp. 133):

But the worst arguments arose over Cin's [DeFreeze] issuing
"death warrants" for three people. One was Colston Westbrook,
the coordinator of the Black Cultural Association at the Vacaville
prison, who had worked with Cin and Cujo [SLA member
William Wolfe] and the others at the prison.... Cin pronounced
the death sentences upon all three because he insisted they were
informing to the FBI. He never explained how he could know
such a thing.

In a taped message, SLA Field Marshall Cinque declared that[115] (pp.134):

Colston Westbrook: male, black, age 35, brown eyes, brown
hair, 5'8", 210 pounds, Berkeley language instructor, resident
of Oakland, is a government agent....

Donald DeFreeze systematically transformed Patty Hearst into a
Manchurian Candidate bank robber. She took on a new identity and
received a new name, Tania. As Tania she was emotionally disconnected
from her past and her family, espoused revolutionary doctrine that was
completely alien to her, and participated in the robbery of the Hibernia
Bank in the Sunset District of San Francisco on April 15, 1974. A bank
surveillance camera recorded her while she identified herself as Tania and
held an M-1 rifle. The SLA got away with $16,000.00. There was gunfire
during the robbery.

The SLA hid out as fugitives from the time of the kidnapping of Patty
Hearst until five of them died in Los Angeles, burned to death during
a shootout with the FBI. Emily and Bill Harris and Patty Hearst were not with

the other SLA members at the time. They traveled around the country on the run for over a year until they were captured by the FBI in the fall of 1975.

Patty Hearst was charged with two crimes, the bank robbery and a holdup of a sporting goods store. She served two years in jail before her sentence was commuted by President Carter on February 1, 1979. One of the most active members of the Committee for the release of Patricia Hearst was Congressman Leo Ryan, who corresponded with the Deputy Director of the CIA about CIA mind control research at Vacaville.

The expert witnesses for Patty Hearst during her trial were Dr. Louis Jolyon West, Dr. Martin Orne, Dr. Margaret Singer, and Dr. Robert Lifton. Dr. West and Dr. Orne were MKULTRA contractors with TOP SECRET clearance. Dr. Singer was a co-author of Dr. West's[329] and Dr. Singer[289] and Dr. Lifton[162, 163, 164, 166] both interviewed American POWs returning from the Korean War. Dr. Lifton[166] wrote the classic text on mind control based on his experience with victims of Korean brainwashing, *Thought Reform and the Psychology of Totalism: A Study of "Brainwashing" in China*.

Dr. Lifton[163] contributed to a special issue of *The Journal of Social Issues* entitled, "Brainwashing." The Issue Editors were Raymond Bauer and Edgar Schein[279], who was a research psychologist at Walter Reed Army Institute of Research. Other contributors included Julius Segal[281] who was a research psychologist at the Air Force's Human Relations Research Laboratory.

Dr. Lifton[164] also participated in a Panel Meeting on "Communist Methods of Interrogation and Indoctrination" moderated by MKULTRA contractor Dr. Harold Wolff and Human Ecology Foundation Board Member, Lawrence Hinkle. Lifton[165] attended a meeting on November 11, 1956 on "Methods of Forceful Indoctrination" which was moderated by Dr. John Lilly, who later reported at a CIA-sponsored LSD symposium that he had given LSD to dolphins[169]. MKULTRA contractor, Dr. Louis Jolyon West, Edgar Schein, and Lawrence Hinkle attended this November 11, 1956 meeting. An earlier meeting on "Factors Used to Increase the Susceptibility of Individuals to Forceful Indoctrination" had been held on April 8, 1956, moderated by Dr. Lilly[167] and attended by Dr. Wolff[334]. Dr. Robert Lifton was firmly imbedded in the MKULTRA mind control network.

There was a connection between the Patty Hearst kidnapping, the Stanford Research Institute, Dr. West, MKULTRA and STARGATE. Remote viewers at Stanford Research Institute were asked by the Berkeley police to track Patty Hearst after her abduction by the Symbionese Liberation

Army[280]. Remote viewer Pat Price picked a photograph of one of the SLA abductors out of several volumes of photographs shown to him by Berkeley police, and identified the man as Lobo. This later proved to be SLA member William Wolfe, who was known as Willie the Wolf, or Cujo. Dr. West was a member of the medical oversight board for remote viewing research at Science Applications International Corp. into the 1990s, and therefore must have been aware of STARGATE. He must have known about the use of Stanford Research Institute remote viewers in the Patty Hearst case.

Dr. West testified that Patty Hearst had a new identity deliberately created by Donald DeFreeze. All four expert witnesses testified that Patty Hearst had been brainwashed using classical mind control techniques. She did not meet the full criteria for a Manchurian Candidate because she did not have amnesia. By the diagnostic rules of the American Psychiatric Association, she developed dissociative disorder not otherwise specified (DDNOS) rather than full dissociative identity disorder (DID). Since 1994, dissociative identity disorder has been the official name for multiple personality disorder in American Psychiatry[12].

DDNOS is a category that includes incomplete or partial forms of dissociative identity disorder. DDNOS cases either do not have amnesia, or the identity states are not fully formed and crystallized. A full Manchurian Candidate meets the American Psychiatric Association criteria for dissociative identity disorder. A Manchurian Candidate without amnesia would meet criteria for DDNOS.

Drs. West, Singer, and Orne are Board Members of the False Memory Syndrome Foundation, and Drs. West and Singer were Board Members of the Cult Awareness Network. Dr. Lifton is not connected to either of these organizations. However, all four individuals were experts in the set of mind control techniques used by BLUEBIRD, ARTICHOKE and MKULTRA contractors, Donald DeFreeze and the leaders of destructive cults. Drs. West and Orne are also experts on the dissociative disorders.

Meiers[190] describes numerous documented connections between the CIA, Jim Jones and his Peoples Temple, the SLA, the Patty Hearst kidnapping, the University of California at Berkeley, and Congressman Leo Ryan, who was killed at the Jonestown airport in South America on November 18, 1978. For instance, prior to a 12-man advance party arriving in Jonestown in Guyana in December, 1973, the site was the location for the SHALOM PROJECT, in which 200 CIA-supplied black ex-Green Beret Special Forces experts trained mercenaries for warfare in Angola.

According to one member of the People's Temple interviewed by the San Francisco Police Department's Intelligence and Antiterrorist Division in connection with the Patty Hearst kidnapping, SLA leaders Donald DeFreeze and Nancy Ling, and Patty Hearst's boyfriend, Steven Weed, were onsite together at the People's Temple headquarters in Ukiah, California prior to the kidnapping. Jim Jones was directly involved in the administration of a $2 million dollar food giveaway arranged by William Randoph Hearst in response to ransom demands by Donald DeFreeze.

These relationships between the SLA, Vacaville State Prison, Jim Jones, the Patty Hearst kidnapping, the CIA and Congressman Leo Ryan require further investigation and documentation. For the purposes of this book, Patty Hearst provides a well-documented example of the deliberate creation of a DDNOS-level Manchurian Candidate.

Chorover[59] describes another mind control program at Vacaville State Prison that was aborted because of public protest. A Maximum Psychiatric Diagnostic Unit was set up at Vacaville in February, 1972 to deal with selected inmates out of the 700 held in solitary confinement in California prisons. A program was approved for this Unit in which prisoners would have electrodes implanted in their brains to monitor them and control their behavior after discharge, using radio transmitters. Due to public protest, the California Department of Corrections called a press conference on December 30, 1971 to announce that the project had been "temporarily abandoned for administrative reasons," repeating the pattern of the Tuskeegee Syphilis Study and the Lafayette Clinic aggression project, both of which were run by physicians, and shut down due to negative public reaction.

The motives for transformation of Patty Hearst into a Manchurian Candidate bank robber are uncertain but her case is publicly documented and confirmed by four of the twentieth century's leading experts on mind control, Drs. West, Orne, Singer and Lifton. The methods used to turn Patty Hearst into a Manchurian Candidate are similar to those in the Palle Hardrup case. Palle Hardrup was controlled by a lone criminal, and Patty Hearst was brainwashed in a similar fashion, except that Donald DeFreeze had the support of six other members of the SLA.

20

CANDY JONES

The Control of Candy Jones[23] is about the creation of a Manchurian Candidate by U.S. mind control doctors, none of whom are identified by their real names in the book. The story has not been independently corroborated, and could be factual, based on sincerely believed false memories, or merely a publicity stunt by Candy Jones and her husband, Long John Nebel. However, hypnosis expert Dr. Herbert Spiegel[296], who examined Candy Jones in person, is quoted[23] (pp. 201) as saying, "I have no doubt that she's been brainwashed."

The only independent documentation relevant to the Candy Jones story I have obtained is the fact that the boxer, Gene Tunney, who was involved indirectly in the recruitment of Candy Jones, was the man who introduced William Stephenson, The Man Called Intrepid[302], to J. Edgar Hoover. William Stephenson was the boss of Ernest William Bavin, who corresponded with both G.H. Estabrooks and J. Edgar Hoover. Estabrooks and Hoover corresponded extensively with each other, and Estabrooks referred Dr. Hudson Hoaglund of the Worcester Foundation for Experimental Biology (MKULTRA Subproject 8) to Hoover.

Candy Jones was born Jessica Wilcox in Wilkes-Barre, Pennsylvania on December 31, 1925. Her mother separated from her father when Candy was three years old. She was brought up by her mother and grandmother. During a visit by her father when she was four, she was abused psychologically and physically. This involved threats and manipulation by her father, and his squeezing her fingers hard enough in a nutcracker to cause bruising. The father's rationale for the abuse was to demonstrate that he could make her cry. This was done in retaliation for her not crying about his imminent departure from the household as a visit was drawing to an end.

There is no evidence of childhood sexual abuse in the biography, but Jessica Wilcox was a lonely, isolated girl and was physically abused by her mother. Methods of physical abuse included beating with a leather riding crop. She was locked in a small bedroom on the third floor of the house, at night with all light bulbs removed from the room. On one occasion, her mother took her to an orphanage, and appeared to be dropping her off there, then suddenly she took her back home again without explanation. There was an inconsistent tug-of-war between mother and grandmother for Jessica's affection. Grandmother would often release Jessica from her sensory deprivation room prematurely.

Grandmother, always called "Ma-Ma" by Jessica, was a powerful figure. She had divorced her husband late in the nineteenth century, survived the Depression on her own, and completed training at an osteopathic college in Philadelphia. Jessica would watch Ma-Ma combing her hair for hours, then go to her own room and do the same, pretending to be her beloved grandmother. Ma-Ma died when Jessica was eleven, leaving her alone with her mother.

During the school term, Jessica had to come directly home from school, then do all her homework. She had to dress formally for dinner, which was served at 5:00, and was in bed every night at 6:00. At age eleven her bedtime was extended to 7:00. During the winter months of her childhood, her only outside playmate, whom she saw only occasionally, was the daughter of the family's laundress.

In order to cope with this combination of abuse and neglect, Jessica Wilcox developed imaginary friends in childhood, to keep her company in the lonely isolation of her home. These included Arlene, Dottee, Pansy, Willy, and possibly an identity named Doll. She would see them in Ma-Ma's mirror, and they would come to tea. Donald Bain, author of *The Control of Candy Jones*, believed that Dr. Jensen, Candy's mind control doctor, amplified Arlene from an imaginary playmate into an alternate identity who did courier work for the CIA. According to the description in the biography, though, Arlene was already a fully formed alter personality before Candy met Dr. Jensen. She took executive control of the body on many occasions during childhood, and had distinct attributes separate from Jessica (pp. 101):

> *Once Jensen had become aware of Candy's imaginary childhood*
> *friends, he set out to bring back into her adult life some of those*
> *fanciful characters, particularly Arlene. She had been according*

to Candy, the dominant personality in the "club." Arlene could run faster, climb higher and swim better than any other club members, including Candy, and took over whenever Candy was engaged in difficult physical activities. Both Candy and Arlene, in various hypnotic sessions with Nebel, freely discussed Arlene's superiority in these areas. From Jensen's point of view, Arlene could be the most useful as a "second personality," if, from his retrospective position, he can be given the benefit of the doubt and assumed to have been in search of another person within Candy Jones with whom to accomplish something tangible. That tangible goal would be to create what G.H. Estabrooks termed "the perfect spy."

The biography describes clear switching of alter personalities observed by Candy's husband, Long John Nebel prior to the discovery of Arlene Grant. Nebel didn't understand what was going on, and thought Candy was incomprehensibly moody. Arlene describes watching the verbal abuse of Jessica by her mother during childhood, and verbal abuse by Candy's first husband. Jessica Wilcox had complex, fully formed multiple personality disorder as a child, not simple imaginary companions, according to the description in the biography.

In late 1936, Jessica's mother moved to Atlantic City, at which time Jessica was five feet tall. By the time she finished high school, she had grown eight inches, and was strikingly beautiful. At the end of high school, Jessica wanted to be a doctor. She wrote to her father asking for money to help with her education. He sent $200.00, but her mother used it to pay bills. Her mother wanted her to enter secretarial school, but Jessica had different plans, which lead to her winning the Miss Atlantic City contest in 1941, at age sixteen. Her mother's reaction to her triumph was critical and condescending.

One of the judges of the Miss Atlantic City contest was John Robert Powers, a famous modeling agent. Jessica went to New York at Powers' invitation, but never signed with his agency. While there, she went to the offices of Powers' biggest rival, Harry Conover, at 52 Vanderbilt Avenue. After a brief wait, Jessica was introduced to Conover, who immediately gave her the name Candy Johnson. He hired her at a pay rate of $5.00 an hour. The name was soon changed to Candy Jones.

A major campaign to market Candy Jones was launched, starting with a printing of 10,000 engraved, red-and-white striped business card bearing the statement, *Candy Jones Was Here*. She appeared regularly on magazine covers, including eleven covers in one month in 1943. One of these was photographed by Jack Nebel, who later renamed himself Long John Nebel.

Candy was voted Model of the Year in 1943 by a panel of judges that included Loretta Young. Partly to escape from her mother, in 1944 Candy left for the Southwest Pacific to do a USO tour as a troop entertainer. She had just completed an eight-month show on Broadway, and launched her musical tour at a military base in the United States before leaving for the Pacific. Her experiences on that tour are described in one of eleven books she wrote, *More Than Beauty*. Candy Jones and Betty Grable were the leading U.S. troop entertainers in World War II.

In April, 1945 while in Moratai, Candy contracted malaria and brucellosis, the latter from unpasteurized milk flown in from Australia. She was transferred to a hospital in the Philippines, where she developed a fungal infection that made much of her hair fall out. This was treated by a nurse shaving her head. While in the hospital in the Philippines, Candy became friends with a number of different medics, one of whom was Gilbert Jensen. She remained in the Pacific until August, 1945 but it was not until 1946 that her hair and complexion had recovered enough to start modeling again. She took a role in a Broadway musical about Chopin entitled *Polonaise* in the interim, but had to wear a wig and heavy theatrical makeup to cover up the lingering effects of her tropical infections.

On July 4, 1946, Candy Jones and Harry Conover were married in a ceremony attended by 2000 guests. It was an unhappy union that yielded three sons. After these pregnancies, Candy had two abortions at Harry's insistence. It was not until twelve years into the marriage that Candy realized Harry was bisexual. The marriage ended in divorce in 1959. On May 18, 1958, Harry disappeared with $125,000.00 in Candy's modeling fees, none of which Candy ever saw again. He eventually spent two years in prison for theft and non-payment of alimony. These events were headline news in New York. After Harry Conover left with her money, Candy Jones had $36.00 in her business account and three sons to support and educate.

Candy continued to run the modeling school out of 52 Vanderbilt, spending most of her time in room 808, across the hall from offices rented by the former heavy-weight boxing champion, Gene Tunney. During this period Long John Nebel, born Jack Zimmerman on June 11, 1911, became the most successful talk show host in New York radio. In 1960 he divorced his first wife, Lillian. After a 28-day courtship, Long John Nebel and Candy Jones were married on December 31, 1972.

Not realizing what was going on, Long John Nebel observed a switch from Candy to Arlene and back to Candy again at the wedding. He observed another switch on his wedding night, which Arlene later confirmed. He said it was as if another woman had walked out of the bathroom, Candy having just gone in. This other woman had a different voice, manner, and look, and Candy appeared to be amnesic for her when she regained control of the body. Candy carried on as if nothing had happened. Another switch to Arlene occurred on January 1, 1973. As Arlene, Candy suddenly became inexplicably angry. She reverted to her usual warm, pleasant manner when Candy came back. This switching back and forth caused much marital conflict. Candy could not remember or account for her changed behavior, and Long John could not understand the inconsistency.

On June 3, 1973 John Nebel suggested to Candy that he should try to treat her chronic insomnia with hypnosis. He was not qualified as a hypnotist or psychotherapist. His efforts were successful, though,with a large reduction in Candy's sleeplessness. During one of the hypnosis sessions, Candy spontaneously regressed to childhood, a common occurrence during hypnosis, and relived events from childhood. During subsequent sessions, under hypnosis, Candy spoke from a persona identified as Doll, while age regressed back to age eleven. Such age regression can occur in good hypnotic subjects who do not have a dissociative disorder, and is not by itself evidence of multiple personality disorder.

During the hypnotic work, Nebel was gradually introduced to the various club members, whom he thought were imaginary friends reactivated in the trance state. When Candy described visiting Dr. Jensen in California as part of her CIA work, Nebel took little interest in this at first. He was not looking for or expecting anything like the mind control story that would unfold. One day in June, Arlene spontaneously took executive control during hypnosis, and spoke to Nebel for a lengthy period of time. Once Nebel had met Arlene, and knew her by name, the story of her mind control came to the surface.

Long John Nebel sought consultation with Dr. Herbert Spiegel, who confirmed that Candy was highly hypnotizable. Dr. Spiegel[295] does not state in his Foreword to *The Control of Candy Jones* that he believes in the reality of the mind control, nor does he state that he disbelieves it. That is the correct position to take on the matter, because the reality of the story can be confirmed only by independent documentation and evidence, and disproving it was beyond the resources or role of Dr. Spiegel.

The mind control part of the tale begins across the hall from 808 - 52 Vanderbilt Avenue, in the office rented by Gene Tunney One night when Candy was working late, at about 7:30 P.M., she observed a middle-aged woman trying a series of keys on Tunney's door. This was unusual because the cleaning woman used a single master key. The woman entered the suite, did not turn on the light, and shone a flashlight around the office. Candy was wondering whether to intervene when she was interrupted by a modeling student. When her attention returned to Tunney's office, the woman was just leaving. The next day, Candy learned that the office had been burglarized, but Gene Tunney told her that nothing important had been stolen.

Two nights later, a young couple began trying different keys in Tunney's door, and this time Candy approached them, spoke with them briefly, and they left. When she mentioned this incident to Tunney the next day, his reply was, "Oh, really?"

A week later, Candy met a retired Army general with whom she was acquainted in front of her office building. As they rode up the elevator together, the general mentioned that he was visiting Gene Tunney. Candy, the general, and Tunney talked briefly before she went on with her afternoon's business.

A few days after this, an FBI agent appeared at Candy Jones' office, presented identification, and asked her about the burglary across the hall. He asked her about a microphone she had purchased from Allen Funt, who was doing a radio version of what would become Candid Camera on television, and then asked to borrow it for a long-term surveillance assignment on West 157th Street. The reason he offered for wanting her microphone was its high quality. Candy agreed.

A month later, the agent returned with a second agent and the microphone. The two proposed to Candy that she allow mail for them to be delivered at her office. Again she agreed. The arrangement was that mail addressed to fictitious names at Candy's agency would be received and held for pickup by the agent. As well, there might be mail from Europe addressed to Candy or a specific man's name. In response, she was supposed to phone a number and report its arrival.

Two weeks later, Gene Tunney moved out of the suite across the hall. The Army general maintained contact with Candy throughout the year she used her office as a mail drop for whatever agency was employing her. Late in the summer of 1960, Candy received a latter from the FBI saying that she should expect a call within a few days. This turned out to be from the Army general. He asked her to deliver a letter to a man who would be her contact at the St. Francis Hotel in San Francisco during a trip she had scheduled there. The contact was Gilbert Jensen, whose name she didn't recognize when the general gave it to her.

On November 16, 1960, Candy Jones and Gilbert Jensen had dinner at the Mark Hopkins Hotel. Her first visit to Dr. Jensen's office in Oakland was in November, 1960, and the next two were in late 1960 and early 1961.

Dr. Jensen asked in detail about Candy's group of childhood imaginary friends, and asked her to choose one as a fictitious name for her CIA passport. He recruited her for the CIA as a courier prior to starting mind control. He had her choose a last name for her fake passport, which she did using Ma-Ma's married name, Rosengrant. This is how Arlene Grant acquired her last name. Dr. Jensen explained that she would do courier assignments in the United States, in conjunction with her business trips. She would switch to Arlene Grant for occasional overseas trips that were not linked to her personal or business travel.

Jensen also asked Candy about Arlene's appearance in the mirror, when she had seen Arlene there during childhood. He then provided Candy with a brunette Arlene Grant wig to match the description. He had a photographer come to her hotel room to take the Arlene Grant passport photograph. Candy kept a copy of this photo, which appears in the biography. In the biography, there is a signed statement from lawyer William J. Williams, dated February 27, 1976, confirming that early in the 1960's, Candy had given him an envelope to open in the event of her dying or disappearing under unusual circumstances, particularly if she died under a different name. She specified the name Arlene Grant in the letter.

Candy disclosed to her editor at Harper and Row, Joe Vergara, that she was involved in national and international courier assignments for a secret government agency. Vergara confirmed this to Donald Bain at a lunch at Anatolli's restaurant on December 12, 1974. She told her friend, columnist Mel Heimer, some vague details about her activities, but he had died before Donald Bain began writing *The Control of Candy Jones*. According to Candy, Jensen used to interrogate her about what she had told Heimer, read his books, and made a point of watching him during media appearances.

Candy Jones maintained a box number 1294 at Grand Central Station from August, 1961 to 1968 or 1969, which she used for CIA mail and to receive messages from Jensen. According to the memories uncovered during hypnosis, Jensen met Arlene by chance. She spontaneously took control of the body at his office and identified herself by name. By her account, she already had fully formed multiple personality before Jensen started his mind control.

Dr. Jensen capitalized on his discovery immediately. He had Arlene describe herself, and instructed her that he could call her out in the future by calling, "A.G.!, A.G.!" He also told Arlene that she would always come up through Candy's stomach, a suggestion that apparently caused the nausea she experienced on switching. Dr. Jensen conditioned Arlene and Candy through repeated use of hypnosis, sodium amytal, possibly Thorazine, and sexual abuse. She remembered him inserting a lighted candle in her vagina as a demonstration of Arlene's ability to control pain. This occurred during a demonstration conducted at Camp Peary, Virginia, the CIA training facility where Yuriy Nosenko was held in solitary confinement (see Chapter 4). Dr. Jensen also inserted a post-hypnotic suggestion that Candy would get sick and might even have a convulsion if she ever consulted a psychiatrist. He administered mind control drugs used by OSS, CIA and U.S. Army doctors in mind control experiments, and by the ARTICHOKE team, giving them to her either in orange juice or intravenously.

Dr. Jensen reported to the senior CIA mind control doctor, who is identified in the biography as Dr. Marshall Burger, a pseudonym. Dr. Burger had hypnotized Candy during a phone conversation in 1946, when he had been consulted because of an attack of severe chills. This was odd, because Dr. Burger was either a psychiatrist or a psychologist. Candy was staying in a hotel in Chicago in order to appear on a radio talk show, Don McNeill's Breakfast Club, the next day. A staff assistant from the show advised her that a doctor would be calling to talk to her, which turned out to be Dr. Burger. He became actively involved in her mind control in the 1960's, and may have implanted preliminary post-hypnotic suggestions in 1946.

Both Dr. Jensen and Dr. Burger worked intensively with Candy Jones implanting suggestions designed to convert her into a racist, and to make her avoid close personal involvement. They suggested to her that certain people, including blacks, Jews, and Italians, smell bad. The purpose of this programming seemed to be to socially isolate her. Candy was deliberately instructed while under the influence of hypnosis and drugs not to make friends and not to get married.

Candy described being transported to a rural laboratory-like facility in Texas just inside the Louisiana border. There she attended lectures given by Dr. Burger along with eight or nine other mind control subjects. Dr. Burger was introduced by Dr. Jensen at these lectures, which focused on anti-black racism and world power. Candy remembered being trained in combat, espionage, and surveillance techniques at Camp Peary in 1971. She also remembered being trained at a CIA facility in Florida that had been involved in preparation for the Bay of Pigs invasion. She claimed to have become involved in a mission into Son Toy prison camp in North Vietnam, which she was to have participated in under cover of a USO entertainment tour. This mission was scrubbed at the last minute.

Another memory involved a scene straight out of *The Manchurian Candidate*, and took place at CIA headquarters in Langley, Virginia. Dr. Jensen prepared her for a demonstration in front of twenty-four doctors by giving her an intravenous drug, which he did frequently. The drugs were usually called "vitamins." She was the first of eight mind control subjects to be demonstrated that day, and considered going first to be particularly stressful. The demonstration took place in an amphitheater. It was there that Dr. Jensen allegedly inserted a lighted candle in her vagina. Several of the doctors tried unsuccessfully to break Dr. Jensen's mind control, before the demonstration came to an end. Although the date is uncertain, the demonstration seems to have taken place in 1971, prior to termination of MKSEARCH in 1972.

Part of Candy Jones' motivation for participating in the mind control and courier assignments included direct payments by the CIA for her sons' schooling and to cover large hospital bills. She couldn't have afforded these herself in the years after the divorce. Her first foreign trip for the CIA was in 1965, and in 1966 she went to Taiwan. The Taiwan trip appears to have been a variant of the courier trip to Tokyo described by G.H. Estabrooks (see Chapter 15).

Candy was switched to Arlene Grant in Dr. Jensen's office using intravenous drugs. He told her that her destination was Taiwan, and that she would be met there by a man who would recognize her. The man was a prominent Chinese businessman. On the first trip she was treated well, being met at the airport, where she handed over her courier envelope. She was then escorted to a large mansion on big grounds about twenty miles outside of Taipei. At the house, Candy observed two young Chinese women in white lab coats, but they were said by the businessman to be domestic workers. She slept late, ate well, and returned to San Francisco well rested after a three-day stay.

The second trip to Taiwan began like the first one, with Arlene being called out at Dr. Jensen's office following administration of vitamins. There is confusion, according to Donald Bain, about whether the torture Candy Jones experienced occurred in two further missions, or only the second, with the third being relatively benign.

On the second trip, the Chinese businessman and his associates used a variety of physical torture techniques to attempt to extract information from Arlene. She had no information to give them beyond that in the envelopes she had turned over. She was given electric shocks to her wrists, shoulders and fingers, and was threatened with shocks to her breasts. Much of this occurred with Candy strapped in a chair. Following the torture, the torturers became very friendly and explained that the purpose of the shocks was to help jog her memory in a scientific way. On her return to San Francisco, Dr. Jensen gave her another injection and explained that the torture was a mistake. He said it was due to a typographical error.

On the third trip to Taiwan, Candy delivered an envelope to a woman in an art gallery, who spat in her face after she accepted it. She was then met by the Chinese businessman, and again taken to the mansion in the countryside. Donald Bain (pp. 208) quotes Candy Jones' own words from an audio tape transcript to describe another incident in Taiwan:

> *I was in this place that wasn't too far from the second airport. It was on Taiwan, but to the south. I can't think of the name of the airport, but it's where you go out of Taiwan, not come into it. It was a house about a ten or fifteen minute drive from the airport.*

> *I was coming back (to the United States) and you don't always leave from the same airport. The weather was bad and the flight was not going to be taking off. A man told me to come back to the house with him and wait for the flight. I can't think of his name. He was American, and he was going to be on the same flight... I met him at the airport. He came over to me. He told me that I looked very familiar and asked whether he had seen me there before.*

I was Arlene Grant when he came up to me. The flight was going to be delayed two hours, and he told me the house he was going to was actually part of an American installation, like an officer's club or something like that. I stupidly said, "Okay, okay."

So we went outside and he got us a rickety-tin old cab. We chatted in the cab and he told me he was in Taiwan surveying American business interests there, and had done a report on American holdings. He was wearing civilian clothes, and was very pleasant.

The house was very nice and looked like a club. Lots of entertainment went on in houses on Taiwan that were turned into nightclubs. I don't like the look of those big Chinese houses, but some people do. It was a tacky place. We walked in and the same goddam oriental music was playing (Candy was triggered by this music, apparently an aspect of her mind control). There were little tables in the lobby,; it was like an inn. There were a few people around. He asked me what I wanted to drink, and they served anything you wanted. They even had American drinks. We were sitting talking and he asked me whether I would like to see the rest of the place. I agreed. He told me there was a beautiful view that he enjoyed every time he stopped there. There was a very large and beautiful staircase leading upstairs.

We went in one large room that could have been a dining room or a conference room. He asked me whether I knew a certain man, who had his offices in that house. I don't know what his name was. He told me this man was an old friend of his and suggested we step in and say hello.

I followed him into a room. The man behind the desk was middle-aged -- forty-eight or forty-nine. He introduced me to the man. The man looked Chinese to me. He was sitting and reading a magazine.

The man with me told his friend that he had adopted me like an orphan and taken me out of the storm. The man behind the desk spoke English quite well. He invited me to sit down, and told me he had heard about me. I had been introduced to him as Arlene Grant. He asked me where I had been, and obviously I couldn't tell him the truth. He offered me tea, but I declined. He insisted, however, that I have a drink. I pointed out that I had own downstairs at the table. He suggested I have a fresh one and asked me what I was drinking. I told him vodka on the rocks. He served a fresh drink. He talked a great deal about San Francisco and how wonderful it was that the American woman was free to travel and do things.

I don't know what was in that drink but I suddenly became very dizzy. He asked me what was wrong, and I told him that I was dizzy and hot. He asked me if I wanted to relax, but I told him I had to leave because I had to catch a plane. I thought I was going to be sick, and I told him that. He called in a woman who took me to the ladies room. It looked more like an infirmary to me than a ladies room. There were two beds in the room. There was a bathroom, but the beds were in a little room separated from the toilet by a curtain. I was drenched with sweat, and very weak. The woman, who was Chinese and spoke very little English, told me that she would take care of my clothes. The sweat was pouring from me, and I could feel my heart beating a mile a minute. I was wearing a suit, and she asked me to give her my jacket. Even the shoulders of my jacket were wringing with sweat. I took off my skirt, jacket and blouse and handed them to the woman. She said she would bring me a gown, and suggested I lie down on the bed. I did and waited for her, but she didn't come back. She had also taken my shoes. My foot began to ache in the spot where I had broken it a few years before. I was wearing an Ace bandage on it as I often did when I traveled.

A man came into the room. He introduced himself as a doctor. Right behind him was the man who had given me the drink in his coffee. The doctor told me I looked terrible. I must have because my hair was soaking wet. I said I thought something had been put into my drink, and the man became very offended. The man introduced to me as a doctor took my pulse. He seemed very professional, and he looked into my eyes. He told the other man that I was going to sleep and that I needed rest. The doctor had a much heavier Chinese accent than the other man.

I asked them what had happened to me. The doctor said he didn't know but asked if I had ever had malaria. I agreed that I had, but said that this was not malaria and I knew that it wasn't. He assured me that I would shake and get chills, just like malaria. I asked him for my pocketbook, and told them that I had to get the plane back to the United States. They brought my pocketbook to me, and when I looked into it I knew someone had gone through it. I began to become very frightened.

The doctor asked if I felt sick to my stomach. I said that I did, and he began to pull the covers off me to examine my stomach. I told him not to. My sheets and pillowcase were soaking wet, and the doctor suggested I get into another bed so that they could change this one. I refused to move. A woman entered the room and grabbed my arms and literally dragged me out of one bed and into the other. I was embarrassed at only having my bra and pants under the gown. Someone asked me what was wrong with my foot, and I told them that I had tripped.

The man who had given me the drink asked me who I had seen while I was in Taiwan. I could barely answer because I was so sleepy. Suddenly, the doctor gave me a shot in the arm. He tried to roll me over on the bed, and although I tried to fight him, I was too weak to resist. He told the woman to pull me over, which she did. I suddenly was afraid I was going to be murdered right there. They had me on my stomach and examined my buttocks, and the doctor commented that I hadn't received any injections there.

My voice was growing very weak. The man told the doctor to let me sleep it off, and said he didn't think I knew anything. He then asked me where the papers were. I told him that I didn't have any papers. He asked me who I had given the papers to. I didn't answer, and the men left the room. The woman asked me if I wanted to sit up, but I was so weak I couldn't manage it, and my muscles felt like jelly. The woman tried to pull me up by my arms, and although I wanted to hit the woman, I couldn't muster the strength.

The woman pinched me, and asked me where the papers were. She kept pinching me all over my body. She eventually began to pinch my breasts, and I fell back on the bed from the pain. She kept pulling me up, and every time she did, she continued to pinch me viciously. I felt myself passing out, and I believe I actually did black out. The woman left the room and I tried to get up, but I simply fell on the floor. I tried to reach up to pull the sheet down over me but I couldn't raise my arm. The last thing I remember was trying to crawl underneath the bed.

I must have been out for a long time, and when I woke up I was again in the bed. The doctor came in and gave me a shot in my other arm. I stopped perspiring, and I feel into a deep, deep sleep, waking up the next day. My clothes were in the room and had all been cleaned. I never saw that woman again. A younger girl came into the room, asked me how I felt and gave me some orange juice. I was afraid to drink anything, but asked the girl for some water. When she brought the water, I made her drink some first before I would take it. She also brought me coffee, which I had her taste first. The girl told me I better hurry if I was going to make my flight home. She could barely speak English. The girl said I'd had a bad dream and had been very sick. I pulled up the sleeve on my gown and looked at my arms. There was injection mark on each one.

The girl left the room, and when I tried to get up, I had to grab a chair to support myself on my wobbly legs. I used the chair like a crutch to move across the room. I locked the door, got dressed, rinsed out my mouth in the bathroom, washed my face and looked in the mirror. I don't think I'd ever seen myself look quite so terrible. I realized that I was not wearing the black wig any longer, and discovered it lying on the other bed.

After I was cleaned up and dressed, I unlocked the door and went to the staircase. I looked down and saw there were people having drinks at small tables. They didn't pay any attention to me as I started to come down, but then I tripped and tumbled down the entire staircase. People ran over and picked me up and put me in a chair. I told them I was all right and had just had a fainting spell.

Someone drove me to the airport and I flew home. I immediately went to see Gilbert Jensen and told him about the incident. He seemed very concerned and wanted to see my arms. My breasts were all black and blue from being pinched, but I refused to show them to him.

This account by Candy Jones is the only published description of an ARTICHOKE interrogation. Whether it was conducted by the CIA or a foreign intelligence service, is unknown. Whether it is fact or fiction is unknown. It is possible that there was another personality behind Arlene Grant who was carrying classified information, and it could be that the purpose of the interrogation was to contact that level of her personality system. Whatever the historical facts, the account provides the subjective flavor of such interrogations.

The last intelligence contact reported in *The Control of Candy Jones* occurred on July 3, 1973. Candy and Long John Nebel received a message from Japan Airlines that a ticket was being held for her on Japan Airlines flight 5, for the sixth of July, leaving Kennedy Airport for Tokyo, with an open ticket on to Taipei. She never made the trip. The message said that the booking had been made by "Cynthia." *Cynthia* was the code name of an actual female OSS operative, whose real name was Amy Elizabeth Thorpe[139], but Thorpe died on December 1, 1963, so could not have been involved in the Japan Airlines booking. The Cynthia who made that booking in 1973 could have been an individual or an operation using the code name Cynthia.

During their hypnotic work, Candy Jones and Long John Nebel uncovered suicide programming implanted by Dr. Jensen. Candy was to have gone to the Paradise Beach Hotel in the Bahamas and jumped off a cliff there. The trip was canceled because of their wedding on December 31, 1972.

The book closes with the impression that Arlene Grant was still involved in intelligence activities on a limited scale at the time of writing, in 1976. If Candy Jones actually was a CIA Manchurian Candidate courier, documentation of that fact must be on file somewhere in intelligence archives. The mind control techniques she describes are similar to those used by the ARTICHOKE team, Bjorn Neilsen, leaders of destructive cults, and interrogators around the world.

21

SIRHAN SIRHAN

Sirhan Sirhan, a Palestinian Arab refugee, shot Robert Kennedy in the pantry of the Ambassador Hotel in Los Angeles at 12:15 A.M. on June 5, 1968. Kennedy was at the hotel as part of his campaign for the Democratic Presidential nomination. He had just won the California primary that evening. The shooting was observed by many witnesses, and Sirhan was wrestled to the ground and disarmed immediately. He was found guilty of first-degree murder at trial.

The opinion of expert witness Dr. Bernard L. Diamond is that Sirhan acted alone while in a self-induced trance state. In an interview with Dr. Diamond, the following exchange occurred[114]:

> *Harris:*   *Is there a clear division in him between two states of consciousness, a controlled cool state and a dissociated state of violence, fear and rage?*
>
> *Diamond:*   *Yes, in the hypnotic state he can relive childhood horrors; he can remember writing in the notebook and he can reproduce the automatic writing; he remembers the killing and also remembers his experiences under hypnosis. He can remember none of these things when he is not in hypnosis.*
>
> *His mind is truly split, with part of his life on one side and part on the other.*

For this book, the assumption is that Sirhan Sirhan was a self-created Manchurian Candidate at the dissociative disorder not otherwise specified (DDNOS) level. The dissociated assassin state did not have a fully formed separate identity, and therefore the clinical diagnosis would be DDNOS instead of multiple personality disorder. Sirhan Sirhan corresponds to the auto-hypnotic sub-pathway of the factitious pathway to dissociative identity disorder I describe in the second edition of my textbook[258]. He was a self-created assassin, but not consciously so.

For this book, I will ignore conspiracy evidence concerning the girl in the polka dot dress, the number of entry holes in Robert Kennedy and the surrounding walls and door jambs, possible contact between Sirhan Sirhan and William Jennings Bryan, technical consultant on the movie *The Manchurian Candidate*, and other reasons to suspect that Sirhan Sirhan may have been controlled by someone[303]. Roger LaJeunesse, the FBI agent in charge of the Sirhan investigation, is quoted[143] as saying, "The case is still open. I'm not rejecting the Manchurian Candidate aspect of it."

When he was a child in Jerusalem, Sirhan Sirhan was traumatized by the war and especially by several bombings. On one occasion a soldier was blasted to pieces near the Sirhan home. Young Sirhan Sirhan saw the soldier's foot hanging from a church steeple. His mother described him as going pale, being unable to move for a while, and fainting in response.

On another occasion a bomb went off across the street from the Sirhan home (it might have been a mortar shell). Bystanders thought Sirhan had been hit. When his mother brought him into their home, Sirhan was, in his mother's words, in a trance state: "When we got in, he was just - gone - blacked out." He was very pale, his fists were clenched, and he had not fainted.

Another time when he was seven, Sirhan saw a nine-year old girl who was bleeding profusely from the knee from shrapnel. He fainted. These "faints" were actually dissociative episodes because his body would not go limp. During some of the spells his eyes would be open. Some days he would "faint" twice, especially if he ever saw any blood on the street after a bombing.

Mrs. Sirhan said of her son, "One night, living in Old Jerusalem, I felt him and he was cold like stick. More than any of his brothers, he had less blood and more fear."

In the spring of 1948, when Sirhan was four, a group of Zionist commandos attacked a British radio station located above the Sirhan home. They dynamited the upper floor and converted the family bathroom into a machine-gun nest, while the family retreated to the basement. Another time, Sirhan was found screaming because a bucket of water he was carrying had a hand floating in it. Besides describing the trauma of being in a refugee camp, Sirhan's mother also recounted serious beatings of him by his father.

Six months after the family emigrated to America, Sirhan's father, Bishara Sirhan, returned to Jerusalem alone, taking with him the money that had been earned by Sirhan's mother and brothers since they arrived on January 12, 1957. The physical abuse of Sirhan by his father was corroborated by an independent witness, Ziad Hasheimeh, who knew the family.

Mrs. Sirhan is quoted as saying[143] (pp. 204):

> *In the street the boys shout and kick away a stuffed soccer ball. The ball squirts away from the pack. They chase it and leave Sirhan standing in a kind of trance. Later they return and Sirhan is still standing and staring. They take him home where he remains for several days.*

Sirhan Sirhan experienced severe war trauma, physical abuse, abandonment by his father, and the stress of refugee camp and moving to America as a child. His mother describes frequent dissociative states occurring prior to age ten. He was highly hypnotizable when examined by Dr. Diamond.

Sirhan Sirhan initially admired Robert Kennedy and saw him as a defender of the politically oppressed and poor, with whom he undoubtedly identified. This changed when Kennedy became identified with the Israeli enemy who bombed and killed the Arabs. Kennedy stated his intent to send fifty jet bombers to Israel in late May, 1968. Although Sirhan may not have known about the fifty bombers until after the assassination, Kennedy became aligned with the Jewish enemy in his mind, and probably with the father who abandoned and betrayed him, and returned to Jerusalem. Robert Kennedy died on the anniversary of Israel's victory in the Six-Day War, which ended with an Israeli attack on Egyptian airstrips on June 5, 1967.

Sirhan learned self-hypnosis from mail order materials he obtained from the Rosicrucians. He attended a meeting of the Akhvaton Chapter of the Ancient Mystical Order of Rosae Crucis in Pasadena on May 28, 1968 and signed their guest book. He had been studying their materials for some time before that. From these materials Sirhan learned techniques for self-hypnosis and automatic writing that he practiced for hours.

Sirhan's notebooks were introduced as evidence at trial. They contained many pages of trance writing that are obviously disturbed. Single pages include many different hand writing styles and repetitions of dissociated fragments of language. In the notebooks he writes repeatedly about shooting Robert Kennedy. One page includes numerous repetitions of,

"R.F.K. must die," "Robert F. Kennedy must be assassinated," and "Robert F. Kennedy must be assassinated before 5 June 68." These are followed by references to, "please pay to the order of" and cash payments to Sirhan.

The assassination was definitely premeditated, but only within a dissociated state. My expert opinion, if I were testifying in such a case, would be that the self-induced dissociative state is irrelevant. It is not grounds for diminished criminal capacity. Just as clinical patients with dissociative identity disorder (multiple personality disorder) are held responsible for the actions of all their alter personalities, being a self-created Manchurian Candidate should not diminish one's criminal responsibility. This is so despite the real amnesia in such cases.

Dr. Diamond demonstrated Sirhan's high hypnotizability many times in audio taped sessions with a variety of witnesses. On one occasion, he introduced a post-hypnotic suggestion that on his signal Sirhan would start climbing on his cell bars like a monkey. Sirhan did that in response to the post-hypnotic signal, then explained his behavior with the rationalization that he was getting some exercise. When confronted with an audiotape of Dr. Diamond's implantation of the post-hypnotic instruction, for which Sirhan was amnesic, Sirhan stated that Dr. Diamond was trying to trick him. He insisted that he had decided on his own to climb the bars for exercise.

This kind of rationalization for obedience to post-hypnotic suggestion is typical of the highly hypnotizable individual. Kaiser[143] presents evidence that the political motivation Sirhan claimed for the assassination was a post-hypnotic rationalization, one that occurred after the shooting.

The major trance technique Sirhan used was staring at candles and mirrors for long periods of time. This is an important detail because there were lights and mirrors in the area of the Ambassador Hotel where Sirhan stood immediately before shooting Robert Kennedy. In combination with four Tom Collins drinks, the lights and mirrors probably helped trigger Sirhan into his dissociated assassin state.

At about 10:30 P.M. on June 4, 1968, Mrs. Mary Grohs, a teletype operator for Western Union was working in the Colonial Room of the Ambassador Hotel when she saw Sirhan "stare fixedly" at her teletype machine. Kaiser[143] (pp. 531) quotes her as saying:

Well, he came over to my machine and started staring at it. Just staring. I'll never forget his eyes. I asked him what he wanted.

*He didn't answer. He just kept staring. I asked him again.
No answer. I said that if he wanted the latest figures on Senator
Kennedy he'd have to check the other machines. He still didn't
answer. He just kept staring.*

Mrs. Grohs did not testify at trial and told Kaiser that the police had
instructed her not to say anything about the incident. This would be
expected of investigators and prosecutors who feared that such information
would support an insanity defense. It is only necessary to reject, suppress
or discredit such information if one assumes that amnesia is grounds for
diminished criminal responsibility or an insanity defense.

Dr. Martin Schorr, an expert witness for the prosecution, stated at trial
that Sirhan had two distinct personalities, which dissociated under stress.
He compared Sirhan to "Jekyll-Hyde" and Eve White-Eve Black of *The
Three Faces of Eve*[300]. Dr. Schorr said that Sirhan was "unaware of the
killer in himself, but is aware of his own ambivalence."

Dr. Simson-Kallas, who examined Sirhan at San Quentin prison after
his conviction, concluded that Sirhan had multiple personality and had
been programmed by someone else, but his grounds for this conclusion
are unclear. Although he never interviewed Sirhan directly, Dr. Herbert
Spiegel, who interviewed Candy Jones, reviewed extensive case material
provided to him by assassination researchers William Turner and John
Christian[303]. Dr. Spiegel concluded that Sirhan was highly hypnotizable
and not suffering from schizophrenia. On this point, he agreed with Dr.
Simson-Kallas.

Many of the expert witnesses in the Sirhan case, including Dr. Diamond
and the prosecution psychiatrists, concluded that Sirhan's thought
processes were always organized and coherent outside the dissociated
trance state. In the 1960's, the term *schizophrenia* was overused and
used loosely by American psychiatrists. There is no reason to think that
Sirhan Sirhan would receive a diagnosis of schizophrenia if interviewed
with the more scientific and reliable diagnostic procedures of the early
twenty-first century.

The prosecution expert witnesses included Dr. Seymour Pollack. He did
his psychiatry training at the New York Psychiatric Institute, where Harold
Blauer was killed with an injection of U.S. Army mescaline in 1953. Dr.
Pollack recommended at trial that Sirhan be sent to the medical facility
at Vacaville State Prison, where drug research was conducted under

MKSEARCH Subproject 3, and where Donald DeFreeze was contacted by Colston Westbrook. MKSEARCH ran from 1964 to 1972, the time period of the Sirhan trial and DeFreeze's imprisonment at Vacaville.

Sirhan Sirhan was a self-created Manchurian Candidate. He carried out an actual assassination. He illustrates the point that the term *Manchurian Candidate* could be expanded to include self-created variants. The self-created assassins help us to understand the mind of the Manchurian Candidate; one might think of them as naturally-occurring analogs.

22
MARK DAVID CHAPMAN

Mark David Chapman, the man who shot John Lennon, was born at Harris Hospital in Fort Worth, Texas on May 10, 1955. His father, David Curtis Chapman, was a staff sergeant in the Air Force. His mother, Diane, was a homemaker. Shortly after Mark's birth, his father left the Air Force and moved the family to Indiana. There he worked for American Oil Company and took a degree in engineering at Purdue. From Indiana, the family moved to Decatur, Georgia where Mark's father worked in the credit department at American Oil. After two years, the family was transferred to Roanoke, Virginia where Mark's sister, Susan Jill, was born. She is seven years younger than Mark.

Like Sirhan Sirhan, for the purposes of this book Mark David Chapman is assumed to be a self-created Manchurian Candidate level assassin.

From Virginia, the Chapman family moved back to Georgia. It was there that Mark first became aware of the Little People inside his mind. Chapman's biographer, Jack Jones[142] (p. 115) quotes Mark describing his father as living "by very rigid patterns, doing the same things day after day. He was very meticulous, very unemotional.... I don't recall that my father ever hugged me or told me he loved me.... He was just a shell who swallowed everything. And then, when it finally came out, God help you."

According to Mark, his father beat his mother regularly. Mark also recalls his mother coming into his bed at night to escape her husband. He recalls physically interfering when his father was beating his mother. When his parents separated, Mark believes, his father cut his mother out of much of their joint marital property.

While Mark was in prison for the murder of John Lennon, from 1981 to 1992, his father never visited him once. During that period David

Chapman was married twice, and suffered a series of heart attacks and a stroke, from which he recovered.

There is no evidence that Mark was ever sexually abused. In a 1987 interview in *People* magazine, his mother minimized the amount of conflict and spousal abuse in her home. It does seem that Mark's childhood was traumatic. His early years were filled with loneliness, emotional neglect by his father, a rigid unemotional home atmosphere, and hypersensitivity to taunting and rejection by other children. Mark felt like an empty nobody, except that he was full of anger.

To fill up the emptiness, to create a sense of power and control in his life, to escape from the outside world, and to create secure attachment figures for himself, Mark created an inner world in which he was the boss. He followed primarily the neglect pathway to a dissociative disorder not otherwise specified I describe in my textbook[258]. His biographer quotes him as saying[142] (pp. 122):

> *The Little People adored me. I got my respect and adulation from an imaginary source, rather than confronting the kids and the things that hurt me and earning it on my own. When I got really angry about something, I would take it out on the Little People. Sometimes if somebody had hurt me at school or I was angry with my father, I would get revenge by killing some of the Little People. I had a button on the arm of the couch in the den. When I pushed it, it would blow up the houses where the Little People lived. Sometimes I would kill hundreds or thousands of them. Then, after I calmed down later, I would apologize. They would always forgive me.*

Mark Chapman sang Beatles songs to the Little People. His problem was that his surface self had no real identity, despite his interactions with the Little People. It was a shell. The first transformation in surface identity occurred after Mark started taking LSD at age fourteen. He also smoked marijuana and sniffed glue. Over the summer between eighth and ninth grades he changed from being "aloof, solicitous, and clean-cut," a student government representative and YMCA counselor, to being a drug head. This was a sudden religious conversion. The "religion" was psychedelia.

In March, 1970, Mark ran away from home to join the circus. His brief stay on the beach in Florida with hippies and drug abusers did not bring happiness. He returned home to high school, and on October 25, 1970 attended a religious retreat with other teenagers. This sowed the seeds of his next transformation.

In the summer of 1971, while on vacation at his grandmother's home in Ormand Beach, Florida, Mark's wallet was ransacked by a group of hippie friends. Chapman described his reaction to this event as follows (pp. 149):

> *And I remember, when I realized that my buddies had gone through my wallet, feeling the lowest I had ever felt. I felt like nobody. Like nothing. Nothing at all. . . at some point I lifted my hands and I said, 'Jesus, come to me. Help me.' And that was my time of true spiritual rebirth.*

It was not a true rebirth. It was just another change in persona. There was no depth to the rebirth. Mark David Chapman's spiritual problem, his emptiness and rage, was not solved. It was merely glossed over temporarily. On return to high school for his junior year, Mark was completely disconnected from his druggie identity of the previous two years. His longtime friend, Miles McManus, said of Chapman's transformation to born-again Christian, "It was a true personality split."

Shortly after his religious conversion to Christianity, Chapman began to think of his idol John Lennon as a Communist and a blasphemer. He would sing out loud to his friends, to the tune of John Lennon's song, *Imagine*, "Imagine John Lennon is dead."

After transforming John Lennon into the enemy, Chapman began to worship the pop singer Todd Rundgren. Prior to killing John Lennon on December 8, 1980, Chapman left a copy of *The Ballad of Todd Rundgren* in his hotel room. Lennon and Rundgren feuded in public while Chapman was in high school - at one point, John Lennon called Rundgren "Todd Runtgreen." Lennon was already being transformed from beloved idol into murder victim in Chapman's mind while he was in high school. This transformation parallels the devaluation of Robert Kennedy in the mind of Sirhan Sirhan.

Chapman's Christian fundamentalism was fleeting, like his other identities and enthusiasms. Soon it was replaced by an obsession with Todd Rundgren. The next shift in identity was triggered by work Mark did as a counselor and assistant program director at the South De Kalb County YMCA from 1970 to 1975. The children called him "Captain Nemo." This became his new identity. Everyone in the YMCA thought Chapman was an excellent counselor.

In 1975 Mark went to Beirut, Lebanon with the YMCA's international program. He was evacuated after several weeks due to the war conditions there. He got a job instead at the YMCA resettlement camp for Vietnam refugees at Fort Chaffee, Arkansas. It was in 1975, after his first experience with sexual intercourse, that he began masturbating up to seven times per day.

For his first twenty years, Chapman was aware of a dissociated internal child who was not one of the Little People. While the fake adult persona experimented with drugs, Christianity, masturbation and being Captain Nemo, the little child became the inner container for all Chapman's anger and resentment. He, the child, eventually became the killer of John Lennon. Chapman's account of the process is as follows (pp. 57):

> *My child was always conflicting with my fake adult, my phony adult that I had erected around it.*
>
> *All that rage came spilling out and I killed the hero of my childhood. All the rage at the world and in my myself and in my disappointments and disillusions. All those feelings I kept pent up, feelings that the child couldn't handle... but I didn't, like a child, know how to kill anybody. So I summoned the forces of evil to do it, to help me do it. I did what I thought you could do to get the evil forces. You chant and you take your clothes off. You get angry and you say horrible things. I had to pump up to do it...*
>
> *The adult was just a front for an act of evil that was carried out by a child. It was a child's anger, a child's jealousy, a child's rage. But the adult was so undeveloped, he didn't know what to do with it.*
>
> *The adult was all surface, anyway. It was a front. It couldn't handle anything. It diverted everything to the child, and the child put it in his black toy box, because he couldn't handle adult feelings either.*
>
> *He would, the adult would take each feeling and say some words and then give it to the child. The child would put it in the toy box he never opened, except to put something new in it.*
>
> *The child would play with his new toys. But one day he opened the box to put something new inside, he came across a toy that he had played with years ago. It had once been his hero, but it wasn't the same. He showed it to the fake adult, the phony*

adult.... Then the adult knew what to do. And they conspired together, the child and the child's fake adult, to kill a hero. To kill the phony. To kill phoniness. To take some kind of a stand for the first time in our lives. To do something. To do something real. I was going to stamp out phoniness....

Then John Lennon got out of the limousine. He had something in his hands. Some cassette tapes. The child looked at his hero - his broken toy - and his hero looked back at him. It was a hard look. The child was sure that his hero recognized him from earlier in the day, when he signed the album. Neither one smiled. Nobody said a word. There was dead silence in my brain and John Lennon walked past me.... His back was to the child and the voice said: Do it! Do it! Do it! Do it! Do it!

I aimed at his back. I pulled the trigger five times. And all hell broke loose in my mind.

It was like everything had been stripped away then. It wasn't a make-believe world anymore. The movie strip broke.

Mark David Chapman was diagnosed by the psychiatrist who examined him in jail as schizophrenic. He was actually suffering from dissociative disorder not otherwise specified, and was a self-created Manchurian Candidate assassin. Chapman's inner word became real when he pulled the trigger five times, because then it had a real effect in the outside word.

In the spring of 1976, Chapman went to a fundamentalist college in Lookout Mountain, Tennessee called Covenent College. He dropped out in the spring semester and returned to De Kalb County YMCA, like he returned home after failing to create a new circus identity as a teenager.

Shortly after returning home, Chapman suffered another identity collapse (pp. 168): "And then, when my YMCA identity fell apart, when I was stripped of that is when the clouds really started getting dark and I slipped into an abyss that ended in murder, of someone I didn't even know."

Despondent, Chapman went to Hawaii to kill himself in 1977, but his spirits lifted so he returned home to pursue his relationship with his girlfriend, Jessica Blankenship. When this relationship failed, he returned to Hawaii in May. Soon he tried to kill himself by carbon monoxide poisoning, using his car. The attempt was foiled because the hose he had connected to his exhaust pipe melted.

Chapman was admitted to Castle Memorial Hospital, a Seventh Day Adventist facility, on June 21, 1977 where he received a diagnosis of depression. During that admission the psychiatrist discovered nothing about the Little People, the inner child, or the dissociated phony adult. In 1977, virtually all psychiatrists would have missed all of that, or misinterpreted it as schizophrenia.

After discharge on July 5, 1997 Chapman moved in with the Reverend Peter Anderson and his wife, to whom he had been introduced by Dennis Mee-Lee from Castle Memorial Hospital.

On July 6, 1978 Chapman took a hastily planned trip to Japan, Hong Kong, Thailand, India, Iran, Israel, Switzerland, England, Georgia and then back to Hawaii. He was met at the airport on August 20, 1978 by his girlfriend, Gloria Abe. They became engaged in early 1979 and married on June 2, 1979. Mark worked at the hospital again but was fired in late 1979 due to hostility towards co-workers and excessive perfectionism. At this point, he started talking to the Little People again, for the first time since his adolescence.

Early in 1980, Chapman began to think more intently about killing John Lennon. He also explained the Little People to his wife, Gloria. One night Gloria awoke to hear what seemed like two voices shouting and arguing about killing John Lennon, but Mark was the only other person in the house.

During 1980, Chapman put himself in trance while sitting naked listening to Beatles songs on headphones. He did this in a ritualistic manner and called upon Satan to give him power to kill John Lennon. This is very similar to the trance exercises Sirhan Sirhan performed with mirrors and candles, in order to create a dissociated assassin state within himself. It is curious that Dr. Bernard Diamond diagnosed Sirhan Sirhan as a self created multiple personality, but considered Mark David Chapman to be schizophrenic, when the mental processes of the two are so similar.

During 1980 Chapman called on the Little People to help him plan and carry out the murder. The killing of John Lennon was carefully premeditated by the phony adult. Mark David Chapman's inner world was not chaotic, disorganized or psychotic; it was controlled at a high level of precision. Chapman rightly refused to mount an insanity defense even when encouraged to do so by defense psychiatrists who considered him schizophrenic.

Chapman described his Little People this way (pp. 289):

> *But anyway, that's what it was: a board and people were formed into committees. It's exactly like I had when the Little People returned before I killed John Lennon. One committee worked on my finances. And every night or once a week they would give me these reports on how we were doing. And these were all highly trained, efficient people. I even sensed their personalities. One of them even had a name. He was like the chief of staff. He was very aloof and efficient. I would often see him sitting by the window alone in the boardroom, just looking out the window and thinking. We had on the board the equivalent of like a military general, who was head of the defense department, a defense committee and the financial committee, the relationship committee. Just maybe five or six committees that worked there to help me and I would turn to them and they would tell me what to do. Of course they were answerable to me, but they would often give me advice.*

The Little People did not participate in the murder of John Lennon. In fact they actively tried to talk the phony adult out of it, without success. When the phony adult talked to the Little People, including Robert, his most trusted advisor, the phony adult's face would be displayed on a video screen in the inner boardroom. This is typical of the inner worlds of people with dissociative identity disorder or dissociative disorder not otherwise specified[255, 256, 258]. So is referring to oneself as "we" or "us," which schizophrenics do not usually do.

After discussion with "Mr. President," the phony adult, about the plan to kill John Lennon, the Little People maintained their integrity by departing (pp. 237):

> *One by one, beginning with his defense minister, the Little People rose from their seats and walked from the secret chamber inside the mysterious mind of Mark David Chapman. Alone in his dangerous world at last, abandoned even by the endlessly forgiving Little People whom he had created within himself, the face of Mark David Chapman faded from the screen.*

The Little People and the murderous inner child had evolved into much more than inner fantasies. They had their own separate, dissociated feelings, motives and points of view. They monitored and interacted with the outside world, took executive control of the body, made decisions and carried out internal actions independently of the control of the phony adult. They feared his retaliation, but they did not bend to his will.

Chapman went to New York twice in late 1980, the first time for reconnaissance, the second to carry out the murder in front of the Dakota apartments late on the evening of December 8. Afterwards, in jail, in 1981, Robert returned to the phony adult when he was awaiting trial (pp. 279):

> *Robert briefly explained that he could reconvene the government to try to help Chapman cope with the aftermath of the tragedy that he had allowed the small, Evil One inside him to create. Chapman considered the offer, but decided against it. He was too ashamed, he said.*

During his imprisonment, Chapman became possessed by demons, a not uncommon occurrence in people with dissociative disorders. The demons went away in response to exorcisms conducted by Chapman alone and by Chapman and a prison minister in 1985. The demons must have been disavowed, angry parts of his mind.

Mark David Chapman was not a full Manchurian Candidate because there was no amnesia and because he was self-created. He did carry out an assassination, though. He was not schizophrenic - if he had been correctly diagnosed at Castle Memorial Hospital in 1977, and provided skilled psychotherapy, John Lennon might be alive today.

By the time he killed John Lennon, Chapman had transformed his identity into Holden Caulfield from *The Catcher in the Rye*[262]. This was but one more in a long series of transformations of identity, none permanent or successful. The psychological processes of Mark David Chapman are closely related to those of Sirhan Sirhan; he provides another example of the self-created Manchurian Candidate assassin.

IV. CONCLUSIONS

23

IATROGENIC MULTIPLE PERSONALITY DISORDER

As I describe in my 1997 textbook[258], there are four pathways to multiple personality disorder, now officially named dissociative identity disorder by the American Psychiatric Association: (1) childhood abuse; (2) childhood neglect; (3) factitious; and, (4) iatrogenic. Iatrogenic means created by the therapist. The same four pathways may result in partial or incomplete forms of multiple personality called dissociative disorder not otherwise specified.

Dissociative identity disorder may arise as (1), a natural response to severe, chronic childhood abuse, which may include any combination of physical, sexual, emotional and verbal abuse. It may be a response to (2), severe, chronic childhood neglect. It may be (3), a factitious disorder, that is, the symptoms may be self-created by a person who wants to get into the patient role. Finally, (4), the disorder may be iatrogenic, which means created by a doctor or therapist. In civilian therapies, iatrogenic dissociative identity is created unwittingly and is malpractice, while in Manchurian Candidate Programs it is created on purpose.

Civilian iatrogenic dissociative identity disorder is grounds for a successful malpractice lawsuit: this fact alone establishes that the Manchurian Candidate Programs were harmful, unethical and a violation of human rights. They were designed to create an enduring psychiatric disorder, which is the opposite of what doctors are supposed to do under the Hippocratic Oath and the Nuremberg Code.

Sirhan Sirhan and Mark David Chapman correspond to the factitious pathway, while Palle Hardrup, Candy Jones and Patty Hearst correspond to the iatrogenic pathway.

Controversies concerning the percentage of multiple personality cases that are due to the different pathways have been analyzed in my other writings[258, 259, 260]. In clinical work, I rarely encounter pure factitious or iatrogenic cases. Instead, most cases contain elements of all four causal pathways, in ratios that vary from case to case.

The reality of iatrogenic multiple personality and the reality of the Manchurian Candidate prove each other. If iatrogenic multiple personality actually occurs, and individuals in such cases experience real but iatrogenic amnesia, auditory hallucinations and posttraumatic stress disorder, then the disorder has been created unwittingly by incompetent, misguided therapists. If therapists can create multiple personality disorder unintentionally, then a skilled mind control doctor should be able to create a Manchurian Candidate on purpose. The therapies in which multiple personality is created unwittingly should mimic the conditions and techniques used by Palle Hardrup, Bjorn Neilsen, Donald DeFreeze and BLUEBIRD/ARTICHOKE doctors to create Manchurian Candidates.

Inversely, if Manchurian Candidates are real and have been used in actual operations, and if their locking mechanisms, amnesia barriers and post-hypnotic suggestions present a serious barrier to counter-intelligence detection and penetration, then one would expect iatrogenic cases to occur in therapies that mimic the conditions of mind control.

Additionally, if iatrogenic multiple personality and Manchurian Candidates are real, then cases should arise naturally and spontaneously under conditions that mimic misguided therapies and mind control programs. The fundamental condition is inescapable control by adults with power and authority who behave in contradictory, unintegrated ways, at times kind and protective, at others abusive and hateful. This is the classic good cop-bad cop method of interrogation. It is also the experience of children in abusive, traumatic and neglectful families.

If cases of multiple personality disorder never arose spontaneously in abusive and neglectful families, I would expect Manchurian Candidates to be difficult or impossible to create, and I would not expect to encounter iatrogenic cases of multiple personality disorder. I would conclude that the human mind just doesn't work that way, and doesn't split off new identities under difficult circumstances, except perhaps in extremely rare cases.

All four pathways to multiple personality depend on the core features of the condition, amnesia and dissociated executive control, being universal aspects of normal human psychology, a view for which I present the evidence and logic in my other writings[258-260]. I am not trying to prove anything about iatrogenic dissociative identity disorder in this chapter. My goal is to explain why the Manchurian Candidate programs could help us better understand clinical dissociative disorders.

In the course of my work as an expert witness, I have encountered five cases of relatively pure iatrogenic multiple personality disorder. In each case I have reviewed medical records, interviewed the person directly, and administered a battery of self-report, computer-scored and structured interview measures, and in several I analyzed the opinions, affidavits and testimony of the defendants. In one case, I listened to audiotapes of therapy sessions. Additionally I have attended workshops and talks by some of the defendants and reviewed their published writings.

The conclusion that each of the five cases was iatrogenic was reached in several ways. Each litigant was making that claim. In all five cases, there was no evidence of a dissociative disorder existing prior to therapy in the medical records or in the histories I took. There was abundant evidence of treatment techniques and boundary violations that mimicked the mind control techniques used by destructive cults, Bjorn Neilsen, Donald Defreeze, Gilbert Jensen, and BLUEBIRD/ARTICHOKE doctors.

Subsequent to retracting their multiple personality and false memories, all five litigants experienced spontaneous stable remission of their multiple personality disorder without any therapy designed to achieve that goal. The multiple personality melted away quickly once the litigants escaped the control of their therapists.

I compared the five iatrogenic cases to twelve cases I judged to be examples of the childhood abuse and neglect pathways to multiple personality disorder. Each of these twelve individuals had participated in specific psychotherapy for multiple personality for a period of years and had reached stable integration according to criteria accepted in the field[258]. None of the childhood trauma pathway cases had retracted her diagnosis or trauma history.

At the time of interview, the two groups did not differ on any of the measures I used. These included the Dissociative Experiences Scale, the Dissociative Disorders Interview Schedule, the Structured Clinical Interview for DSM-III-R (SCID), the Millon Clinical Multiaxial Inventory II and III, the Hamilton Rating Scale for Depression, the Symptom Checklist-90-Revised, and the Beck Mood Inventory. Four of the iatrogenic subjects also completed the posttraumatic stress disorder section of the Diagnostic Interview Schedule. All these measures are commonly used in the field and are referenced and discussed in my writings[258, 81, 82].

The two groups did not differ on their lifetime psychiatric profile on the Structured Clinical Interview for DSM III-R. They did not differ on demographic features or childhood histories of physical and sexual abuse as reported on the Dissociative Disorders Interview Schedule, the text of which is available in my textbook[258] and on my web page at www.rossinst.com. The iatrogenic cases had retracted much of their trauma, but their non-retracted trauma histories were still substantial.

Dissociative symptoms prior to diagnosis of the multiple personality were mild in intensity and low in frequency in the iatrogenic cases; the dissociative symptoms appeared to be components of other disorders such as depression and bulimia. The iatrogenic patients' involvement in the mental health system prior to the iatrogenic therapy was minimal. In contrast, the childhood onset cases had long, complicated mental health histories prior to diagnosis of their multiple personality, including chronic, complex dissociative symptoms.

In the five iatrogenic cases, pre-existing diagnoses of bipolar mood disorder were made in three, and major depressive disorder in the other two. Self-defeating and/or dependent personality disorder were present in all five cases. Three of the four iatrogenic cases tested were positive for posttraumatic stress disorder, and in each case the PTSD was caused by false memories and the trauma of therapy.

The iatrogenic cases provided extreme examples of massive overutilization of treatment techniques and boundary violations. As I describe in a composite case in my textbook[258], the treatments mimicked the mind control techniques used by destructive cults[289], and by the mind control doctors who created Manchurian Candidates. The treatments included prolonged inpatient admissions lasting as long as two years which imposed conditions of sensory deprivation, sleep and food deprivation; repeated trance induction; isolation from the outside world; control of information; and altered states of consciousness due to drugs.

The patients' families of origin were defined as Satanic and all doubts about the reality of the multiple personality or the false memories of Satanic ritual abuse were defined as symptoms of cult programming or resistance to treatment. The treatment team had a hierarchical organizational structure with a charismatic leader at the top, just like destructive cults. The treatment violated the methods and principles I recommend in my book, *Satanic Ritual Abuse: Principles of Treatment*[256], and it did so to an extreme degree.

Boundary violations by the therapists ranged from minor problems to sexual involvement. There was excessive personal disclosure by therapists, and the patients often knew the names of therapists' spouses and children. The personal beliefs of the therapists about "the cult," and the therapists' fear and paranoia, were well known to the patients. In many cases, the treatment plan was modified to protect the therapist and patient from the cult. Mail was opened by hospital staff and reviewed for secretly implanted triggers. Control of the patient's life space, thoughts, beliefs, behaviors and interactions was extensive or complete for prolonged periods of time.

Serious medical problems were ignored or interpreted as cult programming. For instance, a pneumonia was said to be an attempt to sabotage therapy; an extreme elevation in blood pressure during a voluntary physical restraint session was not treated; a purulent discharge went untreated for a week while being interpreted as the workings of a cult alter personality; and the importance of other medical problems was minimized. Serious untreated medical problems included multiple sclerosis, epilepsy, hypothyroidism, an abscessed tooth, and hypertension.

The medical records were extremely unusual. There were no target symptoms or problems that could be treated in an acute setting. The charts were full of comments about the cult, programming, Satanic holidays and the like. These were reported as facts, not allegations of the patient, and were the primary concern of the staff. Stabilization, return to the outside world, building daily coping skills, employment, and the quality of outside relationships all took second place to the cosmic battle with the powers of evil, as represented by the cult, the cult alter personalities, and the cult programming. There was no evidence that any of the Satanic ritual abuse was real.

The five cases show that the threshold for creation of iatrogenic multiple personality is set very high. The degree of control and social influence required to create an iatrogenic case of multiple personality is comparable to the brainwashing conditions required by destructive cults, Communist

Chinese interrogators, and creators of Manchurian Candidates. An hour or two of outpatient therapy per week is not enough. In the five iatrogenic cases I reviewed as an expert witness, there was massive over-involvement of the therapist and massive over-utilization of standard treatment techniques. In the most severe cases, total control of the patient was exerted in an inpatient environment for months or years.

Creating a Manchurian Candidate requires intrusion into the subject's life space on the scale experienced by Palle Hardrup and Patty Hearst. G.H. Estabrooks said that months of training were required, even though subjects had been carefully selected.

I have also served as an expert witness for the defense in iatrogenic multiple personality cases. In several of these cases I judged the complaint of iatrogenic multiple personality to be fake. I call this condition *false false memory syndrome*. These people do not really have iatrogenic multiple personality; they are faking it. In these cases, there was a prolonged history of faking all kinds of medical conditions prior to the factious multiple personality arising. The conditions of extreme social influence and control by the therapist were absent.

The plaintiffs in these cases had faked multiple personality and now were suing for damages, blaming the therapist for their own deceptive behavior. It is possible that Candy Jones' story was fake; the information necessary to make a decision about causal pathway in Candy Jones' case is contained in still-classified documents not available under the Freedom of Information Act.

If more information about the Manchurian Candidate was declassified by the CIA and other intelligence agencies, this would help me in my clinical study of multiple personality disorder. The available Manchurian Candidate documents were declassified in the 1970's. It is time, I think, for another round of declassification. I close this chapter of *The CIA Doctors* with a request for more documents.

24

THE REALITY OF THE
MANCHURIAN CANDIDATE

What does it mean to say that the Manchurian Candidate is real? "Real" or childhood-onset dissociative identity disorder is never literally real. There is never really more than one person there. According to the diagnostic rules of the American Psychiatric Association[12], psychiatric diagnoses must be based on observed behaviors and reported symptoms. This is true for all psychiatric diagnoses. Multiple personality disorder is an *observed behavior*. The person with multiple personality acts *as if* he or she has different people inside who take turns being in control of the body. This is a behavior, not a literal fact.

The causal pathway of the multiple personality is not relevant to making the diagnosis by American Psychiatric Association rules. Multiple personality, on the one hand, is never literally real. On the other hand, one "really" has multiple personality if one exhibits the behavior of switching and amnesia, unless the condition is being consciously faked, in which case the diagnosis is factitious disorder. By American Psychiatric Association rules, multiple personality is equally "real" if the causal pathway is childhood abuse, childhood neglect or iatrogenic. Therefore a Manchurian Candidate has "real" multiple personality.

The clinical reason to be interested in etiological pathway is not to decide if a case is "real" or not, but to help in treatment planning. The controversy about "real" versus iatrogenic multiple personality is based on a misconception. The disorder is never literally or concretely real, which is why it can be treated with psychotherapy. Despite the fact that it is not literally real, multiple personality can have very real consequences. There are no better examples of this fact than Mark David Chapman and Sirhan Sirhan. The separate identities and amnesia barriers in multiple personality are *symptoms*, not literal facts. When I speak of an *amnesia barrier*, for instance, I realize that there is no physical wall inside the mind.

People actually do find themselves in strange locations, unaware of how they got there, because of multiple personality. These things really happen. Study of the Manchurian Candidate helps us understand the sense in which multiple personality disorder is real. The amnesia barriers, locking mechanisms, and layers of personalities in the Manchurian Candidate actually do provide a barrier to counter-intelligence penetration, as G. H. Estabrooks described. Like the Manchurian Candidate, the person with iatrogenic multiple personality actually experiences the symptoms of the disorder, and actually has dissociative identity disorder by American Psychiatric Association rules.

Consider the hypnotized patient in the middle of gallbladder surgery. The patient is awake, alert and reporting no pain or discomfort. His pulse, blood pressure, muscle tension, and all other physiological measures are normal. What does it mean to say that the pain control isn't "real," that the person is "only hypnotized?" Nothing.

Likewise, a debate about whether Manchurian Candidates are "real" is meaningless. What matters is whether the Manchurian Candidate can escape detection and, if caught, whether the classified information he or she holds can be hidden from interrogators. Similarly, for the traumatized child, what matters is whether the multiple personality works as a way to cope with trauma, not whether it is literally real.

In the interests of national security, it is important that the CIA and military intelligence agencies have mind control programs in place. This is true, for one reason, because mind control methods are being used by leaders of destructive cults, dictators and terrorists. There is nothing wrong with the intelligence agencies seeking the assistance of physicians in such programs. The problem is the conflict between the National Security Act and the Hippocratic Oath.

To date, organized medicine has behaved as if this conflict does not exist. That needs to change. The doctors who create Manchurian Candidates need to be governed not just by the National Security Act, but also by the Hippocratic Oath. How this conflict should be resolved, and how it should be regulated by civilian, organized medicine, is uncertain The problem requires study and discussion. Whatever the outcome of such discussion,we will always need an effective, functioning intelligence community. The CIA stands between me and Gulag.

The Manchurian Candidate is fact, not fiction. The degree of control and coercive persuasion required to create a Manchurian Candidate sets the threshold for creation of iatrogenic multiple personality disorder at a high level.

Study of the Manchurian Candidate leads to the conclusion that creation of iatrogenic multiple personality requires much more control and influence than is possible in one or two hours of outpatient therapy per week. When the necessary degree of control and influence is missing, the causal pathway to multiple personality is more likely to be childhood abuse, childhood neglect, or factitious. The relevance of the Manchurian Candidate to clinical psychiatry is the light it sheds on pathway differentiation. That is one reason I have studied the Manchurian Candidate for thirteen years, despite attacks on me in medical journals[79, 191], books[213], and magazines[3], and on CBC and BBC television.

There have been extensive human rights violations by American psychiatrists over the last 70 years. These doctors were paid by the American taxpayer through CIA and military contracts. It is past time for these abuses to stop, it is past time for a reckoning, and it is past time for individual doctors to be held accountable.

The Manchurian Candidate Programs are of much more than "historical" interest. ARTICHOKE, BLUEBIRD, MKULTRA and MKSEARCH are precursors of mind control programs that are operational in the twenty first century. Human rights violations by psychiatrists must be ongoing in programs like COPPER GREEN, the interrogation program at Abu Ghraib prison in Iraq. Such programs must be carried out within CIA units like Task Force 121 (*The Dallas Morning News*, December 1, 2004, p. 1A). Information pointing to ongoing human rights violations by psychiatrists is available in publications like *The New Yorker* (see article by Seymour M. Hersh, May 24, 2004). Yet the indifference, silence, denial, and disinformation of organized medicine and psychiatry continue. One purpose of *The CIA Doctors: Human Rights Violations By American Psychiatrists* is to break that silence.

IV. REFERENCES

SENATE HEARINGS AND GOVERNMENT REPORTS

Biomedical and Behavioral Research, 1975. Joint Hearings Before the Subcommittee on Labor and Public Welfare and the Subcommittee on Administrative Practice and Procedure of the Committee on the Judiciary, United States Senate, Ninety-Fourth Congress, First Session on Human-Use Experimentation Programs of the Department of Defense and Central Intelligence Agency.

Biological Testing Involving Human Subjects by The Department of Defense, 1977. Hearings Before the Subcommittee on Health and Scientific Research of the Committee on Human Resources United States Senate, Ninety-Fifth Congress, First Session on Examination of Serious Deficiencies in the Defense Department's Efforts to Protect the Human Subjects of Drug Research.

Final Report. Advisory Committee on Human Radiation Experiments. Pittsburgh: U.S. Government Printing Office, 1995.

Human Drug Testing by the CIA, 1977. Hearings before the Subcommittee on Health and Scientific Research of the Committee on Human Resources, United States Senate, Ninety-Fourth Congress, First Session.

Project MKULTRA, The CIA's Program of Research in Behavioral Modification. Hearings Before the Select Committee on Intelligence, and Subcommittee on Health and Scientific Research of the Committee on Human Resources, United States Senate, Ninety-Fourth Congress, Second Session, 1977.

Quality of Health Care - Human Experimentation, 1973. Hearings Before the Subcommittee on Health of the Committee on Labor and Public Welfare, United States Senate, Ninety-Third Congress, First Session.

The Nelson Rockefeller Report to the President by the Commission on CIA Activities. New York: Manor Books, 1975.

BOOKS AND PAPERS

1. Abramson, H. *The Use of LSD in Psychotherapy.* New York: Josiah Macy, Jr. Foundation, 1960.

2. Abramson, H. *The Use of LSD in Psychotherapy and Alcoholism.* New York: Bobbs-Merrill, 1967.

3. Acocella, J. The politics of hysteria. *The New Yorker*, April 6, 1998, 64-79.

4. Adey, W.R. Sensitivity of brain tissue to intrinsic and environmental oscillating fields. *Electroencephalography and Clinical Neurophysiology*, 38, 547, 1975.

5. Adey, W.R., Bawin, S.M. (Eds.). *Brain Interactions with Weak Electric and Magnetic Fields. Neurosciences Research Program Bulletin*, 15, 1-129, 1977.

6. Adey, W.R., Tokizane, T. (Eds.). *Structure and Function of the Limbic System.* New York, Elsevier, 1967.

7. Adey, W.R., Bell, F.R., & Dennis, B.J. Effects of LSD-25, psilocybin, and psilocin on temporal lobe EEG patterns and learned behavior in the cat. *Neurology*, 12, 591-602, 1962.

8. Adey, W.R., Porter, R., Walter, D.O., & Brown, T.S. Prolonged effects of LSD on EEG records during discriminative performance in cat: Evaluation by computer analysis. *Electroencephalography and Clinical Neurophysiology*, 18, 25-35, 1965.

9. Agee, P. *Inside the Company. CIA Diary.* New York: Bantam, 1975.

10. Allen, J.R., West, L.J. Flight from violence: Hippies and the green rebellion. *American Journal of Psychiatry*, 125, 364-370, 1968.

11. American Psychiatric Association. *Diagnostic and Statistical Manual of Mental Disorders, Third Editon.* Washington, D.C. American Psychiatric Association, 1980.

12. American Psychiatric Association. *Diagnostic and Statistical Manual of Mental Disorders, Fourth Edition.* Washington, DC American Psychiatric Association, 1994.

13. Ames, A. Aniseikonic glasses. In F.P. Kilpatrick (Ed.), *Explorations in Transactional Psychology* (pp. 119-147. New York: New York University Press, 1961.

14. Andreasen, N.A. Daniel X. Freedman, M.D. 1921-1993. A Memoriam to a scientist in the service of the ill. *American Journal of Psychiatry*, 151, 799-801, 1994.

15. Anonymous. In Memoriam. Donald Ewen Cameron - 1901-1967. *Canadian Psychiatric Association Journal*, 12, 475, 1967.

16. Author. Clues to biochemistry of schizophrenia: May lead to rational therapy of disease. *Factor*, December, 1959, pp. 8-9.

17. Azima, H. Sleep treatment in mental disorders. *Diseases of the Nervous System*, 19, 523-530, 1958.

18. Azima, H. Psilocybin disorganization. *Recent Advances in Biological Psychiatry*, 5, 184-198, 1962.

19. Azima, H., Cramer, F.J. Effects of partial perceptual isolation in mentally disturbed individuals. *Diseases of the Nervous System*, 17, 117-122, 1956.

20. Azima, H., Vispo, R.H. Imipramine: A potent new antidepressant compound. *American Journal of Psychiatry*, 115, 245-247, 1958.

21. Azima, H., Wittkower, E.D., & LaTendresse, J. Object relations therapy in schizophrenic states. *American Journal of Psychiatry*, 115, 60-62, 1958.

22. Azrin, N.H., Lindsley, O.R. The reinforcement of cooperation between children. *Journal of Abnormal and Social Psychology*, 51, 100-102, 1955.

23. Bain, D. *The Control of Candy Jones*. Chicago: Playboy Press, 1976.

24. Baldwin, M., Bach, S.A., & Lewis, S.A. Effects of radio-frequency energy on primate cerebral activity. *Neurology*, 10, 178-187, 1960.

25. Baldwin, M., Lewis, S.A., & Bach, S.A. The effects of lysergic acid after cerebral ablation. *Neurology*, 9, 469-474, 1959.

26. Bamford, J. *The Puzzle Palace. Inside the National Security Agency, America's Most Secret Intelligence Organization*. New York: Penguin Books, 1982.

27. Barker, E.T., Buck, M.F. LSD in a coercive milieu therapy program. *Canadian Psychiatric Association Journal*, 22, 311-314, 1977.

28. Barker, E.T., Mason, M.H. Buber behind bars. *Canadian Psychiatric Association Journal*, 13, 61-72, 1968.

29. Barker, E.T., McLaughlin, A.J. The total encounter capsule. *Canadian Psychiatric Association Journal*, 22, 355-360, 1977.

30. Barker, E.T., Mason, M.A., & Wilson, J. Defence-disrupting therapy. *Canadian Psychiatric Association Journal*, 14, 355-359, 1969.

31. Bender, L. Children's reactions to psychotomimetic drugs. In D.H. Efron (Ed.), *Psychotomimetic Drugs*, pp. 265-271. New York: Raven Press, 1970.

32. Bender, L., Faretra, G., & Cobronik, L. LSD and UML treatment of hospitalized disturbed children. *Recent Advances in Biological Psychiatry*, 5, 84-92, 1962.

33. Berkhout, J., Walter, D.O., & Adey, W.R. Autonomic responses during a replicable interrogation. *Journal of Applied Psychology*, 54, 316-325, 1970.

34. Berlin, L., Guthrie, T., Weider, A., Goodell, H., & Wolff, H.G. Studies in human cerebral function: The effects of mescaline and lysergic acid on cerebral processes pertinent to creative activity. *Journal of Nervous and Mental Disease*, 122, 487-491, 1955.

35. Blake, A.F. To 'sleep:' perchance to kill? *Providence Evening Bulletin*, May 13, 1968.

36. Blum, W. *The CIA. A Forgotten History*. London: Zed Books, 1986.

37. Boslow, H.M., Kohlmeyer, W.A. The Maryland defective delinquency law: An eight-year follow-up. *American Journal of Psychiatry*, 119, 118-124, 1963.

38. Bowart, W. *Operation Mind Control*. New York: W.W. Norton, 1978.

39. Bower, T. *The Paperclip Conspiracy. The Hunt for the Nazi Scientists*. Boston: Little Brown and Company, 1987.

40. Bradley, P.B., Elkes, J.B. A technique for recording the electrical activity of the brain in the conscious animal. *Electroencephalography and Clinical Neurophysiology*, 5, 451-458, 1953.

41. Brauchi, J.T., West, L.J. Sleep deprivation. *Journal of the American Medical Association*, 171, 11-14, 1959.

42. Breutsch, W.L. Translation of Wagner-Jauregg, J. The history of the malaria treatment of general paralysis. *American Journal of Psychiatry*, 151, 231-234, 1994.

43. Brown, A.C. *Wild Bill Donovan. The Last Hero*. New York: Times Books, 1982.

44. Brussell, M. Why was Patty Hearst kidnapped? *Paranoia Annual*, 1, 97-112, 1974/1996.

45 Budiansky, S., Goode, E.E., & Gest, T. The cold war experiments. *U.S. News and World Report*, January 24, 1994, pp. 32-38.

46. Bursten, B., Delgado, J.M.R. Positive reinforcement induced by intracerebral stimulation in the monkey. *Journal of Comparative and Physiological Psychology, 51, 6-10, 1958.*

47. Cahill, B. New 'personalities' made to order. *Montreal Gazette*, June 18, 1956.

48.   Cahill, B.   Psychic driving: repeated statements may influence glands. *Toronto Globe and Mail*, October 31, 1956.

49.   Cahill, B.   "Two month sleep, shock new schizophrenic cure", *Montreal Gazette*, September 2, 1957

50.   Cameron, D.E.   Red light therapy in schizophrenia. *British Journal of Physical Medicine*, 10, 11, 1936.

51.   Cameron, D.E.   Psychic driving. *American Journal of Psychiatry*, 112, 502-509, 1956.

52.   Cameron, D.E.   Production of differential amnesia as a factor in the treatment of schizophrenia. *Comprehensive Psychiatry*, 1, 26-34, 1960.

53.   Cameron, D.E., Lohrenz, J.G., & Handcock, K.A.   The depatterning treatment of schizophrenia. *Comprehensive Psychiatry*, 3, 65-76, 1962.

54.   Cameron, D.E., Levy, l., Ban, T., & Rubenstein, L.   Repetition of verbal signals in therapy.   In J.H. Masserman (Ed.), *Current Psychiatric Therapies: 1961* (pp. 100-111).   New York: Grune & Stratton, 1961.

55.   Cameron, D.E., Levy, L., Rubenstein, L. & Malmo, R.B. Repetition of verbal signals: Behavioral and physiological changes. *American Journal of Psychiatry*, 115, 985-991, 1959.

56.   Case, R.G.   Goodbye, Mr. Estabrooks! *Syracuse Herald American*, January 6, 1974.

57.   Chess, S.   Lauretta Bender, M.D. 1899-1987. *American Journal of Psychiatry, 152, 436, 1995.*

58.   Chodoff, P., Mercer, E.   A response to psychiatric abuse.   In E. Stover, E.O. Nightingale (Eds.), *The Breaking of Bodies and Minds. Torture, Psychiatric Abuse and the Health Professions* (pp. 223-228).   New York: W.H. Freeman, 1985.

59.   Chorover, S.L.   *From Genesis to Genocide. The Meaning of Human Nature and the Power of Behavioral Control.*   Cambridge: The MIT Press, 1979.

60.   Clare, A.   *Medicine Betrayed. The Participation of Doctors in Human Rights Abuses.*   British Medical Association, London: Zed Books, 1992.

61.   Cleghorn, R.A.   D. Ewen Cameron, M.D. F.R.C.P. [C]. *Canadian Medical Association Journal*, 97, 984-985, 1967.

62.   Cohen, B.D., Luby, E.D., Rosenbaum, G., & Gottlieb, J.S. Combined Sernyl and sensory deprivation. *Comprehensive Psychiatry*, 2, 345-348, 1961.

63. Cohen, B.D., Rosenbaum, G., Dobie, S.I., & Gottlieb, J.S. Sensory isolation: Hallucinogenic effects of a brief procedure. *Journal of Nervous and Mental Disease*, 129, 486-491, 1959.

64. Cohen, B.D., Rosenbaum, G., Luby, E.D., & Gottlieb, J.S. Comparison of phencyclidine (Sernyl) with other drugs. *Archives of General Psychiatry*, 6, 395-401, 1962.

65. Collins, A. *In The Sleep Room. The Story of CIA Brainwashing Experiments in Canada.* Toronto: Lester & Orpen Dennys, 1988.

66. Condon, R. *The Manchurian Candidate*. New York: Jove Books, 1959/1988.

67. Davis, E. Illusion-producing drug now on black market. *Atlanta Journal*, July 13, 1962.

68. Deckert, G.H., West, L.J. Hypnosis and experimental psychopathology. *American Journal of Clinical Hypnosis*, 5, 256 276, 1963.

69. Delgado, J.M.R. Evaluation of permanent implantation of electrodes within the brain. *Electroencephalography and Clinical Neurophysiology, 7, 637-644, 1955.*

70. Delgado, J.M.R. Electronic command of movement and behavior. *Transactions of the New York Academy of Sciences*, 21, 689-699, 1959.

71. Delgado, J.M.R. Prolonged stimulation of brain in awake monkeys. *Journal of Neurophysiology*, 22, 458-475, 1959.

72. Delgado, J.M.R. Emotional behavior in animals and humans. *Psychiatric Research Reports*, 12, 259-266, 1960.

73. Delgado, J.M.R. Social rank and radio-stimulated aggressiveness in monkeys. *Journal of Nervous and Mental Disease*, 144, 383-390, 1967.

74. Delgado, J.M.R. Limbic system and free behavior. In W.R. Adey & T. Tokizane (Eds.), *Structure and Function of the Limbic Sytem*, pp. 48-68. New York: Elsevier, 1967.

75. Delgado, J.M.R. *Physical Control of the Mind.* New York: Harper & Row, 1969.

76. Delgado, J.M., Mark, V., Sweet, W., Ervin, F., Weiss, G., Bach-Y-Rita, G., & Hagiwara, R. Intracerebral radio stimulation and recording in completely free patients. *Journal of Nervous and Mental Disease*, 147, 329-340, 1968.

77. Demarr, E.W., Williams, H.L., Miller, A.I., & Pfeiffer, C.C. Effects in man of single and combined oral doses of reserpine, iproniazid, and d-lysergic acid diethylamide. *Clinical Pharmacology and Therapeutics*, 1, 23-30, 1960.

78. Ditman, K.S., Moss, T., Forgy, E.W., Zunin, L.M., Lynch, R.D., & Funk, W.A. Dimensions of the LSD, methylphenidate and chlordiazepoxide experiences. *Psychopharmacologia*, 14, 1-11, 1969.

79. Einspruch, B.C. Review of *Stranger Than Fiction: When Our Minds Betray Us*, by Feldman M.D., Feldman, J.M., & Smith, R. *Journal of the American Medical Association*, 279, 1918-1919, 1998.

80. Elkes, J. Some effects of psychotomimetic drugs on the experimental animal, and in man. *Neuropharmacology. Transactions of the Third Conference* (pp. 205-295). Josiah Macy Jr. Foundation, 1957.

81. Ellason, J.W., Ross, C.A. Millon Clinical Multiaxial Inventory II follow-up of patients with dissociative identity disorder. *Psychological Reports*, 78, 707-716, 1996.

82. Ellason, J.W., Ross, C.A. Two-year follow-up of inpatients with dissociative identity disorder. *American Journal of Psychiatry*, 154, 832-839, 1997.

83. Estabrooks, G.H. *Man the Mechanical Misfit*. New York: MacMillan Company, 1941.

84. Estabrooks, G.H. *Hypnotism*. New York: E.P. Dutton, 1943.

85. Estabrooks, G.H. *Spiritism*. New York: E.P. Dutton, 1947.

86. Estabrooks, G.H. (Ed.). *Hypnosis: Current Problems*. New York: Harper & Row, 1962.

87. Estabrooks, G.H. Hypnosis comes of age. *Science Digest,* April, 1971, 44-50.

88. Estabrooks, G.H., Gross, N.E. *The Future of the Human Mind*. New York: E.P. Dutton, 1961.

89. Faden, R.R. *Final Report. Advisory Committee on Human Radiation Experiments*. Washington, DC: U.S. Government Printing Office, 1995.

90. Farber, I.E., Harlow, H.F., & West, L.J. Brainwashing, conditioning, and ddd (debility, dependency, and dread). In R. Ulrich, T. Stachnik, & J. Mabry (Eds.), *Control of Human Behavior*, pp. 322-330. Glenview: Scott, Foresman and Company, 1966.

91. Faretra, G, Bender, L. Autonomic nervous system responses in hospitalized children treated with LSD and UML. *Recent Advances in Biological Psychiatry*, 7, 1-8, 1964.

92. Feldman, M.D., Feldman, J.M., & Smith, R. *Stranger Than Fiction: When Our Minds Betray Us*. Washington, DC: American Psychiatric Press, 1998.

93. F.J.B.   D. Ewen Cameron 1901-1967. *American Journal of Psychiatry*, 124, 168-169, 1967.

94. Frankel, F.H., Orne, M.T. Treatment of anxiety and panic disorders: Strategies of relaxation, self-control, and fear-mastery. *Task Force on the Treatment of Anxiety Disorders* (pp. 2007-2009). Washington, DC: American Psychiatric Association, 1989.

95. Frazier, H. *Uncloaking the CIA*. New York: The Free Press, 1975.

96. Freedman, D.X. Effects of LSD-25 on brain serotonin. *Journal of Pharmacology and Experimental Therapeutics*, 134, 16-166, 1961.

97. Freedman, D.X. Psychotomimetic drugs and brain biogenic amines. *American Journal of Psychiatry*, 119, 843-850, 1963.

98. Freedman, D.X., Giarmin, N.J. LSD-25 and the status and level of brain serotonin. *Annals of the New York Academy of Sciences*, 96, 98-107, 1962.

99. Fremont-Smith, F. Preface. In H. Abramson (Ed.), *The Use of LSD in Psychotherapy and Alcoholism*, pp. xv-xvi. New York: Bobbs-Merrill, 1967.

100. Frohman, C., Luby, E.D., Tourney, G., Beckett, P.G.S., & Gottlieb, J.S. Steps towards isolation of a serum factor in schizophrenia. *American Journal of Psychiatry*, 117, 401-408, 1960.

101. Fulcher, J.H., Gallagher, W.J., & Pfeiffer, C.C. Comparative lucid intervals after amobarbital, CO_2, and arecoline in the chronic schizophrenic. *Archives of Neurology and Psychiatry*, 78, 392-395, 1957.

102. Galanter, M. *Cults and New Religious Movements*. Washington, DC: American Psychiatric Press, 1989.

103. Gaylin, W.M. Joel S. Meister, and Robert C. Neville. *Operating on the Mind. The Psychosurgery Conflict*. New York: Basic Books, 1975.

104. Gilbert, G., Wagner-Jauregg, T., & Steinberg, G.M. Hydroxamic acids: Relationship between structure and ability to reactivate phosphate-inhibited acetylcholinesterase. *Archives of Biochemistry and Biophysics*, 93, 469-475, 1961.

105. Gillmor, D. *I Swear By Apollo. Dr. Ewen Cameron and the CIA Brainwashing Experiments*. Montreal: Eden Press, 1987.

106. Goldberger, L. Cognitive test performance under LSD-25, placebo and isolation. *Journal of Nervous and Mental Disease*, 142, 4-9, 1966.

107. Goldby, S. Experiments at the Willowbrook State School. *The Lancet*, April 10, 749, 1971.

108. Goldstein, L., Murphree, H.B., & Pfeiffer, C.C. Quantitative electroencephalography in man as a measure of CNS stimulation. *Annals of the New York Academy of Sciences*, 107, 1045-1056, 1963.

109. Goldstein, L., Murphree, H.B., Sugarman, A.A., Pfeiffer, C.C., & Jenney, E.H. Quantitative electroencephalographic analysis of naturally occurring (schizophrenic) and drug-induced psychotic states in human males. *Clinical Pharmacology and Therapeutics*, 4, 10-21, 1963.

110. Hanley, J., Zweizig, J.R., Kado, R.T., Adey, W.R., & Rovner, L.D. Combined telephone and radiotelemetry of the EEG. *Electroencephalography and Clinical Neurophysiology*, 26, 323-324, 1969.

111. Harriman, P.L. The experimental induction of a multiple personality. *Psychiatry*, 5, 179-186, 1942.

112. Harriman, P.L. The experimental production of some phenomena related to multiple personality. *Journal of Abnormal and Social Psychology*, 37, 244-255, 1942.

113. Harriman, P.L. A new approach to multiple personalities. *American Journal of Orthopsychiatry*, 13, 638-643, 1943.

114. Harris, T.G. Sirhan B. Sirhan. *Psychology Today*, 3, 48-55, 1969.

115. Hearst, P. *Patty Hearst. Her Own Story.* New York: Avon Books, 1982.

116. Heath, R.G. Electrical self-stimulation of the brain in man. *American Journal of Psychiatry*, 120, 571-577, 1963.

117. Heath, R.G. Factors altering brain function and behavior in schizophrenia. *Psychiatric Research Reports*, 19, 178-191, 1964.

118. Heath, R.G. Pleasure and brain activity in man. Deep and surface electroencephalograms during orgasm. *Journal of Nervous and Mental Disease*, 151, 3-18, 1972.

119. Heath, R.G. Modulation of emotion with a brain pacemaker: Treatment for intractable psychiatric illness. *Journal of Nervous and Mental Disease*, 165, 300-317, 1977.

120. Heath, R.G., Guerrero-Figueroa, R. Psychotic behavior with evoked septal dyrythmia: Effects of intracerebral acetylcholine and gamma aminobutyric acid. *American Journal of Psychiatry*, 121, 1080-1086, 1965.

121. Heath, R.G., John, S.B., & Fontana, C.J. Stereotaxic implantation of electrodes in the human brain: A method for long-term study and treatment. *IEEE Transactions on Biomedical Engineering*, 23, 296-304, 1976.

122. Heath, R.G., Monroe, R.R., & Lief, H.I. The integration of psychiatric and psychoanalytic training at Tulane: A ten-year review. *Journal of Medical Education*, 36, 857-874, 1961.

123. Heath, R.G., Martens, S., Leach, B.E., Cohen, M., & Angel, C. Effect on behavior in humans of the administration of taraxein. *American Journal of Psychiatry*, 114, 14-24, 1957.

124. Heath, R.G., Martens, S., Leach, B.E., Cohen, M., & Feigley, C.A. Behavioral changes in nonpsychotic volunteers following the administration of taraxein, the substance obtained from serum of schizophrenics. *American Journal of Psychiatry*, 114, 917-920, 1958.

125. Heims, S.J. *The Cybernetics Group*. Massachusetts: The MIT Press, 1991.

126. Hinkle, L.E., & Wolff, H.G. Communist interrogation and indoctrination of "enemies of the state." *Archives of Neurology and Psychiatry*, 76, 115-174, 1956.

127. Hinkle, L.E., Kane, F.D., Christenson, W.N., & Wolff, H. Hungarian refugees: Life experiences and features influencing participation in the revolution and subsequent flight. *American Journal of Psychiatry*, 116, 16-19, 1959.

128. Hinkle, L.E., Plummer, N, Metraux, R., Richter, P., Gittinger, J.W., Thetford, W.N., Ostfeld, A.M., Kane, F.D., Goldberger, L., Mitchell, W.E., Leichter, H., Pinsky, R., Goebel, D., Bross, I.D.J., and Wolff, H.G. Studies in human ecology. *American Journal of Psychiatry*, 114, 212-220, 1957.

129. Hoagland, H. Donald Ewen Cameron 1901-1967. *Recent Advances in Biological Psychiatry*, 10, 321322, 1967.

130. Hoch, P.H. Remarks on LSD and mescaline. *Journal of Nervous and Mental Disease*, 125, 442-444, 1957

131. Hoch, P.H., Cattell, J.P, & Pennes, H.H. Effects of mescaline and lysergic acid. *American Journal of Psychiatry*, 108, 579-584, 1952.

132. Hoffer, A. A program for treatment of alcoholism: LSD, malvaria and nicotinic acid. In H. Abramson (Ed.), *the Use of LSD in Psychotherapy and Alcoholism*, pp. 343-406. New York: Bobbs-Merrill Company, 1967.

133. Hoffer, A., Osmond, H. the adenochrome model and schizophrenia. *Journal of Nervous and Mental Disease*, 128, 18-35, 1959.

134. Howard, J. *Margaret Mead. A Life.* New York: Simon and Schuster, 1984.

135. Hunt, L. *Secret Agenda. The United States Government, Nazi Scientists, and Project Paperclip, 1945 to 1990.* New York: St. Martin's Press, 1991.

136. Hunter, E. *Brain Washing in Red China. The Calculated Destruction of Men's Minds.* New York: Vanguard Press, 1951.

137. Huxley, A. *Brave New World.* New York: Harper, 1932/1998.

138. Hyde, H.M. *Room 3603. The Story of the British Intelligence Center in New York During World War II.* New York: Farrar, Straus and Giroux, 1962.

139. Hyde, H.M. *Cynthia.* New York: Farrar, Straus and Giroux, 1965.

140. Jeffreys-Jones, R. *The CIA and American Democracy.* New York: Yale University Press, 1989.

141. Jones, J.H. *Bad Blood.* New York: The Free Press, 1981.

142. Jones, J. *Let Me Take You Down. Inside the Mind of Mark David Chapman, The Man Who Shot John Lennon.* New York: Villard Books, 1992.

143. Kaiser, R.B. *R.F.K. Must Die. A History of the Robert Kennedy Assassination and Its Aftermath. New York: E.P. Dutton, 1970.*

144. Kallman, F.J. Review of psychiatric progress 1947. Heredity and eugenics. *American Journal of Psychiatry*, 105, 448-451, 1948.

145. Kallman, F.J. Review of psychiatric progress 1948. Heredity and eugenics. *American Journal of Psychiatry*, 105, 497-500, 1948.

146. Keith, J. *Secret and Oppressed. Banned Ideas and Hidden History.* Portland, OR: Feral House, 1993.

147. Kelly, G.A. *A Theory of Personality. The Psychology of Personal Constructs.* New York: W.W. Norton, 1955.

148. Kessler, R. *Inside the CIA. Revealing the Secrets of the World's Most Powerful Spy Agency.* New York: Pocket Books, 1992.

149. Kety, S.S., Woodford, R.B., Harmel, M.H., Freyhan, F.A., Appel, K.E., & Schmidt, C.F. Cerebral blood flow and metabolism in schizophrenia. The effects of barbiturate semi-narcosis, insulin coma and electroshock. *Journal of Clinical Investigation*, 27, 476 483, 1948.

150. Kiev, A. (Ed.). *Magic, Faith and Healing.* New York: Collier-Macmillan, 1964.

151. Knapp, A.G., Anderson, J.A. Theory of categorization based on distributed memory storage. *Journal of Experimental Psychology*, 10, 616-637, 1984.

152. Kochakian, C.P. *Hopkins class is told of drugs.* Baltimore Sun, September 9, 1970.

153. Krugman, S. Experiments at the Willowbrook State School. *The Lancet*, May 8, 966-967, 1971.

154. Krugman, S., Giles, J.P., & Hammond, J. Infectious hepatitis. Evidence for two distinctive clinical, epidemiological, and immunological types of infection. *Journal of the American Medical Association*, 200, 365-373, 1967.

155. Lane, M. *Plausible Denial. Was the CIA Involved in the Assassination of JFK?* New York: Thunder's Mouth Press, 1991.

156. Lapon, L. *Mass Murderers in White Coats. Psychiatric Genocide in Nazi Germany and the United States.* Springfield, MA: Psychiatric Genocide Research Institute, 1986.

157. Lawrence, L. *Were we Controlled? The Assassination of President Kennedy.* New Hyde Park, New York: University Books, 1967.

158. Lee, M., & Shlain, B. *Acid Dreams. The Complete Social History of LSD: The CIA, the Sixties, and Beyond.* New York: Grove Weidenfeld, 1985.

159. Lewis, B.M., Sokoloff, L., Wechsler, R.L., Wentz, W.B., & Kety, S.S. Determination of cerebral blood flow using radioactive krypton. *Report No. NADC-MA-5601* (pp. 1-34). Johnsville, PA: U.S. Naval Air Development Command, Feb. 20, 1956.

160. Li, C-L., Baldwin, M. Implanted electrodes in the human brain. *Electroencephalography and Clinical Neurophysiology*, 13, 464-466, 1961.

161. Lief, H.I., Lief, V.F., Warren, C.O., & Heath, R.G. Low dropout rate in a psychiatric clinic. *Archives of General Psychiatry*, 5, 200-211, 1961.

162. Lifton, R.J. Home by ship: Reaction patterns of American prisoners repatriated from North Korea. *American Journal of Psychiatry*, 110, 732-739, 1954.

163. Lifton, R.J. Thought reform of Chinese intellectuals: A psychiatric evaluation. *Journal of Social Issues*, 3, 5-20, 1957.

164. Lifton, R.J. Chinese Communist "thought reform:" Confession and re-education of western civilians. *Bulletin of the New York Academy of Sciences*, 33, 626-644, 1957.

165. Lifton, R.J. Psychiatric aspects of Chinese Communist thought reform. *Group for the Advancement of Psychiatry, Symposium No. 4*, 234-249, 1957.

166. Lifton, R.J. *Thought Reform and the Psychology of Totalism.* Chapel Hill: University of North Carolina Press, 1961.

167. Lilly, J.C. Factors used to increase the susceptibility of individuals to forceful indoctrination: Observations and experiments. *Group for the Advancement of Psychiatry*, 3, 89-90, 1956.

168. Lilly, J.C. Mental effects of reduction of ordinary levels of physical stimuli on intact, healthy persons. *Psychiatric Research Reports*, 5, 1-9, 1956

169. Lilly, J.C. Dolphin-human relation and LSD. In H. Abramson (Ed.), *The Use of LSD in Psychotherapy and Alcoholism*, pp. 47-52. New York: Bobbs-Merrill Company, 1967.

170. Lilly, J.C. *Programming and Metaprogramming in the Human Biocomputer.* New York: Julian Press, 1967.

171. Lilly, J.C. *The Deep Self. Profound Relaxation and the Tank Isolation Technique.* New York: Warner Books, 1978.

172. Lipton, M.A. The relevance of chemically-induced psychoses to schizophrenia. In D.H. Efron (Ed.), *Psychotomimetic Drugs*, pp. 231-239. New York: Raven Press, 1970.

173 Litman, R.E., West, L.J. Research on violence: The ethical equation. In N. Burch & H.L. Altshuler (Eds.), *Behavior and Brain Electrical Activity*, pp. 525-539, 1975.

174. MacLean, J.R., MacDonald, D.C., Ogden, F., & Wilby, E. LSD 25 and mescaline as therapeutic adjuvants. In H. Abramson (Ed.), *The Use of LSD in Psychotherapy and Alcoholism*, pp. 4070429. New Yorl: Bobbs-Merrill Company, 1967.

175. Malamud, W., Overholser, W. Multidisciplinary research in schizophrenia. *American Journal of Psychiatry*, 114, 865-872, 1958.

176. Malamud, W., Hoaglund, H., & Kaufman, I.C. A new psychiatric rating scale. *Psychosomatic Medicine*, 8, 243-245, 1946.

177. Malitz, S. The role of mescaline and DO lysergic acid in psychiatric treatment. *Diseases of the Nervous System*, 27, 39-42, 1966.

178. Malitz, S. Paul Hoch, 1902-1964. *American Journal of Psychiatry*, 153, 1339, 1996.

179. Malitz, S., Esecover, H., Wilkens, B., & Hoch, P.H. Some observations on psilocybin, a new hallucinogen, in volunteer subjects. *Comprehensive Psychiatry*, 1, 8-17, 1960.

180. Malmo, R.B., Smith, A.A., & Kohlmeyer, W.A. Motor manifestations of conflict in interview: A case study. *Journal of Abnormal and Social Psychology*, 52, 268-271, 1956.

181. Mandell, A., West, L.J. Hallucinogens. In A.M. Freedman & H.I. Kaplan (Eds.), *Human Behavior: Biological, Psychological, and Sociological*, pp. 480-491. New York: Athenium, 1967.

182. Mangold, T. *Cold Warrior. James Jesus Angleton: The CIA's Master Spy Hunter.* New York: Published by Simon & Schuster, 1991.

183. Mark, V.H., & Ervin, F.R. *Violence and the Brain.* New York: Harper & Row, 1970.

184. Marks, J. *The Search for the Manchurian Candidate.* New York: W.W. Norton, 1988.

185. Marrazzi, A.S. An experimentalist looks at psychiatry. *Recent Advances in Biological Psychiatry*, 7, 143-161, 1965.

186. Marrazzi, A.S., Meisch, R.A., Pew, W.L., & Beiter, T.G. Quantified LSD effects on ego strength. *Recent Advances in Biological Psychiatry*, 2, 197-207, 1959.

187. McHugh, P.R., Smith, G.P. Negative feedback in adrenocortical response to limbic stimulation in Macaca Mulatta. *American Journal of Physiology*, 213, 1445-1450, 1967.

188. McHugh, P.R. Resolved: Multiple personality disorder is an individually and socially created artifact. *Journal of the American Academy of Child and Adolescent Psychiatry*, 34, 957-959, 1995.

189. McHugh, P.R. Foreword. In A. Piper, *Hoax and Reality. The Bizarre World of Multiple Personality*, pp. ix-x. Northvale, NJ: Jason Aronson, 1997.

190. Meiers, M. *Was Jonestown a CIA Medical Experiment?* Lewiston: Edwin Mellen Press, 1988.

191. Merskey, H. Multiple personality disorder and false memory syndrome. *British Journal of Psychiatry*, 166, 281-283, 1995.

192. Minsky, M. *The Society of Mind.* New York: Touchstone, 1985.

193. Moan, C.E., Heath, R.G. Septal stimulation for the initiation of heterosexual activity in a homosexual male. *Journal of Behavior Therapy and Experimental Psychiatry*, 3, 23-30, 1972.

194. Monroe, R.R., Heath, R.G., Mickle, W.A., & Llewellyn, R.C. Correlation of rhinencephalic electrograms with behavior. A study on humans under the influence of LSD and mescaline. *Electroencephalography and Clinical Neurophysiology*, 9, 623-642, 1957.

195. Moore, J. Canadian psychiatrists develop beneficial brain-washing. *Weekend Magazine*, 5, 40, 1955.

196. Moore, M. Winfred Overholser, M.D. President 1947-1948. A biographical sketch. *American Journal of Psychiatry*, 105, 10-14, 1948.

197. Morehouse, D. *Psychic Warrior. The True Story of the CIA's Paranormal Espionage Programme.* Michael Joseph, 1996.

198. Morganfield, R. LSD tested at Baylor's med school. *Houston Chronicle*, October 1, 1994, pp. 29.

199. Moss, T. ESP over long distance. *Proceedings of the 11th Parapsychology Conference*, Freiberg, Germany, p. 176-196, 1968.

200. Moss, T. ESP effects in "artists" contrasted with "non-artists." *Journal of Parapsychology*, 33, 57-69, 1969.

201. Moss, T. Telepathy in the waking state. In R. Cavanna (Ed.), *International Conference on Methodology in Psi Research*, pp. 121 142. New York: Parapsychology Foundation, 1970.

202. Moss, T., Gengerelli, J. The effect of belief on ESP success. In J.B. Rhine (Ed.), *Progress in Parapsychology*, pp. 152-169. North Carolina: Seeman, 1971.

203. Moss, T., Johnson, K. Is there an energy body? *Osteopathic Physician*, 39, 27-43, 1972.

204. Moss, T., Schmeidler, G. Quantitative investigation of a "haunted house." *Journal of the American Society of Psychical Research*, 62, 399-410, 1968.

205. Moss, T., Hubacher, J., & Gray, J. Skin vision and telepathy in a blind subject. *Proceedings, Parapsychology Association.* Edinburgh, 1972.

206. Moss, T., Paulson, M., Chang, A., & Levitt, M. Hypnosis and ESP: A controlled experiment. *American Journal of Clinical Hypnosis*, 13, 46-56, 1970.

207. Murphree, H.B., Pfeiffer, C.C., Goldstein, L., Sugerman, A.A., Jenney, E.H. Time-series analysis of the effects of barbiturates on the electroencephalograms of psychotic and nonpsychotic men. *Clinical Pharmacology and Therapeutics*, 8, 830-840, 1967.

208. Myers, W.A., Heath, R.G. Cannabis sativa: Ultrastructural changes in organelles of neurons in brain septal region of monkeys. *Journal of Neuroscience Research*, 4, 9-17, 1979.

209. Narabayashi, H. Stereotaxic amygdalotomy for behavioral and emotional disorders. *Brain Nerve* (Japan) 16 800-804, 1964.

210. Naylor, D. *Mind Control.* Los Angeles: ZM Productions, 1998.

211. Nemeroff, C.B. Morris A. Lipton, M.D., Ph.D. 1915-1989. *American Journal of Psychiatry*, 156, 941-942, 1999.

212. Nickson, E. *The Monkey Puzzle Tree.* Toronto: Alfred A. Knopf, 1994.

213. Ofshe, R., Watters, E. *Making Monsters. False Memories, Psychotherapy, and Sexual Hysteria*. New York: Charles Scribner's, 1994.

214. Ofshe, R.J., Singer, M. Attacks on peripheral versus central elements of self and the impact of thought reforming techniques. *Journal of Cultic Studies*, 3, 3-24, 1986.

215. Orne, M.T. The potential uses of hypnosis in interrogation. In A.D. Biderman (Ed.), *the Manipulation of Human Behavior* (pp. 169-215). New York: John Wiley & Sons, 1961.

216. Orne, M.T. Antisocial behavior and hypnosis: Problems of control and validation in empirical studies. In G.H. Estabrooks (Ed.), *Hypnosis: Current Problems* (pp. 137-192). New York: Harper & Row, 1962.

217. Orne, M.T. Hypnotically induced hallucinations. In L.J. West (Ed.), *Hallucinations* (pp. 211-219). New York: Grune & Stratton, 1962.

218. Orne, M.T. Can a hypnotized subject be compelled to carry out otherwise unacceptable behavior? *International Journal of Clinical and Experimental Hypnosis*, 20, 101-117, 1972.

219. Orne, M.T. Psychotherapy in contemporary America: Its development and context. In D.X. Freedman (Ed.), *American Handbook of Psychiatry, Volume 5, Treatment* (pp. 1-33). New York: Basic Books, 1975.

220. Orne, M.T. The significance of unwitting cues for experimental outcomes: Toward a pragmatic approach. *Annals of the New York Academy of Sciences*, 364, 152-168, 1981.

221. Orne, M.T., Bates, B.L. Reflections on multiple personality disorder: A view from the looking glass of hypnosis past. In A. Kales (Ed.), *Mosaic of Contemporary Psychiatry in Perspective* (pp. 247-260). New York: Springer-Verlag, 1992.

222. Orne, M.T., Dinges, D.F., & Orne, E.C. On the differential diagnosis of multiple personality in the forensic context. *International Journal of Clinical and Experimental Hypnosis*, 32, 118-169, 1984.

223. Orne, M.T., Dinges, D.F., Orne, E.C., & Evans, F.J. *Voluntary Self-Control of Sleep to Facilitate Quasi-Continuous Performance*. Fort Detrick, MD: U.S. Army Medical Research and Development Command. (NTIS No. AD-A102264), 1980.

224. Orne, M.T., Kihlstrom, J.F., Evans, F.J., & Orne, E.C. Attempting to breach posthypnotic amnesia. *Journal of Abnormal Psychology*, 89, 605-616, 1980.

225. Orne, M.T., Pettinati, M.H., Evans, F.J., & Orne, E.C. Restricted use of success cues in retrieval during posthypnotic amnesia. *Journal of abnormal Psychology*, 90, 345-353, 1981.

226. Osmond, H. A comment on some uses of psychotomimetics in psychiatry. In H. Abramson (Ed.), *The Use of LSD in Psychotherapy and Alcoholism*, pp. 430-433. New York: Bobbs-Merrill, 1967.

227. Osmond, H., Cheek, F., Albahary, R., & Sarett, M. Some problems in the use of LSD 25 in the treatment of alcoholism. In H. Abramson (Ed.), *The Use of LSD in Psychotherapy and Alcoholism* (pp. 434-457, 1967.

228. Ostfeld, A., Benjamin, B., Gittinger, J., Goldberger, L., Kane, F.O., Leichter, H.J., Metraux, R., Mitchell, W.E., Pinsky, R.H., Richter, P., Thetford, W.N., Hinkle, L.E., & Wolff, H.G. Factors relative to the occurrence and distribution of illness in a homogeneous population of ostensibly healthy individuals. *Journal of Nervous and Mental Disease*, 124, 405-412, 1956.

229. Overholser, W. Presidential address. *American Journal of Psychiatry*, 105, 1-9, 1948.

230. Overholser, W., Elkes, J. A collaborative research program between Saint Elizabeth's Hospital and National Institutes of Mental Health. *American Journal of Psychiatry*, 116, 465-466, 1959.

231. Overholser, W., Werkman, S.L. Etiology, pathogenesis, and pathology. In *Schizophrenia: A Review of the Syndrome* (pp.82-106). New York: Logos Press, 1958.

232. Pam, A. Biological psychiatry: Science or pseudoscience? In C.A. Ross & A. Pam (Eds.), *Pseudoscience in Biological Psychiatry* (pp. 1-84). New York: John Wiley & Sons, 1995.

233. Pasternak, D. Wonder weapons. *U.S. News and World Report*, July 7, 1997, pp. 38-46.

234. Penfield, W., Baldwin, M. Temporal lobe seizures and the technic of subtotal temporal lobectomy. *Annals of Surgery*, 136, 625-634, 1952.

235. Persinger, M.A. Elicitation of "childhood memories" in hypnosis-like settings is associated with complex partial epileptic-like signs for women but not men: Implications for the false memory syndrome. *Perceptual and Motor Skills*, 78, 643-651, 1994.

236. Pfeiffer, C.C. Parasympathetic neurohumors: Possible precursors and effect on behavior. *International Review of Neurobiology*, 1, 195-244, 1959.

237. Pfeiffer, C.C., Jenney, E.H. The inhibition of the conditioned response and the counteraction of schizophrenia by muscarinic

stimulation of the brain. *Annals of the New York Academy of Sciences*, 96, 753-764, 1962.

238. Pfeiffer, C.C., Smythies, J.R. (Eds.). *International Review of Neurobiology*. New York: Academic Press, 1959.

239. Pfeiffer, C.C., Groth, D.P., & Bain, J.A. Choline versus dimethylyaminoethanol (Deanol) as possible precursors of cerebral acetylcholine. *Recent Advances in Biological Psychiatry*, 1, 259-271, 1958.

240. Pfeiffer, C.C., Goldstein, L., Munoz, C., Murphree, H.B., & Jenney, E.H. Quantitative comparisons of the electroencephalographic stimulant effects of deanol, choline, and amphetamine. *Clinical Pharmacology and Therapeutics*, 4, 461-466, 1963.

241. Pfeiffer, C.C., Murphree, H.B., Jenney, E.H., Robertson, M.G., Randall, A.H., & Bryan, L. Hallucinatory effects in man of acetylcholine inhibitors. *Neurology*, 9, 249-250, 1958.

242. Pinard, G., Young, S.N. McGill University, Department of Psychiatry 50th anniversary. *Journal of Psychiatric Neuroscience*, 4, 141-142, 1993.

243. Piper, A. *Hoax and Reality. The Bizarre World of Multiple Personality Disorder*. Northvale, NJ: Jason Aronson, 1997.

244. Plum, F. Harold G. Wolff 1898-1962. *Journal of Nervous and Mental Disease*, 135, 283-285, 1962.

245. Prange, A.J., Breese, G.R., Jahnke, G.D., Martin, B.R., Cooper, B.R., Cott, J.M., Wilson, I.C., Alltop, L.B., Lipton, M.A., Bissette, G., Nemeroff, C.B., & Loosen, P.T. Modification of pentobarbital effects by natural and synthetic polypeptides: Dissociation of brain and pituitary effects. *Life Sciences*, 16, 1907-1914, 1975.

246. Prince, M. Indigenous Yoruba psychiatry. In A. Kiev (Ed.), *Magic, Faith and Healing* (pp. 84-120). New York: Collier-Macmillan, 1964.

247. Prince, M. *The Dissociation of a Personality*. New York: Oxford University Press, 1905/1978.

248. Prince, R. The Central Intelligence Agency and the origins of transcultural psychiatry at McGill University. *Annals of the Royal College of Physicians and Surgeons of Canada,* Volume 28, Number 7, 407-413, 1995.

249. Prouty, F. *JFK. The CIA, Vietnam, and the Plot to Assassinate John F. Kennedy*. New York: Birch Lane Press, 1992.

250. Reiter, P.J. *Antisocial or Criminal Acts and Hypnosis: A Case Study*. New York: Charles C. Thomas, 1958.

251. Regis, E. *The Biology of Doom. The History of America's Secret Germ Warfare Project*. New York: Henry Holt, 1999.

252. Rinkel, M., Hyde, R.W., Solomon, H.C., & Hoaglund, H. Clinical and physio-chemical observations in experimental psychosis. *American Journal of Psychiatry*, 111, 881-895, 1955.

253. Rockwell, D.H., Yobs, A.R., & Moore, M.B. The Tuskeegee study of untreated syphilis. The 30th year of observation. *Archives of Internal Medicine*, 114, 792-798, 1964.

254. Rogers, C.R. A study of psychotherapeutic change in schizophrenics and normals: the design and instrumentation. *Psychiatric Research Reports*, 15, 51-60, 1962.

255. Ross, C.A. *The Osiris Complex. Case Studies in Multiple Personality Disorder*. Toronto: University of Toronto Press, 1994.

256. Ross, C.A. *Satanic Ritual Abuse. Principles of Treatment*. Toronto: University of Toronto Press, 1995.

257. Ross, C.A. Multiple personality disorder and false memory syndrome. *British Journal of Psychiatry*, 167, 263-264, 1995.

258. Ross, C.A. *Dissociative Identity Disorder. Diagnosis, Clinical Features, and Treatment of Multiple Personality, Second Edition*. New York: John Wiley & Sons, 1997.

259. Ross, C.A. Subpersonalities and multiple personalities: A dissociative continuum? In J. Rowan & M. Cooper (Eds.), *The Plural Self. Multiplicity in Everyday Life* (pp. 183-197). Thousand Oaks, CA: Sage Publications, 1999.

260. Ross, C.A. Dissociative disorders. In T. Millon, P. Blaney, & R. Davis (Eds.), *Oxford Textbook of Psychopathology*. New York: Oxford University Press, in press.

261. Rosvold, H.E., Delgado, J.M.R. The effect of delayed-alternation test performance of stimulating or destroying electrical structures within the frontal lobes of the monkey's brain. *Journal of Comparative and Physiological Psychology*, 49, 365-372, 1956.

262. Salinger, J.B. *Catcher in the Rye*. New York, Bantam Books, 1964.

263. Sands, S.L., Malamud, W. A rating scale analysis of the clinical effects of lobotomy. *American Journal of Psychiatry*, 106, 760-766, 1949.

264. Saltzberg, B., Burch, N.R. Period analytic estimates of moments of the power spectrum: A simplified EEG time domain procedure. *Electroencephalography and Clinical Neurophysiology*, 30, 568-570, 1971.

265. Saltzberg, B., Heath, R.G. Electroencephalographic waveform analyses and data compression: Computer technics. *Bulletin of the Tulane Medical Faculty*, 25, 255-265, 1966.

266. Saltzberg, B., Heath, R.G., & Edwards, R.J. EEG spike detection in schizophrenic research. *Digest of the Seventh International Conference on Medical and Biological Engineering* (pp. 266). Stockholm, August 1967.

267. Saltzberg, B., Lustick, L.S., & Heath, R.G. Detection of focal depth spiking in the scalp EEG of monkeys. *Electroencephalography and Clinical Neurophysiology*, 31, 327-333, 1971.

268. Saltzberg, B., Burton, W.D., Barlow, J.S., & Burch, N.R. *Electroencephalography and Clinical Neurophysiology*, 61, 89-93, 1985.

269. Saltzberg, B., Burton, W.D., Burch, N.R., Ewing, C.L., Thomas, D.J., Weiss, M., Berger, M.D., Jessop, E., Sances, A., Walsh, P.R., Myklebust, J., & Larson, S.J. Evoked potential studies of the effects of impact acceleration on the motor nervous system. *Aviation, Space, and Environmental Medicine*, 54, 1100-1110, 1983.

270. Saltzberg, B., Burton, W.D., Burch, N.R., Fletcher, J., & Michaels, R. Electrophysiological measures of regional interactive coupling. Linear and non-linear dependence relationships among multiple channel electroencephalographic recordings. *International Journal of Bio-Medical Computing*, 18, 77-87, 1986.

271. Saltzberg, B., Heath, R.G., Fortner, C.M., & Edwards, R.J. Coded stimulation of the eighth nerve as a means of investigating auditory memory. *Recent Advances in Biological Psychiatry*, 10, 240-248, 1967.

272. Sarbin, T.R. On the belief that one body may be host to two or more personalities. *International Journal of Clinical and Experimental Hypnosis*, 43, 163-183, 1995.

273. Sargant, W. *Battle For the Mind*. Garden City, NY: Doubleday, 1957.

274. Sarwer-Foner, G.J. On the mechanisms of action of neuroleptic drugs: A theoretical psychodynamic explanation. The Hassan Azima Memorial Lecture. *Recent Advances in Biological Psychiatry*, 6, 244-257, 1963.

275. Savage, C.W., Harman, W., Savage, E., & Fadiman, J. Therapeutic effects of the LSD experience. *Psychological Reports*, 14, 111-120, 1964.

276. Schachter, D.L. *Searching for Memory. The Brain, The Mind, and the Past*. New York: Basic Books, 1996.

277. Scheflin, A. Freedom of the mind as an international human rights issue. *Human Rights Law Journal*, 3, 3-63, 1982.

278. Scheflin, A.W., & Opton, E.M. *The Mind Manipulators*. New York: Paddington Press, 1978.

279. Schein, E.H. Epilogue: Something new in history? *Journal of Social Issues*, 13, 56-60, 1957.

280. Schnabel, J. *Remote Viewers: The Secret History of America's Psychic Spies*. New York: Dell, 1997.

281. Segal, J. Correlates of collaboration and resistance behavior among U.S. army POWs in Korea. *Journal of Social Issues*, 13, 31-40, 1957.

282. Shapiro, S. Experiments at the Willowbrook State School. *The Lancet*, May 8, 967, 1971.

283. Shor, R.E. On the physiological effects of painful stimulation during hypnotic analgesia: Basic issues for further research. In G.H. Estabrooks (Ed.), *Hypnosis: Current Problems* (pp. 54-75). New York: Harper & Row, 1962.

284. Shor, R.E., Orne, M.T. (Eds.). *The Nature of Hypnosis: Selected Basic Readings*. New York: Holt, Rinehart & Winston, 1965.

285. Siegel, R.K., West, L.J. *Hallucinations. Behavior, Experience, and Theory*. New York: John Wiley & Sons, 1975.

286. Silva, F., Heath, R.G., Rafferty, T., Johnson, R., & Robinson, W. Comparative effects of the administration of taraxein, d-LSD, mescaline, and psilocybin to human volunteers. *Comprehensive Psychiatry*, 1, 370-376, 1960.

287. Simpson, C. *Blowback. The First Full Account of America's Recruitment of Nazis, and its Disastrous Effect on Our Domestic and Foreign Policy*. New York: Weidenfeld and Nicolson, 1988.

288. Simpson, C. *The Splendid Blonde Beast. Money, Law, and Genocide in the Twentieth Century*. New York: Grove Press, 1993.

289. Singer, M. *Cults in Our Midst. The Hidden Menace in Our Everyday Lives*. San Francisco: Jossey-Bass, 1995.

290. Singer, M.T., Ofshe, R. Thought reform programs and the production of psychiatric casualties. *Psychiatric Annals*, 20, 188-193, 1990.

291. Smith, R.H. *OSS. The Secret History of America's First Central Intelligence Agency*. Berkeley: University of California Press, 1972.

292. Smith, R.J. *The Unknown CIA. My Three Decades with the Agency*. New York: Berkeley Books, 1989.

293. Sokoloff, L., Perlin, S., Kornetsky, C., & Kety, S.S. Effects of lysergic acid diethylamide on cerebral circulation and metabolism in man. *Federation Proceedings*, 15, 174, 1956.

294. Sokoloff, L., Perlin, S., Kornetsky, C., & Kety, S.S. The effects of d-lysergic acid diethylamide on cerebral circulation and over-all metabolism. *Annals of the new York Academy of Sciences*, 66, 468-477, 1957.

295. Spiegel, H. Foreword. In D. Bain, *The Control of Candy Jones* (pp. ix-xi). Chicago: Playboy Press, 1976.

296. Spiegel, H. , Spiegel, D. *Trance and Treatment*. New York: Basic Books, 1976

297. Stevenson, W. *A Man Called Intrepid: The Secret War*. New York: Harcourt Brace Jovanovich, 1976.

298. Stover, E. & Nightingale, E.O. *The Breaking of Bodies and Minds. Torture, Psychiatric Abuse, and the Health Professionals -* New York: W.H. Freeman, 1985.

299. Tapscott, M. DOD, intel agencies look at Russian mind control technology, claims. *Defense Electronics*, July 13, 1993, pp. 17.

300. Thigpen, C.H., Cleckley, H.M. *The Three Faces of Eve*. New York: McGraw-Hill, 1957.

301. Thomas, G. *Journey into Madness. The Secret Story of Secret CIA Mind Control and Medical Abuse*. New York: Bantam, 1989.

302. Troy, T.F. *Wild Bill and Intrepid. Donovan, Stephenson, and the Origin of the CIA*. New Haven: Yale University Press, 1996.

303. Turner, W. & Christian, J. *The Assassination of Robert F. Kennedy. The Conspiracy and the Coverup*. New York: Thunder's Mouth Press, 1993.

304. Tyhurst, J.S. Individual reactions to community disaster. *American Journal of Psychiatry*, 107, 764-769, 1951.

305. Tyhurst, J.S., Richman, A. An evaluation of the clinical significance of reserpine. *Journal of Nervous and Mental Disease*, 122, 492-497, 1955.

306. Valentine, D. *The Phoenix Program*. New York: Avon Books, 1990.

307. Vankin, J. *Conspiracies, Crimes, and Coverups. Political Manipulation and Mind Control in America*. New York: Paragon House, 1991.

308. Volkman, E. & Baggett, B. *Secret Intelligence. The Inside Story of America's Espionage Empire*. New York: Berkeley Books, 1989.

309. Vonderlehr, R.A., Clark, T., Wenger, O.C., & Heller, J.R. Untreated syphilis in the male Negro. A comparative study

of treated and untreated cases. *Journal of the American Medical Association*, 107, 856-859, 1936.

310. Wasson, R.G. *Soma: Divine Mushroom of Immortality.* San Diego: Harcourt Brace Jovanovich, 1973.

311. Watson, R., Glick, D., Hosenball, M., McCormick, J., Murr, A., Begley, S., Miller, S., Carroll, G., & Keene-Osborn, S. America's nuclear secrets. *Newsweek*, December 27, 1993, pp. 14-18.

312. Weberman, A.J. & Canfield, M. *Coup D'Etat in America. The CIA and the Assassination of John F. Kennedy.* San Francisco: Quick American Archives, 1992.

313. Weinstein, H. *Psychiatry and the CIA: Victims of Mind Control.* Washington, DC: American Psychiatric Press, 1990.

314. Weissman, M.M. Daniel X. Freedman, MD August 17, 1921 to June 3, 1993. *Archives of General Psychiatry*, 50, 665-668, 1993.

315. West, L.J. United States Air Force prisoners of the Chinese communists. Methods of forceful indoctrination: Observations and interviews. *Group for the Advancement of Psychiatry Symposium*, 4, 270-284, 1957.

316. West, L.J. Brainwashing. In A. Deutsch (Ed.), *The Encyclopedia of Mental Health, Volume 1*, pp. 250-257. New York: Franklin Watts, 1963.

317. West, L.J. Sensory isolation. In A. Deutsch (Ed.), *the Encyclopedia of Mental Health, Volume 1*, pp. 1837-1841. New York: Franklin Watts, 1963.

318. West, L.J. Hypnosis in medical practice. In H.I. Lief, V.F. Lief, & N.R. Lief (Eds.), *The Psychological Basis of Medical Practice*, pp. 510-520. New York: Harper & Row, 1963.

319. West, L.J. Monkeys and brainwashing. In H. Harlow (Ed.), *Psychiatric Spectator*, 2, 21-22, 1964.

320. West, L.J. Psychiatry, "brainwashing," and the American character. *American Journal of Psychiatry*, 120, 842-850, 1964.

321. West, L.J. Dissociative reactions. In A.M. Freedman & H.I. Kaplan (Eds.), *Comprehensive Textbook of Psychiatry*, pp. 885-889. Baltimore: Williams and Wilkins, 1967.

322. West, L.J. Psychobiology of racial violence. *Archives of General Psychiatry*, 16, 645-651, 1967.

323. West, L.J. Campus unrest and the counter culture. *The Academy*, 14, 7-8, 10-11, 1970.

324. West, L.J. Contemporary cults: Utopian image, infernal reality. *The Center Magazine*, 15, 10-13, 1982.

325. West, L.J. Cults, liberty, and mind control. In D.C. Rapoport & Y. Alexander (Eds.), *The Rationalization of Terrorism*, pp. 101-108. Frederick, MD: Alethia Books, University Publications of America, 1982.

326. West, L.J. Persuasive techniques in contemporary cults. In M. Galanter (Ed.), *Cults and New Religious Movements*, pp. 165-192. Washington, DC: American Psychiatric Press, 1989.

327. West, L.J., Allen, J.R. Hippie culture. *Psychiatric Spectator*, 5, 8-9, 1968.

328. West, L.J., Martin, P. Pseudo-identity and the treatment of personality change in victims of captivity and cults. In S.J. Lynn & J.W. Rhue (Eds.), *Dissociation. Clinical and Theoretical Perspectives*, pp. 268-288. New York: Guilford, 1994.

329. West, L.J., Singer, M.T. Cults, quacks, and nonprofessional psychotherapies. In H.I. Kaplan, A.M. Freedman, & B.C. Sadock (Eds.), *Comprehensive Textbook of Psychiatry*, pp. 3245-3258. Baltimore: Williams and Wilkins, 1980.

330. West, L.J., Pierce, C.M., & Thomas, W.D. Lysergic acid diethylamide: Its effects on a male asiatic elephant. *Science*, 138, 1100-1103, 1962.

331. Westbrook, C.R. *The Dual Linguistic Heritage of Afro-Americans*. M.A. Thesis, Berkeley: University of California, Berkeley, 1971.

332. Wheat, R.P., Zuckerman, A., & Rantz, L.A. Infection due to chromobacteria. *Archives of Internal Medicine*, 88, 461-466, 1951.

333. Winn, D. *The Manipulated Mind*. London: The Octagon Press, 1983.

334. Wolff, H.G. Factors used to increase the susceptibility of individuals to forceful indoctrination: Observations and experiments. *Group for the Advancement of Psychiatry*, 3, 123-129, 1956.

IV. APPENDICES

APPENDIX A

G.H. ESTABROOKS DOCUMENTS

JOHN EDGAR HOOVER
DIRECTOR

Federal Bureau of Investigation
United States Department of Justice
Washington, D. C.

July 12, 1939.

Dr. G. H. Estabrooks
Placement Bureau
Colgate University
Hamilton, New York

Dear Dr. Estabrooks:

Permit me to acknowledge receipt of your letters of June 19th and 27th and July 6th, 1939. I read with great interest the hypothesis which you put forth concerning the sinking of submarines. I realize, of course, that you are only suggesting things that could conceivably happen upon the basis of your experiments and the experimentation of others and that you are not suggesting that such a situation actually did occur in any of the recent submarine disasters.

I appreciate your interest in forwarding these theories to me and your letters are being retained in file for possible future reference in connection with the general subject matter of hypnotism.

Sincerely yours,

J. E. Hoover

OFFICE OF THE DIRECTOR

UNITED STATES DEPARTMENT OF JUSTICE

FEDERAL BUREAU OF INVESTIGATION

WASHINGTON 25, D.C.

March 7, 1962

Dr. G. H. Estabrooks
Department of Psychology
Colgate University
Hamilton, New York

Dear Dr. Estabrooks:

Your letter of February 27th, with enclosures, has been received, and it was good of you to advise me of the symposium you have scheduled. I appreciate your inviting us to participate; however, the pressure of official business will not permit me to designate a representative to attend.

Sincerely yours,

J. Edgar Hoover

JRM NO. C.P.—17

WAR DEPARTMENT
OFFICE OF THE SECRETARY
WASHINGTON, D. C.

Oath. March 19/42

Date: February 20, 1942

Name   George H. Estabrooks

NATURE OF ACTION: Excepted Appointment

Effective Date:

	From	To
Position		Expert Consultant to the Secretary of War without other compensation, with the payment of actual transportation expenses and not to exceed $10 per diem in lieu of subsistence and other expenses.
..de & Salary		
Bureau		
Org. Unit		
Station		
Payroll		
Departmental or Field		DEPARTMENTAL

Remarks:

By order of the Secretary of War

John H. Martin

jeg—8

CSC Report No.

Pub. 139
77th Cong.

Civil Service or
other Legal
Authority

Regular

Appropriation:

Date of Birth:

Legal Residence

Sex

Male

NATURE OF POSITION

NEW	ADDNL. IDEX.
VICE	VICE VACANCY

REFERENCE (Name, No. etc.)

COORDINATOR OF INFORMATION

WASHINGTON, D. C.

January 27, 1942

Professor G. H. Estabrooks
Department of Psychology
Colgate University
Hamilton, New York

Dear Professor Estabrooks:

We are very willing, indeed, to examine your plans
on the possibility of applying hypnotism to certain
problems of modern warfare. In your previous letter
to Colonel Donovan you mentioned some detailed
plans you have worked out. I would suggest that you
forward them to us and hope that you will not hesitate to go into the technical details necessary for
us to study your proposal.

Sincerely yours

Robert C. Tryon, Chief
Psychology Division

August 22, 1961

Martin T. Orne, M.D., Ph.D., Director
Harvard Medical School
Department of Psychiatry
Studies in Hypnosis Project
74 Fenwood Road
Boston 15, Massachusetts

Dear Martin:

I am sending to thee a special delivery; one halo, pure gold, one pair of wings which you can try on for size, and a credit card for use in the hereafter.

Your article is of course excellent. Upon receipt of your letter, I immediately called Middendorf and he informed me before I could even broach the subject that they would of course grant your request for reprints. Some day I am going to have myself examined and find out why I do not consider these matters before I embarass my friends.

By the way, I will be at the APA meetings Friday and Saturday, September 1 and 2. Then I have to whip back here and head south. If at all possible, I will hold up at the Biltmore. If you and Ron are anywhere in the vicinity, let me sit down and yak at each other. I am not overlooking the fact that our meeting at Cambridge with yourself and Ron sort of crystallized an idea in my mind.

I had a wonderful month's vacation in Canada, Toronto, Ottowa, Quebec City, Murray Bay, St. John, New Brunswick and home. We particularly like the french country. My wife's native language is French, although she speaks Italian, English, and German as well. I find that with her along the red carpet is literally rolled out, and we seek corners of the back country where they would set the dogs on me if I happened to turn up alone.

Thank you tremendously. Hope to see you at the APA. My best regards to Ron.

Sincerely yours,

G. H. Estabrooks

GHE:er

Colgate University Symposium on Hypnosis

APRIL 1 - 2, 1960

HAMILTON, N. Y.

PROGRAM

Friday, April 1, 9 A. M., Symposium opens, welcomed by the Dean or President. Matters of business. Opening address by G. H. Estabrooks, Chairman. (10 minutes).

9:30 A. M. — E. R. Hilgard, "Lawfulness with Hypnotic Phenomena."

10:30 A. M. — Coffee break

11:00 A. M. — R. E. Shor, "Physiological Responses to Painful Stimulation."

12:30 P. M. — Lunch - Colgate Student Union

1:30 P. M. — B. E. Gorton, "Current Status of Physiologic Research in Hypnosis."

2:30 P. M. — Seymour Fisher, "Problems in Interpretation and Controls in Hypnotic Research."

3:30 P. M. — Coffee break

4:00 P. M. — L. R. Wolberg, "The Efficacy of Suggestion in Clinical Situations."

5:30 P. M. — Reception by the University

7:00 P. M. — Dinner

8:00 P. M. — M. T. Orne, "Antisocial Behavior and Hypnosis: Problems of Control and Validation in Empirical Studies."

SATURDAY, APRIL 2

9:00 A. M. — M. E. Wright, "Hypnosis and Rehabilitation."

10:00 A. M. — G. H. Estabrooks, The Military Implications of Hypnosis — Methods of Research

11:00 A. M. — Coffee break

11:30 A. M. — M. H. Erickson, "Basic Psychological Processes in Hypnotic Research."

12:30 P. M. — Lunch

1:00 P. M. — Panel Discussion

5:00 P. M. — Reception by the Department of Psychology

7:00 P. M. — Dinner - Smorgasbord

Evening   — Informal program to be arranged.

APPENDIX B
BLUEBIRD AND ARTICHOKE DOCUMENTS

ARTICHOKE DOCUMENT

7 January 1953

<u>Outline of Special H Cases</u>

In all of these cases, these subjects have clearly demonstrated that they can pass from a fully awake state to a deep H controlled state via the telephone, via some very subtle signal that cannot be detected by other persons in the room and without the other individual being able to note the change. It has been shown clearly that physically individuals can be induced into H by telephone, by receiving written matter, or by the use of code, signals, or word and that control of those hypnotized can be passed from one individual to another without great difficulty. It has also been shown by experimentation with these girls that they can act as unwilling couriers for information purposes and that they can be conditioned to a point where they can believe a change in identity on their part even on the polygraph.

ADDITIONAL NOTES

1   We know the man was unconscious during sleep because you could touch your fingers to his eyes without response.

2   He could not possibly have lied during the _____ (even if he were a pathological liar). Everything he said during that state was true to him: If anything he thus said were actually false to fact, it would show him to have been mistaken, or psychotic <u>not lying!</u>

3   The Subject maintained an honestly friendly attitude toward us - <u>due to his amnesia</u>. If this has since changed, it would have been due to one thing only - someone having told him that we extracted information from him. I hope and pray that this has not happened.

4   From a medical point of view, Subject was definitely under total effect from the medication. In my opinion, he was not faking, acting or any combination thereof.

There was no indication, physically or mentally, that Subject had been "conditioned" either by H processes or via administration of drugs by another agency prior to our interrogation.

TO   :   Director of Security

VIA   :   Deputy Director of Security
VIA   :   Chief, Security Research Staff
FROM   :   ▓▓▓▓▓▓

SUBJECT: Report of ARTICHOKE Operations, 20 to 23 January 1955.

1. Between Thursday, 20 January, and Sunday, 23 January 1955, the SO ARTICHOKE Team conducted a special operation ▓▓▓▓▓▓▓▓▓▓▓▓ In the opinion of team members and participating case officers of the ▓▓▓▓▓▓, the ARTICHOKE operation was successful. Details follow:

2. It should be noted at this point that because these operations were the first ARTICHOKE operations undertaken in the United States the full names of those participating are omitted from this report and will not be revealed without consent of the Security Office. First names, titles or pseudonyms will be used throughout this report.

3. In view of the highly sensitive nature of the ARTICHOKE techniques and in view of the fact that this was the first ARTICHOKE operation carried out in the United States, the operation was conducted ▓▓▓▓▓▓▓▓▓▓▓▓▓▓▓▓▓▓▓▓▓▓▓▓▓▓▓▓▓▓ This safe house is far removed from surrounding neighbors in a large tract of land and is thoroughly isolated. A limited and Security-cleared household staff maintained functions of the house and messing was by unwitting ▓▓▓▓ Actual ARTICHOKE operations were, as usual, carried out in a special area on the second floor of the house and neither the household staff nor the ▓▓▓▓▓▓ were permitted in the area during any of the processing. SSD Division furnished one Security Officer during the entire period of the operation to act as special guard and to handle any unusual situations which arose during the operation. This guard is hereinafter referred to as ▓▓▓ in this report.

4. For matter of record, it should be noted that the Subject was not a confinement problem and has been, at all times, fully cooperative. Guard detail was not present in connection with the Subject except in a general sense.

5. Technical matters in the case were handled entirely by the TS/PSD under the personal supervision of ▓▓▓▓▓▓ Full tape recordings were made of the entire case and tapes are to be turned over to the participating Division in the immediate future. It should be noted that

during this particular operation, a special device was used in connection with the recording. This device, which is easily concealable, worked with remarkable efficiency and at no time during the entire recording was there any break due to technical failure. It should also be noted that a complex two-way transmitting-receiving unit was again used in this ARTICHOKE operation.

6. Cover for the actual operation followed standard procedure. The Subject was informed in general terms that before being sent for further work, it was necessary that certain tests be made on him physically and psychologically for our protection as well as his. Hence, a complete physical and psychiatric/psychological examination was required. Subject readily accepted this medical cover and the ARTICHOKE technique was introduced easily and with full consent of the Subject.

THE CASE

7. Prior to the actual commencement of ARTICHOKE operations, a number of conferences had been held with the various participating personnel involved. All hands had been briefed and procedures had been worked out; a general time schedule was prepared and operating instructions for ARTICHOKE were issued.

8. On the afternoon of 20 January, the Subject and Case Officer were met ██ They of the interested Division. Using a covert car, Subject was taken to the ████████ arriving there at approximately 9:30 PM. Prior to this, that is, during the day of Thursday, 20 January, the technical equipment had been checked out and installed and ████████ had arrived at the covert area at approximately 8:00 PM for operational purposes. By previous arrangement, the ████████ was picked up by ████ at approximately 9:30 PM ████████ was brought to the safe house at 10:50 PM.

9. Shortly after the arrival of ████████ a preliminary conference began at approximately 11:10 PM with the Subject, ████████████████ ████████████ At 11:33 PM, the Subject, ████████████████ went to the operations area and a few minutes later the ████████ started a general interrogation relative to Subject's background. This interrogation lasted until 12:25 when all except the Subject ████████ left the operations room. Tape recording was cut off at this time.

10. As a result of this interview, ████████ stated that Subject's mental and physical condition was good and noted that the pulse at 12:20 PM was 120/80. Doctor also commented he had noted an increased amount of talk after a drink of whisky and although there was some nervousness present, it

-2-

was not excessive. ████████ stated he had given Subject two grams Phenobarbital to use in assisting the Subject to sleep and it was later confirmed the Subject had taken these prior to going to sleep.

11. Subject.

Because of this successful penetration and because of the extremely high quality of information which the Subject was obtaining, the case is regarded as most sensitive and important by the participating Division. Since the Subject's information had been checked and cross-checked many times by the operating Division's case officers, the Division was of the uniform opinion that the Subject was fully legitimate and fully cooperating with our efforts. They, however, desired ARTICHOKE to give added assurances to the Subject's story and to help them determine absolute suitability for further use of the Subject in his work. For the record, it should be noted that no polygraph techniques had been applied in this case since a physical examination in ████████ by apparently a cleared physician, had indicated too much nervousness for successful polygraph testing.

12. Following established patterns and using medical cover as explained above, the ████ began the physical-psychological examination at 10:00 AM on the morning of Friday, 21 January. This examination continued until 1:00 PM when an hour was taken for lunch. At 2:00 PM ██ again continued a general examination of the Subject with ████ being used, as before lunch, as interpreter. This examination lasted until 3:00 PM when the ████ concluded the first medical session and a portable polygraph was taken in by ████ for the purpose of polygraph testing.

13. Between 3:00 PM and 4:25 PM,

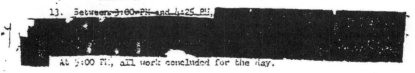

At 5:00 PM, all work concluded for the day.

14. On Saturday, 22 January 1955, Subject had breakfast with ████ and ████ At 9:35 AM, ████ arrived at the gate house and at 9:45 AM, ████ arrived. At 10:35 AM, the Subject, again with ████ acting as interpreter, was examined briefly by

-3-

17. Immediately following the conclusion of the ARTICHOKE treatments, a general conference was held with all hands present and it was agreed at this time that further ARTICHOKE treatments were unnecessary; that results were conclusive and that in view of the Subject's importance, additional work with chemicals or with the H technique might possibly antagonize the Subject and, hence, would be unwarranted and unwise.

18. Following the conclusion of the general discussion, all technical apparatus was removed from the premises and all participating personnel except ██████████ left the area after the ████████ had checked the Subject.

19. On Sunday, 23 January and between 12:00 noon and approximately 1:30 PM, the ████████ returned to the safe house and again re-examined the physical and mental condition of the Subject. At this time, the Subject reported he had slept fairly well but he had a persistent headache. The ████████ pointed out that the headache was a natural consequence of the "examination" and it would gradually disappear. In addition, the ████ wrote a prescription to be picked up in another name which was for future use of the Subject as a general sedative.

20. At 1:50 PM approximately, ██████████████ left the safe house and Subject was turned over for handling to case officers of the participating Division.

CONCLUSIONS

21. In the opinion of the ARTICHOKE team, the operation was profitable and successful. In this case, the Subject was aware that he had been given certain types of solutions but as to what he had been given or amounts given he had no knowledge. Checks made by ████████ and later ████████ apparently indicated that the Subject, although not having specific amnesia for the ARTICHOKE treatment, nevertheless was completely confused and memory was vague and faulty. This vagueness and failure of memory was intensified by the ████████ explanation that the Subject had been dreaming--an opinion which it appears the Subject shared, at least in part.

SPECIAL COMMENTS

22. The work of the case officers of the participating Division in connection with this case was exceptionally good. Their understanding and appreciation of the ARTICHOKE techniques was extremely helpful.

23. The ARTICHOKE team wishes to commend ████████████████ for the expert handling of the support function at the ████████████ which greatly assisted in the development of the ARTICHOKE work.

-5-

MEMO TO THE FILE

1. On 7 January 1955, between 11:00 AM and 12:00 noon, the writer and ████████████████ talked to ████████████████ relative the special case. ████ briefed the writer in detail and answered pertinent questions directed to him by ████████████. At the conclusion of the briefing, ████ stated he would prefer to work on the case the 21st, 22nd, 23rd and 24th of January if a safe area could be arranged. He stated he still preferred working ████████████████████████████████ He also insisted that his name not be mentioned in any way whatsoever since he did not want any leaks in this matter. The writer advised both ████████ and ████████ he felt that as far as security was concerned, those dates were all right and it was proposed the subject be brought ████████████ the evening of Thursday, 20 January with the actual work beginning possibly Friday, the 21st. The writer also asked ████████████ of his feelings in regard to the use of ████████████ for special H work and ████████████ stated he thought that would be interesting and stated he would be willing to assist in connection with this if necessary. The writer informed ████████████ he would brief ████████ Sunday evening at ████████ and check him out as to availability for the 21st, 22nd, 23rd as required.

2. In a subsequent conversation in the writer's car, it was agreed between the writer and ████████████ that it would be necessary for someone to discuss the matter with ████████████████ stated he had to see ████████ for another reason and he would brief him. However, the writer stated he thought it better if ████████ talked with ████████ in connection with briefing ████████ and that ████████ should be present when ████ was briefed.

3. It was agreed that ████████████ would brief in ████████ but that technical details such as ████████████ name, etc. could be omitted from the above mentioned briefing; however, this should be left to the discretion of ████████████. It is suggested that ████████ get in touch with ████████████████████ on Monday and work out details regarding the briefing of both ████████

7 January 1955

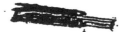

A/0, 2, -/3

TO THE FILES

On 6 April 1954, Tuesday, SI and H experimentation and research was carried on in Building 13 with the following subjects
present: Misses ████████████████████████████   In
addition to Messrs. ████████████████   attended in
a consultant capacity.

The session opened with a slow induction for all hands and
then a subsequent reinduction for M███████████ to enable her to
reconstruct a strange dream she had had the previous week. This
was successful, although in the awake state she could remember no
details.

The major experiment of the evening was then conducted as
follows: Miss ███████ was taken to Room 23 under full hypnosis
and she was instructed by the writer that she would find a Secret
document in or on Mr. ████████████s desk in his room. She was
told she was to conceal this document next to her person and then
return to Room 21 (operation's room), pour herself a drink of water
which she would find on the bookcase and stretch out on the sofa,
face down and go into a deep sleep. She was instructed she would
not awaken under any circumstances. She was told she would only
awaken if someone whispered to her a specific code work and would
recall nothing except sleeping on the couch. ████████ performed
the entire test in exact detail as outlined above and had no subsequent memory whatsoever of any of this activity.

During the experiment, ███████ was taken to the same room
by ███████ and she was told that a person, whom she had never
seen, had taken a Secret document from the Agency. She was told that
this person or the suspected person had been given a drug and was
unconscious on the sofa in Room 21. She was told she was to enter
the room and find the document which would probably be on the person
on the sofa. She was given specific instructions that she must
locate the document. She was told if she found the document to conceal it on her person and return to room 23, sit in the chair and go
at once into a deep sleep. She was further told she would have
no memory of anything except falling asleep. ████████ complied
in specific detail and immediately discovered the document in
████████ sweater sleeve. ████████ concealed the document on
her person, returned to room 23 and at once went into a deep sleep.
Subsequently she was brought back into the operations room and she
and ███████ were awakened. The experiment was carried off
successfully, particularly by ███████ who had entire amnesia

for the work and could not even recall it under hypnosis. ██████ ██████ however, was able to remember certain parts although some of her details seem vague.

This experiment was specifically designed to see if a person ████ ████████ould be disturbed by an unknown person searching her and if a person of a shy retiring nature such as ██████████ould make a body search under hypnosis of another person under hypnosis. Both questions appear to be answered in the affirmative although this, of course, requires additional work.

At the conclusion of this test, another short induction and PH suggestions were removed at this time with the exception that Miss ██████████ was given a PH suggestion that upon awakening she would have an uncontrolled desire to sit in ██████████s lap and all girls, upon entering the cars to go home, would pass into a deep sleep. For matter of record, M██████████did not sit in ██████████ lap and made every effort to avoid so doing. Details are not known why she did not follow through on the suggestion. Insofar as sitting in the cars and going to sleep, everyone with the exception of Miss ██████████responded and again ██████████did not respond to this instruction. An explanation of this cannot be made at present but possibly ██████████did not approve of the idea of sitting in ██████ ██████ap and was refusing all suggestions after the conclusion of the performance. This has not been checked but will be at a later time.

APPENDIX C
MKULTRA CONTRACTS
AND SELECTED DOCUMENTS

The Table of MKULTRA contracts is not complete because some of the information is still classified. The security status of some of the investigators is unknown because it is not clearly stated in the documents. The investigators were probably cleared at TOP SECRET in most or all Subprojects for which security status is not stated.

The amount of money allocated to each Subproject is accurate most of the time. Sometimes the amount is not clear from the documents and a bit of guesswork is required. There are no major errors. The total amount of money funded through MKULTRA was $5,155,623.81.

MKULTRA Contracts

#	Contractor	Status	Institution	Year	Funding Amount	Topic
1		TOP SECRET	Princeton University	1953	$2,000.00	Study of Rivea Corymbosa
2	James Hamilton	TOP SECRET	Stanford University	1953	$4,650.00	Possible synergistic action of drugs which may be appropriate for use in abolishing consciousness
3	George White	TOP SECRET	Bureau of Narcotics	1953	$8,875.00	Construction of a safe house for prostitution
4	John Mulholland		Self-Employed	1953	$4,132.27	Delivery of substances in field operations
5	Alden Sears	TOP SECRET	University of Denver University of Minnesota	1956	$12,139.65	Hypnosis experiments including recall of hypnotically acquired information by very specific signals
6		TOP SECRET	Eli Lilly	1953	$5,000.00	To develop a reliable U.S. source of LSD
7	Harold Abramson	TOP SECRET	Office of Naval Research/ Public Health Service	1953	$90,448.29	LSD
8	Robert Hyde	TOP SECRET	Worcester Foundation for Experimental Biology	1953	$39,500.00	LSD
9	Carl Pfeiffer	TOP SECRET	Emory University/ University of Illinois	1953	$20,889.00	Various sternutatory agents on normal and schizophrenic human beings
10	Robert Hyde	TOP SECRET		1955	$148,515.00	Predicting the effects of LSD
11		TOP SECRET		1953	$11,000.00	Abrus precatorius toxin
12		TOP SECRET		1953	$30,000.00	Erythrina americana/Piscidis erythrina testing on dogs
13			Camp Detrick	1953	$1,000.00	Purchasing of materials/ 'unusual activities'
14	George White	TOP SECRET	Bureau of Narcotics	1953	$3,500.00	Construction of a safe house for prostitution

#	Contractor	Status	Institution	Year	Funding Amount	Topic
15	John Mulholland		Self-Employed	1954	$2,370.00	Continuation of Subproject 4
16	George White	TOP SECRET	Bureau of Narcotics	1953	$7,740.00	Construction of a safe house for prostitution
17	Harold Hodge		University of Denver University of Minnesota	1953	$29,172.00	LSD metabolism
18			Eli Lilly	1953	$400,000.00	Manufacturing LSD
19	John Mulholland		Self-Employed	1954	$1,800.00	Extension of Subproject 4
20		TOP SECRET	Pedlow Nease Chemical Company, Inc.	1953	$205.70	Provide two pounds of Yohimbine
21		TOP SECRET		1955	$5,720.00	Originally to set up a secure pharmacology lab - converted to a study of interrogation of 'returnees'
22	William Boyd Cook	TOP SECRET	Montana State College	1953	$10,261.68	Peyote Studies
23	Charles Geschickter	TOP SECRET	University of Richmond	1953	$42,700.00	Chemical agents which are effective in modifying the behavior and function of the central nervous system
24				1954	$2,900.00	Support for an educational meeting - involved Harold Abramson and Robert Hyde
25	Alden Sears	TOP SECRET	University of Minnesota	1954	$12,360.85	Hypnotic techniques
26	Carl Pfeiffer	TOP SECRET	University of Illinois	1954	$4,781.92	Drugs which may aid in the treatment of the schizophrenic patient
27	Harold Abramson	TOP SECRET	Office of Naval Research	1954	$75,166.40	LSD

#	Contractor	Status	Institution	Year	Funding Amount	Topic
28	Carl Pfeiffer	TOP SECRET	Emory University	1954	$24,996.40	Effects of central nervous system depressant drugs in animals and man
29	Alden Sears	TOP SECRET	University of Denver	1954	$17,388.80	Hypnosis
30			Camp Detrick	1954	$2,699.00	Purchasing material/ unusual activities'
31		TOP SECRET	Pedlow Nease Chemical Company, Inc.	1954	$1,320.00	Production of 2 kg of a rare organic chemical
32		TOP SECRET		1954	$30,000.00	Continuation of Subproject 12
33	Harold Abramson	TOP SECRET	Office of Naval Research	1954	$400.00	Additional costs for Subproject 27
34	John Mulholland		Self-Employed	1954	$1,800.00	Continuation of Subprojects 4,15,19
35	Charles Geschickter	TOP SECRET	Geschickter Fund	1954	$375,000.00	Construction of Gorman annex
36			National Institute of Health/ Public Health Service	1954	$3,000.00	A project involving boarding a freighter and setting up a meeting of some kind with a defector
37				1954	$23,775.00	To provide and grow certain botanicals - macuna/ rhyncosia phaeseolides
38				1954	$1,000.00	Administration of cholorprom-azine, meratron, serpentine, bulbocapnine to humans
39		TOP SECRET	Ionia State Hospital Psychopathic Clinic	1955	$30,000.00	Drug testing on prisoners/ sexual psychopaths including interrogation with hypnosis, LSD, and marijuana

#	Contractor	Status	Institution	Year	Funding Amount	Topic
40	Harold Abramson	TOP SECRET	Office of Naval Research Public Health Service	1955	$41,600.00	Aerosols - blocking of LSD action
41		TOP SECRET	Pedlow Nease Chemical Company, Inc.	1955	$1,500.00	3-6-endoxy-3-methylhexa-hydrophthalic anyhidride N-N-dimethyl-p-phenylene-diamine
42	George White	TOP SECRET	Bureau of Narcotics	1955	$127,110.00	Construction of a safe house for prostitution
43	Louis Jolyon West	TOP SECRET	University of Oklahoma	1956	$20,800.00	Studies of dissociated states
44		TOP SECRET		1955	$16,864.64	Animal models of psychoto-mimetics - human drug testing
45	Charles Geschickter	TOP SECRET	National Institute of Health	1956	$133,000.00	Development of materials and techniques for the production of maximum levels of physical and emotional stress in human beings
46	Harold Hodge	TOP SECRET	Public Health Service	1953	$185,650.00	Radioactive tagging studies of LSD and tetrahydro-cannibinol
47	Carl Pfeiffer	TOP SECRET	New Jersey Neuropsych-iatric Institute/ Emory University/ Atlanta Federal Penitentiary	1955	$45,555.22	LSD testing
48		TOP SECRET	Cornell University	1955	$270,696.00	Study of defector psychology
49	Alden Sears	TOP SECRET	University of Denver	1956	$34,088.60	Hypnosis including hypnotizing unwilling subjects
50			Camp Detrick	1955	$500.00	Petty cash fund related to Subprojects 13 and 30
51	James Moore	TOP SECRET	University of Delaware	1957	$38,502.00	Synthesis and testing of compounds from plants and fungi/ ceremonial mushrooms

#	Contractor	Status	Institution	Year	Funding Amount	Topic
52	James Moore	TOP SECRET	University of Delaware	1958	$57,200.00	Synthesis and consultation on hallucinogens
53		TOP SECRET		1955	$9,300.00	Literature review/ attend a meeting on Russian and U.S. psycho-pharmacology
54		Cleared but level not specified	Office of Naval Research	1955	$62,400.00	A resonance - cavitation model of brain concussion - experiments on cadavers
		Unwitting	National Institutes of Health	1956	$2,808.00	Testing psychoactive drugs
56		TOP SECRET		1956	$$31,616.00	Alcohol intoxication and metabolism
57		TOP SECRET	George Washington University	1956	$32,858.00	Sleep and insomnia studies, including effects of sensory deprivation
58	Gordon Wasson	Unwitting	National Philosophical Society J.P. Morgan and Co., Inc.	1956	$2,080.00	An expedition to collect hallucinogenic mushrooms
59		Unwitting	University of Maryland	1956	$3,900.00	Drug testing
60		TOP SECRET	Human Ecology Fund	1961	$185,607.00	Lip reading/ graphology/a report on "truth drugs"
61	Harold Wolff		Cornell	1956	$138,961.74	Studies of effects of stress on the brain
62	Maitland Baldwin		National Institutes of Health	1956	$9,750.00	Stimulation of monkey's brains by radio frequencies
63	Robert Hyde	TOP SECRET		1961	$5,580.00	Field observations in bars concerning alcohol and psycho-mimetics
64		TOP SECRET		1956	$3,000.00	Drug procurement

#	Contractor	Status	Institution	Year	Funding Amount	Topic
65		TOP SECRET	Cornell University	1956	$76,056.00	Study of defector psychology/ formation of a study group of brainwashing experts
66	Robert Hyde	TOP SECRET	Butler Hospital and Health Center	1956	$24,500.00	Effects of LSD and alcohol
67			University of Indiana	1957	$2,000.00	Library searches
68	Ewen Cameron	Unwitting	McGill University	1957	$38,180.00	The effects upon human behavior of the repetition of verbal signals
69	Ray Stephenson Jay Schulman		Rutgers University	1957	$5,000.00	Sociology of communism Hungarian refugees
70		TOP SECRET	Stanford University	1960	$158,117.93	Fatty acid narcosis/ mechanisms of involuntary sleep
71		TOP SECRET	Stanford University	1959	$9,600.00	Human drug testing - anti interrogation drugs
72		TOP SECRET		1957	$43,037.38	Drug studies
73	Harris Isbell	TOP SECRET	Lexington Kentucky Narcotics Farm	1957	$6,864.00	Hypnosis review - whether drugs can influence hypnotizability
74	Carl Rogers	TOP SECRET	University of Wisconsin	1958	$15,000.00	Biological correlates of emotion in psychotherapy clients
75		Unwitting		1957	$4,160.00	The interaction of personality factors and psychotogenic drugs
76		Unwitting		1957	$10,000.00	A study of anti-authoritarian behavior
77	David Saunders	TOP SECRET	Educational Testing Service	1957	$20,000.00	A study using the Myers-Briggs to determine personality types
78			Bacterial and Pharmaceutical Consultants, Inc.	1962	$70,000.00	Biological warfare research and supply of micro-organisms

#	Contractor	Status	Institution	Year	Funding Amount	Topic
79		TOP SECRET	H.J. Rand Foundation	1957	$1,000.00	To act as a cutout for funding sensitive research
80				1958	$5,000.00	Drug extraction and identification from human tissue
81		Unwitting	Cornell	1958	$5,000.00	A study of immigrant's adjustment
82	H. A. M. Struik	Unwitting	University of Niijmegen Netherlands	1958	$15,000.00	Adaptation of refugees
83		TOP SECRET		1958	$25,000.00	Handwriting analysis
84	Martin Orne	TOP SECRET	Harvard University	1960	$34,000.00	The nature of special states of consciousness and trance states
85		TOP SECRET	Stanford University	1958	$1,040.00	Human blood group research for identification of agents
86		TOP SECRET	Stanford University	1958	$43,734.08	Development of biological response recorders - polygraph/EEG
87			Johns Hopkins University	1958	$3,808.00	Study of potent allergens
88		Unwitting	Princeton University	1958	$5,000.00	An acculturation manual
89		Unwitting		1958	$10,620.00	A study of Hungarian refugees
90		Unwitting	Massachusetts Institute of Technology	1958	$12,000.00	A study of how to recruit foreign scientists as intelligence agents
91		TOP SECRET	Bio-Research, Inc.	1959	$71,760.00	Drug studies on animal models for drugs useful to the CIA based on results of Subprojects 22, 44, 45, 46, 51, 53, 58, 62, 70
92	John Carrol	TOP SECRET	Harvard University	1959	$22,716.62	A teaching machine for foreign languages
93				1959	$14,820.00	Study of bacterial and fungal toxins
94		TOP SECRET	Bio-Research, Inc. Panoramic Research, Inc.	1959	$57,431.82	Brain stimulation studies - remote control of animal behavior

#	Contractor	Status	Institution	Year	Funding Amount	Topic
95	Charles Osgood	TOP SECRET	University of Illinois	1959	$56,500.00	Study of cross-cultural meaning systems
96	George Kelley	TOP SECRET	Ohio State University	1959	$34,465.00	Study of scholarly decision matrices
97	Carl Rogers	TOP SECRET	University of Wisconsin	1959	$8,750.00	Personality change in psychotherapy of schizophrenics
98	Kurt Lang	Unwitting	Queen's College	1959	$9,735.00	Ideological conversion /mass conversion
99		TOP SECRET	Pennsylvania State University	1959	$23,984.00	Studies of drugs active in the central nervous system
100		SECRET	Pennsylvania State University	1960	$271,677.92	Accumulation of pesticides in soil due to rockets and chemical warfare
101		TOP SECRET		1959	$2,000.00	Biologically active materials
102	Muzafer Sherif	Unwitting	University of Oklahoma	1959	$5,750.00	Group psychology of teenage gangs
103	Robert Cormack A.B. Kristofferson	Unwitting	Children's International Summer Villages, Inc.	1959	$1,900.00	Communication in 11-year old children without a common language
104		SECRET	University of Houston	1959	$6,000.00	Isolation of growth factors that greatly increase bacteriological growth useful in time taken to initiate subtle sabotage
105		SECRET	University of Wisconsin	1961	$4,160.00	Studies of staphylococci
106		TOP SECRET	Resources Research, Inc.	1959	$21,855.00	Stimulus - response models in biological systems
107		TOP SECRET	American Psychological Association	1960	$15,000.00	Grant for attending meetings at foreign sites
108		Unwitting		1960	$4,800.00	Ecological factors in a foreign country
109		TOP SECRET		1960	$89,969.60	Drug development of agents to control human behavior

#	Contractor	Status	Institution	Year	Funding Amount	Topic
110			Bacteriological and Pharmaceutical Consultants, Inc.	1960	$210,000.00	Exotic pathogens
111	H.J. Eysenck	Unwitting	University of London	1960	$14,000.00	Measurement of motivation
112	Melvin DeFleur	Unwitting	University of Indiana	1961	$6,056.66	Young children's understanding of occupational roles
113				1960	$3,000.00	Gas-propelled sprays and aerosols
114		COVERT	Butler Hospital and Health Center	1960	$11,280.00	Alcoholic personality
115	Erik Allardt Juhani Mirvas	Unwitting	University of Helsinki	1960	$4,085.50	Interaction of psychiatric patients with the environment
116		SECRET		1961	$74,700.00	Chemical processes/ chemical procurement
117		TOP SECRET	National Institutes of Health	1960	$7,790.00	Cultural influences as brought to bear on children by families
118		COVERT	Pennsylvania State University	1960	$5,000.00	Microbiology consultation
119	Saul Sells	Unwitting	Texas Christian University	1960	$6,370.00	Techniques of activation of the human organism by remote electronic means
120				1964	$21,827.00	Anesthetic agents
121	Raymond Prince	Unwitting	McGill University	1960	$13,850.00	Transcultural study of Yoruba healing methods
122		Unwitting		1960	$2,000.00	Brain studies in cats/neurokinin research
123		Unwitting	Columbia University	1960	$20,000.00	Black male college stereotypes
124	James Hamilton	TOP SECRET	St. Francis Memorial Hospital, San Francisco	1960	$6,500.00	Carbon Dioxide

#	Contractor	Status	Institution	Year	Funding Amount	Topic
125		TOP SECRET	American Psychological Association/ National Institute of Health/ Veterans Administration Center, Martinsburg, West Virginia	1960	$5,102.18	Differential effects of drugs on behavior
126	Charles Fritz	Unwitting	University of Florida/ National Research Council	1960	$4,225.00	Disaster studies
127		Unwitting		1960	$7,490.00	Voting behavior
128				1960	$9,000.00	Rapid hypnotic induction in simulated and real operational settings
129		TOP SECRET	George Washington University Leler University of Georgia	1960	$27,500.00	Bioelectric response patterns
130	William Thetford	TOP SECRET	Columbia University	1960	$13,750.00	Personality theory of conversion hysterics
131				1960	$15,000.00	
132		TOP SECRET	Bureau of Narcotics	1961	$30,000.00	Construction of a safe house for prostitution
133		Unwitting		1961	$10,080.00	Bacteriology Studies
134		Unwitting		1961	$22,000.00	Physique and intelligence
135		Un-witting - David Saunders (Sub-project 77) acted as a consultant under TOP SECRET Clearance		1961	$25,868.00	Skin reactions/ inflammation

#	Contractor	Status	Institution	Year	Funding Amount	Topic
136		Unwitting		1961	$8,579.00	Experimental analysis of extrasensory perception
137		Unwitting		1961	$2,000.00	Graphology
138		Unwitting	University of Texas at Austin	1961	$17,898.00	Biomedical sensors
139		Cleared but level not specified	Pennsylvania State University	1961	$55,670.00	Viral infections - avian vectors
140	James Hamilton	TOP SECRET	St. Francis Memorial Hospital San Francisco	1965	$22,500.00	Human drug tests including cytomel
141				1962	$40,000.00	
142		TOP SECRET		1962	$7,500.00	Electric stimulation of the brain in cold-blooded animals
143	Edward Bennett	TOP SECRET	University of Houston	1963	$41,429.44	Bacterial studies to stimulate bacterial growth
144				1963	$21,000.00	
145				1963	$15,412.80	
146		TOP SECRET		1963	$7,500.00	Anticrop systems - including sugar crops
147				1963	$8,806.72	Cross - tolerance between psychoto-mimetic drugs
148	Harold Hodge	TOP SECRET		1963	$5,000.00	Utilization of professional services of contractor
149	George White	TOP SECRET	Bureau of Narcotics	1964	$10,000.00	Realistic tests of certain development items and delivery systems

50 -12

26 September 1955

MEMORANDUM FOR: THE RECORD

SUBJECT   : MKULTRA Subproject 50

1. This memorandum is written to record the purpose of Subproject 50, the reasons for establishing it, and the mechanics by which it will be administered.

2. The above subproject has been created to continue the support to ███ Division, ████████████ which was previously furnished by Subprojects 13 and 30. Such support will be over and above the yearly financial support of Project MKNAOMI and will fall into two categories: (1) the purchase of certain materials, supplies and equipment where the use of other funds would cause either excessive delay in operations or undue security hazards; and (2) the support of activities in which Agency sponsorship makes it difficult for ██ Division to obtain financial support from normal sources since those sources require an undesirable amount of justification.

3. The subproject has been created at the specific request of Mr. ████████ and with the approval of General ██████ in order to correct undesirable administrative procedures evident in the handling of Subprojects 13 and 30.

4. This subproject will be handled as an imprest fund with an initial grant of $500.00. As expenses are incurred and upon presentation of vouchered proof of expenditure, subsequent grants will be made in the amounts expended. The cash on hand and/or receipts of expenditure will total $500.00 at all times. Instructions to the Fund Custodian are attached.

5. This is a continuing project with no specific amount earmarked per unit time. Budget estimates will be based on experience in Subprojects 13 and 30.

6. Subproject 30 will be closed out and cash on hand will be returned to Finance on receipt of the initial $500.00 grant.

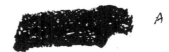

A

Distribution:
  Orig - TSS/CD
    1 - Chrono (b)

TSS/CD ██████ (26 September 1955)

A

Date___9 November 1962___

                                                              IIa, IIIa, IIIb
                                                              IVb, IVc
Branch___BB___   Category__PM Support & Biological ████___( )

Project Title_____N.A.___   Item Classification___Top Secret___

Project Crypto___MKULTRA___   Crypto Classification___Unclassified___

Branch Project No.___N.A.___   Project Engineer___████████___ A

Contractor___████████████████████___ C

Contract No.___Subproject # 78___   Task No.___N.A.___

Type of Contract___MKULTRA___   Date Initiated___September 1958___

Cost___$70,000 00___   Completion Date___Continuing___

Purpose:
     Cut-out for drugs & other materials; development & testing of
anti-material systems, biological hydrogen systems, personnel marking
systems, and BW harassment systems; provides facility for large scale
production of microorganisms; provides general advisory & developmental
service in BW areas.

Status:
     Current in service and fiscal matters.

REQUIREMENT SOURCE:
                Generated by undocumented requests from DDP units
and divisions as well as necessity for TSD to maintain a quick
delivery capability to meet anticipated future operational needs.

MORI ID 17499:17499

96-18
A

DRAFT
22 July 1959

MEMORANDUM FOR: THE RECORD

SUBJECT   : MKULTRA, Subproject No. 96

1. The purpose of this project is twofold: (1) the psychology of personal constructs as developed by Dr ████████ has had successful application in this country and for some time there has been a desire to apply this methodology to foreign cultures; and (2) Dr. ████████ accessibility and acceptability to ████████ psychologists will make it possible to secure invaluable data on ████████ research attitudes and personality information on researchers. MD/OSI, A&E/OTR, and SOB/DDP have expressed an interest in the results of this project and are willing to support it with requirements and technical support.

2. Dr ████████████ is professor of psychology at ████████ c/B ████████ University. He has been a fully cleared consultant to the Agency for four years and has demonstrated unusual sensitivity and perceptivity to Agency needs, particularly in the area of assessment and the psychological support of ████████ He has an excellent national and international professional reputation. He is a member of ████████ ████████ of the ████████ ast-president of the ████████ nd is the leading contender ████████ He is the ████████ and a consistent contributor to leading professional journals.

MORI ID 17402:17402

142-14

22 May 1962

MEMORANDUM FOR: THE RECORD

SUBJECT   : Project MKULTRA, Subproject No. 142

1. The purpose of this subproject is to provide funds to support a small biological program of electrical brain stimulation involving some new approaches to the subject by████████████ *C* The support allows for the rental of minimum space and equipment and the part-time employment of a "pair of hands" to carry out the work planned by████████████ *C*

2. The reason for separating this work financially from the *C* other efforts of████████in the Agency's behalf is to allow him to engage in some very practical experiments at some point in the work which would present security problems if this effort were to be handled in the usual way. Some of the uses proposed for these particular animals would involve possible delivery systems for BW/CW agents or for direct executive action type operations as distinguished from the eavesdropping application of████████████ *H*

3. As indicative in the attached proposal and budget, the total cost of this project for one year will not exceed $7,500.00. Charges should be made against allotment number 2125-1390-3902. *B* The████████████will function as cover and cutout for these funds.

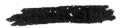

142-14

-2-

4. It is not anticipated that any permanent equipment will be required for this subproject.

5. ▓▓▓▓▓▓ possesses a TOP SECRET clearance for Agency work.

Chief, TSD/Research Branch

APPROVED FOR OBLIGATION
OF FUNDS:

Chief, Technical Services Division

Date: _____ 23 MAY 1962

Attachment:
  Proposal and Budget

Distribution:
  Original only

142-14

22 May 1962

MEMORANDUM FOR: THE RECORD

SUBJECT : Project MKULTRA, Subproject No. 142

1. The purpose of this subproject is to provide funds to support a small biological program of electrical brain stimulation involving some new approaches to the subject by ██████████ The support allows for the rental of minimum space and equipment and the part-time employment of a "pair of hands" to carry out the work planned by ██████████

2. The reason for separating this work financially from the other efforts of ██████████ in the Agency's behalf is to allow him to engage in some very practical experiments at some point in the work which would present security problems if this effort were to be handled in the usual way. Some of the uses proposed for these particular animals would involve possible delivery systems for BW/CW agents or for direct executive action type operations as distinguished from the eavesdropping application of ██████████

3. As indicative in the attached proposal and budget, the total cost of this project for one year will not exceed $7,500.00. Charges should be made against allotment number 2125-1390-3902. The ██████████ will function as cover and cutout for these funds.

142-14

4. It is not anticipated that any permanent equipment will be required for this subproject.

5. ███████ possesses a TOP SECRET clearance for Agency work.

Chief, TSD/Research Branch

APPROVED FOR OBLIGATION
OF FUNDS:

Chief, Technical Services Division

Date: _____ 23 MAY 1963 _____

Attachment:
  Proposal and Budget

Distribution:
  Original only

142-14

PROPOSAL

It is proposed to carry out certain biological studies involving electrical brain stimulation of cold-blooded animals. In addition to the various theoretical reasons for such studies, it appears that certain practical guidance systems involving more detailed behavioral control of both positive and negative sorts may be possible than are presently attainable in the warm-blooded animals being investigated. It is also possible that these simpler systems can accomplish the same operational goals with far less critical demands on the electronic parts of the guidance and control system.

The work to be done will consist of literature search, experimental placement of electrodes, observation of effects of stimulation and collation of information regarding the behavioral effects of stimulation in the various well defined areas. Biologically stable preparations with defined stimulation properties will result from this work.

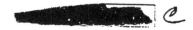 e

APPENDIX D
MKSEARCH CONTRACTS

Subproject	Contractor	Institution	Linked to MKULTRA #
1	Maitland Baldwin	National Institutes of Health	62
2		Bacteriological and Pharmaceutical Consults, Inc.	78, 110
3	James Hamilton	Vacaville State Prison	124, 140
4		Bureau of Narcotics	3, 14, 16, 42
5		An Unidentified Chemical Company	116, 146
6	Charles Geschickter	Georgetown University	23, 25, 26
7	Carl Pfeiffer	New Jersey Neuropsychiatric Institute	9, 26, 28, 47

APPENDIX E
DOCTORS IN THE NETWORK

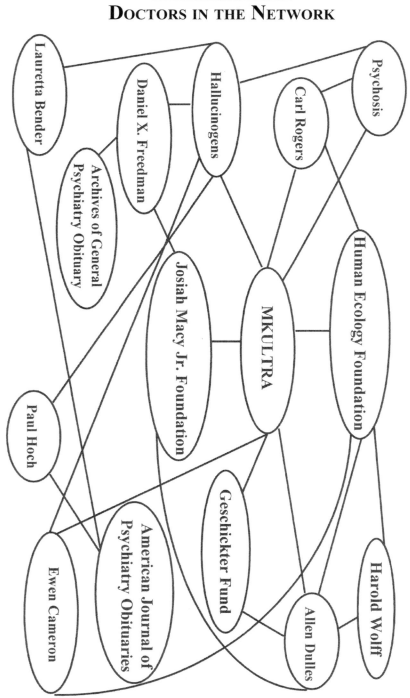

FUNDING FRONTS FOR CIA MIND CONTROL RESEARCH

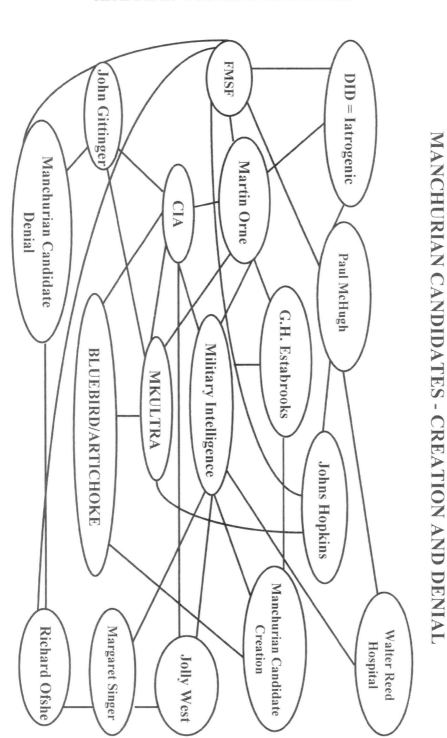

MANCHURIAN CANDIDATES - CREATION AND DENIAL

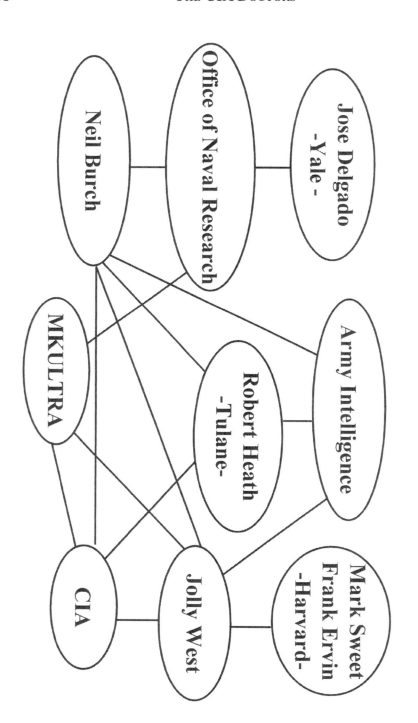

BRAIN ELECTRODE IMPLANT RESEARCH

Appendix F
Martin Orne CIA And Military Contracts

Research Grants

Principal Investigator of contract number AF 49(638) - 72B from the Air Force Office of Scientific Research for an Investigation of the Nature and Uses of Hypnosis as a Control Technique, 19591962.

Principal Investigator of research contract number Nonr - 3952 (00) from the Office of Naval Research for an Empirical Investigation of Basic Research Problems in Hypnosis and Related States, 19621964.

Principal Investigator of research contract number AF-AFOSR-88-63 from the Air Force Office of Scientific Research for a Scientific Investigation of Personality Attributes of Good Subjects, 19621964.

Principal Investigator of research contract number DA-49-193-MD-2480 from the United States Army Medical Research and Development command for Studies in the Detection of Deception, 1963-1964.

Principal Investigator of research contract number DA-49-193-MD-2744 from the United States Army Medical Research and Development Command for an Empirical Investigation of Trance Phenomena, 1966-1967.

Principal Investigator of research grant number AF-AFOSR-707-67 from the Air Force Office of Scientific Research for an Empirical Investigation of the Relationships between Sleep and Hypnosis, 1964-1971.

Principal Investigator of research contract number Nonr-4731(00) from the Office of Naval Research for an Empirical Investigation of Basic Research Problems in Hypnosis and Related States, 19641971.

Principal Investigator of research contract number DA-49-193-MD-2647 from the Unites States Army Medical Research and Development Command for Studies in the Detection of Deception, 1964-1971.

Principal Investigator of research contract number DADA17-71-C-1120 from the United States Army Medical Research and Development Command for the Empirical Investigation of Recovery from Fatigue, 1971-1979.

CIA MKULTRA Subproject 84

APPENDIX G
JOLLY WEST CIA AND MILITARY CONTRACTS

Hospital Appointments

Chief, Psychiatry Service, 3700th USAF Hospital   1952-1956
Lackland Air Force Base, San Antonio, Texas

Psychiatrist-in-Chief, University of Oklahoma   1954-1969

Consultant in Psychiatry, Oklahoma City Veterans   1956-1969

Administration Hospital

Consultant in Psychiatry, United States Air Force Hospital   1956-1966
Force Base, Oklahoma

Consultant in Psychiatry, Palo Alto Veterans Administration Hospital 1966-1967

Consultant in Psychiatry, Veterans Administration Center   1969-?
For Psycho-social Medicine at Brentwood, Los Angeles

Consultant in Psychiatry, Veterans Administration Hospital   1969-?
Sepulveda, California

National and International Appointments

Consultant, United States Air force Aero-Space Medical Center   1961-1966

National Advisory Committee on Psychiatry, Neurology, and   1968-1973
    Psychology, United States Veterans Administration
    Professional Services Subcommittee, 1968-1972,
    Chairman, 1970-1972

Consultant to the Surgeon General, United States Army   1974-1977
    Medical Research and Development Command

Member, United States Army Medical Research and Development   1974-1979
    Advisory Panel

Consultant, V.A. Health Care Committee,   1975-1976
   National Research Council, Division of Medical Sciences,
   Assembly of Life Sciences

Regional and Local Appointments

Dean's Committee, Oklahoma City Veterans Administration Hospital 1954-1969

Dean's Committee, Wadsworth Veterans   1969-1989
   Administration Medical Center

Dean's Committee, Sepulveda Veterans   1970-1989
   Administration Medical Center

CIA-MKULTRA Subproject 43.

APPENDIX H
EWEN CAMERON DOCUMENTS

Partial List of Ewen Cameron Research Grants From Canada's Department of Health and Welfare

604-5-11	The Effect of Senescence on Resistance to Stress	$195,388.00 1950-1957
604-5-13	Research Studies on EEG and Electrophysiology	$60,353.33 1950-1957
604-5-14	Support for a Behavioral Laboratory	$17,875.00 1950-1954
604-5-43	Study of Personal and Social Aspects of Retirement and Retirement Adjustment	$24,450.00 1956-1958
604-5-74	Study of Ultraconceptual Communication	$26,228.08 1959-1963
604-4-76	A Study of the Effects of Nucleic Acid Upon Memory Impairment in the Aged	$18,000.00 1959-1963
604-5-432	A Study of Factors Which Promote or Retard Personality Change in Individuals Exposed to Prolonged Repetition of Verbal Signals	$57,750.00 1961-1964
Total		$395,044.41

Dr. Ewen Cameron's Notes On Linda Macdonald From The Allan Memorial Institute

April 1

When seen a few days ago by Dr. Cameron, this patient showed a very unclear mood. She claimed to be depressed but broke into apparently unmotivated laughter. She showed grimacing in so far that she kept her eyes curiously sealed and flickered them at times. She seemed quite non-logical in her thinking. From this brief interview it would appear that there is a possibility that this patient shows either an hysteria or a pseudoneurotic schizophrenia [an old term for borderline personality disorder]. It does not appear to be a retarded depression.

We are continuing to work her up, and we are asking that special attention be paid to her early parental home.

April 22

The patient said that she occasionally hears a voice talking insider her head. She has difficulty in expressing hostility, and we are encouraging her to do this. The diagnosis is not yet clear; we are still bearing in mind that the psychologists suggest the possibility of underlying schizophrenia. We are carrying on with the present psychotherapeutic approach in order to determine whether this is the case… Recently the patient saw a movie in which the husband and wife started off very happily together. Then the husband had an extramarital affair. The name of the girl in the movie was Linda, just as the patient's is. The patient became very upset and came out complaining of back pain, but she refused to say that it had any connection with the movie. This is also being explored.

July 4

Reviewing the EEG's we find on March 29, 1963 (her admission EEG) that there was no evidence of focal or cerebral damage or epileptiform activity. Fast background rhythm was noted as being due to medication. On May 28, after she had had 31 Page Russells and was on Largactil mgs 50 q.i.d., the EEG was very irregular, showing generalized slow wave dysrhythmia.

July 16

She is quite turbulent. Her speech is very slurred. She shows no definite evidence of delusional ideas. We are starting her on Artane 2t.i.d. today, and this will be raised to Artane 5 t.i.d. in 48 hrs. if she tolerates this well. We are also considering the possibility of raising her sleep medication. In view of the fact that her EEG shows an increase in epileptiform activity, we are going to reduce the ECT to every second day.

July 23

She is not incontinent. Her gait is rather lurching. She is not really concerned with dressing herself at the present time. She is able to feed herself. We do recognize that she is gradually coming out. She knows that she is Linda Macdonald. She cannot recognize her own bed and keeps crawling into others.

September 5

In working over her case on April 5th 1963, the psychologists felt that the general impression was that of a notable hysterical overlay to an early schizophrenic pathology. Our examinations of her clinically, however, have failed this far to show any evidence of schizophrenia. Due to the dangers of neglecting a possible schizophrenia, we put her through intensive therapy. This is now eventuating in quite a good recovery, though with an indication of mild instability in the last day or so.

September 12

She has had a repeat psychological testing. The results, of course, to some extent are influenced by the organic changes produced by the electroshock. Thus far no evidence of a thought disorder can be noted.

Nursing Notes On Linda Macdonald
From The Allan Memorial Insitute

Nursing notes for March 28 - April 11, and May 29 - August 14, 1963 were not forwarded to Linda Macdonald by the Allen Memorial Institute for an unknown reason. Some of the photocopied handwriting is difficult to read, which I have indicated with square brackets.

April 14

When nurse went to wake her up found her crying. Patient stated she felt this coming on for several days and she didn't know why. She said nothing further. Came out on the ward in the afternoon and joined in bingo game and ward party. Much brighter.

April 15

Played cards with husband in early P.M., laughing and talking. Later entertained patient in [?room] playing her guitar. Showed them new chords that her husband had taught her.

Telling other patients how when she was young she had always felt as thought she was adopted. Her brother and sister were like her parents - but not her. She was the black sheep and acted accordingly. Although her father never understood her, she felt that he truly loved her in his own way. Socializing well. Teaching young female patient how to play the guitar.

April 17

Sleeping before dinner. Eager to go to dance downstairs - Participated actively and seemed to enjoy herself. Later played her guitar and sang with a group of other patients. Tea and toast and retired.

April 18

Has difficulty getting to sleep - wandered about the day room for a while - persuaded to go to bed and leave her light on as patient stated she was afraid of the dark. Smoked a cigarette and then noted she turned off her light and was asleep.

April 19

At 7 P.M. patient appeared to experience psychotic breakdown when nurse entered room patient was lying on bed, staring at the ceiling and did not respond to questions. When light was switched on patient blinked, appeared to become markedly anxious and began to scream loudly - she jumped from bed, began banging her head against the wall and whimpered continually - "Don't touch me" - on approach she screamed "Don't touch me" and flung herself on the floor and began to whimper once again.

After injection patient said she heard a voice saying to her, "They're going to frighten you." While patient was dozing she was heard saying - "I'm a mess" - "I'm so mixed up" - "I hit Alex" -I've never hit anyone in my life except my husband and my kids." Patient remained in bed rest of evening, dozing on and off.

April 20

Dressed in a rather juvenile manner, knee socks, flat shoes etc. Saw children this A.M. - very pleased to see them. After visit spent long period singing accompanying herself on a guitar. Came out to dining room later in afternoon - talked about music etc.

Dressed in wool skirt and knee socks, playing rummy with a young female patient before supper. Manner flippant and loud and quite gay. Attended the movie and for the first hour, laughed and appeared to be enjoying it. Grew quite upset after a little domestic scene had been presented, where the young husband comes home drunk and accuses the wife of infidelity. The girl's name in the movie was Linda. Ms. Macdonald left abruptly complaining of headache and backache. Lying in bed with sunglasses on obtained relief from heating pad. Stated "I don't know what I'm going to do if I don't leave here without curing this backache." Ten minutes later was up in the dining strumming her guitar and singing, seeming to have completely forgotten her pains. In one of the happier scenes in the movie she had pointed at the young married couple and said "That's Tom and me all over."

April 21

Gay euphoric manner. Visited by husband and went out for coffee. Manner unchanged upon return. Laughing uproariously and joking and teasing other patients. Asked nurse about depatterning. "It's all that's left for me I guess. But I don't want to forget my children. They are the one good thing in my [?life]."

April 22

Seen by Dr. Briones [the intern] at 5:30P.M. Anxious to go to dance and afraid that her appointment with the doctor will coincide with the dance. "I know I'm here to get help, not to go to dances but it makes me angry when my appointments coincide with the dance." Attended dance and enjoyed it thoroughly. Said to the nurse earlier in the evening "I've heard that they haven't diagnosed me yet. I've been here a month and they don't know what's wrong with me yet?" Went on to say, "I never avoid conflicts I move headlong into them. But none of my wild little escapades have seemed to solve anything. Perhaps this is my escape from my problem. I really want to show my true self to the doctors. I want to know myself as I really am."

April 24

Apparently had a talk with one of the other female patients' ministers. Later seen by Dr. Briones. Returned to ward looking extremely downcast. Nurse asked how it had gone and Ms. Macdonald replied very sarcastically "It went marvelously well, thank you." Later she appeared out on the ward dressed charmingly, ready for the dance. Talked with nurse and a group of female patients. Stated about interview with Dr. Briones "There was a complete lack of communication. I guess it was my fault. But I'm not going to let anything he has said upset me or spoil my evening." She continued to chat gaily discussing art, flowers and other miscellaneous subjects with the nurse. Enjoyed the dance and later entertained a group of patients with her guitar and singing.

April 25

ECT#1.PR DT.O.T.MA   400 x 6 GM Seizure.   [I don't understand all this notation, but it means that she had a grand mal seizure subsequent to her first shock treatment]

Quite apprehensive about treatment. Stated if she knows exactly what things are all about does not mind but was told only that she would have a needle and come straight back upstairs. On return to ward showed no confusion - asked the nurse her husband's name but had no trouble remembering anything else. Complained of headache and started to cry "because of the headache".

May 2

Quite drowsy but no other physical complaints. No memory loss. Stated she hoped she would recover from the effect of the second

E.C.T. in time to attend the dance tonight. Stated her husband would be coming to see her tomorrow night and she would be glad to see him.

May 3

Spent morning strumming guitar and later making sandwiches for party tonight. Mood cheerful, stated she was eager to get her treatments over with - "I don't mind the headaches and sore jaw, I just want to get them finished."

May 3

Visited by husband and went downstairs with him. Does not appear confused, although has forgotten some recent events. Outside walking and on swings. Inquiring about sleep room.

May 9

Patient is aloof, seldom speaks but at times exhibits sudden interest. Post ECT had [?] and watched with interest as nurse persuaded a confused patient to take her meds. Tried to help but said nothing. Smiles when eyes met [?] over patient's head.

Did not dress today, spent time on ward watching T.V. Sits or lies watching T.V. and seems drowsy. When nurse approached she woke up, sat up, smiled, laughs appropriately but says little. Plays cards and picks one string of her guitar but when asked to play a key does not seem to comprehend. 6 P.M. ECT#10 TD.7 MA 400 x 6

May 11

Patient post ECT knew name and city only. Believed she was in hospital having had her first child. Is quite, content to sit on fringe of activities. Answers only direct questions and then only in monosyllables and sometimes just stares. Unable or unwilling to follow directions but cooperative with supervision. Retired without difficulty.

May 12

Following ECT this PM patient was oriented to name only. She smiles but doesn't answer when spoken to and is content to sit watching other patients in room for long periods. Cannot follow directions and when attempts are made in help her or give pills becomes quite negativistic. Spent much time in room and needs much supervision.

May 13

Post ECT she was very confused, oriented only to name Needed much direction about ward and assistance in bathing and dressing. Facies expression [this means a blank expression]. Spent most of day in ICU.

May 14

Disoriented in all spheres [doesn't know who she is, where she is, or the date] following E.C.T. Eventually remembered name only. Eats well with assistance. No anxiety shown over memory loss. Facies blank, passive. Slept for one hour this afternoon then remained lying in bed.

May 16

Facies expressionless and patient confused. Answers to name "Linda" only. Mumbles incoherently and responds only to direct commands slowly. She needs complete direction about ward and complete physical care. Watches other patients on ward. While walking down hall she noticed an open cupboard door, she stopped to close it and continued walking slowly. Manages to feed self.

May 19

Facies flat. Disoriented in all three spheres but looks up when first name is called. Incontinent of urine once only this A.M. Voided this P.M. Needs help bathing and with eating and drinking. Did some doodling with pencil and paper but concentration is very poor. Verbalizing very little and when she does speech is very slurred and slow. Gait a little unsteady and patient needs physical support. A little negativistic at times. Intake 1200 cc.

May 20

Facies remain quite blank, patient remained in ICU - sitting with other patients almost mute - stating "no" to certain directions. Very slow moving - however patient can feed self once started by nurse. No incontinence. Taking fluids well. Intake 600 cc. Output x 2.

May 22

ECT 26 TD 0.7 MA   400 x 6   GM Seizure.   Facies quite blank. Patient disoriented to name, place, and time. When asked her age she replied, "Oh isn't that lovely." Manages to eat and drink when shown. Needs complete direction although she walks much better today. Sits staring at other people. Was found smoking cigarette in day room. Had lunch in ICU. Mumbles incoherently.

Memory span short. Did not accept reassurance or explanation wanting to phone her husband constantly "I don't see why I can't phone, how can he look after my five children?' Borrowing dimes from other patients on ward looking up her number in phone book but could not remember when she went to dial ,talking to nurse this evening about past saying she went to [?] in Ottawa relating how she met her husband and that she has five children very concerned about how her husband would cope with children, short memory span but quite insistent abut phoning, settles down after Largactil 100 mg. Retired early.

May 24

More aware of her surroundings still third stage. Answering simple questions with short simple word answers knows her first name is "Linda" voiding and eating well spending most of time in ICU distinguishing simple objects such as a pen, points to her guitar when asked about it.

May 25

Very good P.M. activity for most part of P.M., played bridge with other patients, pleasant and cheerful on approach, still needs reassurance that what she is doing is right, no somatic complaints.

May 26

Still quite negativistic and resisting direction. However she is very cooperative in taking medications. Intake and output is good. Oriented only to name. Facial expression very blank. Holding her hands up and looking at them - pulling on her fingers. Settled early.

August 17

Friendly and cheerful. Somewhat worried over memory loss, but accepts reassurance very well, Questioned medications. Socializing well with other patients. Requires quite a bit of direction and reassurance.

August 18

Cheerful all day. Socializing well. Dressed somewhat untidily. Still has quite a bit of memory loss but accepts reassurance well. Spoke of looking forward to discharge in the future. Visited by husband and went for a walk with him. Very pleased to see him.

August 20

Fairly good P.M.; socializing well with other patients; played cards for long periods; still seeking constant reassurance in attempts to reeducate herself. Fairly concerned over memory loss.

August 25

Returned to ward about 6 P.M. accompanied by husband; said she had a wonderful weekend and is looking forward to next weekend already.

August 26

Good evening. Very enthusiastic about arranging singing group on the ward. Mixing with the other female patients and displaying protectiveness towards one other female patient. Attended the dance and took an active part. Mood appears elevated and patient [laughing?]. Talking continually. Relates on a superficial level. Neat in appearance. Speaks optimistically about returning home.

September 3

Good evening. Memory loss evident but patient is not disturbed by this. Spent long periods talking and playing cards with other female patients. Cheerful and pleasant on approach, smiling often and talking a great deal.

September 5

Socializing with any patient. Still conversed and appeared less talkative giving the other member of the group to talk. Group with other 4 female patients and when approached by a male patient she started a nice joke and burst everybody into laughter. Went to the dance. Talked much after she came from the dance and other patients complained that Ms. Macdonald is a loud person and always talk much talked more of her appreciation about other patients who are good dancers stated she enjoyed dancing too but she enjoyed more watching good dancers. Anxious to go on weekend tomorrow with husband.

September 8

In from weekend, accompanied by husband. Appeared cheerful relating well. Stated she saw her children and some in-laws whom she had not meet last weekend. Claims she had much enjoyment than the last weekend. Watched the "Ed Sullivan Show" in the T.V. and enjoyed the show very much with a group of patients and staff. Grouped with other patients after tea time till 10 P.M. Seemed to be conversing well at a normal level. Not so talkative as the previous days.

September 10

ECT102

Sept

Appendix I
Agents Tested on Humans by the U.S. Army, Including Viruses, Bacteria, Vaccines and Mind Control Drugs

List Of Agents Used On Human Volunteers
U.S. Army Medical Research Institute Of Infectious Diseases
Fort Detrick, Fredrick, Maryland 21701

12 August 1975

1958 - 1962

Tularemia Vaccine
Rift Valley Fever Vaccine
Venezuelan Equine Encephalomyelitis Vaccine
Western Equine Encephalitis Vaccine
Yellow Fever Vaccine

1963 - 1967

Tularemia Vaccine
Venezuelan Equine Encephalomyelitis Vaccine
Bacterial Endotoxin
Q Fever Vaccine
Antibiotic Therapy
Sandfly Fever
Low Dose Cortisol Administration
Plague Vaccine
Yellow Fever Vaccine
Eastern Equine Encephalitis Vaccine

1968 - 1973

Yellow Fever Vaccine
Eastern Equine Encephalitis Vaccine
Sandfly Fever
Tularemia
Chloromycetin®
Generic Preparation of Choloramphenicol
Venezuelan Equine Encephalomyolitis Vaccine
Adenovirus Vaccine
Western Equine Encephalitis Vaccine
Venezuelan Equine Encephalomyelitis Immune Globulin
Rift Valley Fever Vaccine
Chikungunya Vaccine
Plague Vaccine

No volunteer studies since 1973

1955-1959	1960 to March 1962
Drug	Drug
EA 1778	VX
EA 1476	GB
792	Thorazine
DM	LSD
CS	SNA
CN	PAM-PS
Chloropicrin	CS
GB	BSP
Nasal Toxic Inhala	Atropine
5HTP	Urecholine
Atropine	TMB4
Mustard	GF
Skin Lipids	GA
Stypen Coagula Time	Neostigmine
Malathion Powder	Amphetamine like cpds
Dibenz	BZ
	ThA
	D-tubocurarine
	DMHP
	Creosol/N-ethylmorpholine
	Detran (JB329)
	Dexedrine
	Carare
	Disodiumfluorescinetethylene
	gloycol
	Seco Barbitol
	Dibulaline

March 1962 to PRESENT		
Drug	**Drug**	**Drug**
EA 2233	DFP	Compazine
EA 3148	GB	Dexadrine
Win 19362	GB c PAM	Ditran
18437	Vasoxyl	Dilantin
CS 27349	Valium	Ethanol
EA 3443	GD	Ethanol c Ritalin
EA 3528	1CG	Ethanol c Thorazine
EA 3580	PABA	Ethanol c Scopolomine
EA 3580/VX/PAM	PAH	Ethanol c Valium
CAR 302, 034	APH c PAM	Heparin
302, 089	PAM/ATRO	Inderol
302, 368	P2S	Isuprel
301, 060	THA	Lanoxin
302, 282	VX	
302, 668	VX/SCOP	
302, 582	VX/PAM	
302, 537	Atropine	
302, 196	Homatropine	
220, 548	Methyl Atropine	
226, 086	Amyl Nitrate	
EA 2277 (BZ)	Antipyrine	
EA 3834	BAT	
McN-JR-4929	Benactyzine	
EA 3167	Benac/Atropine	
BSP	Benac/TMB4	
BZ	Caffeine	
CS		

APPENDIX J
OTHER CIA DOCUMENTS

PARTICIPANTS
Conference on d-Lysergic Acid Diethylamide (LSD-25)

PAUL H. HOCH, *Chairman*
Department of Psychiatry, Columbia University, College of Physicians and Surgeons
New York, N. Y.

HAROLD A. ABRAMSON, *Editor*
The Biological Laboratory, Cold Spring Harbor, and the State Hospital
Central Islip, N. Y.

GREGORY BATESON
Ethnology Section, Veterans Administration Hospital
Palo Alto, Calif.

ARTHUR L. CHANDLER
Psychiatric Institute of Beverly Hills
Beverly Hills, Calif.

SIDNEY COHEN
Neuropsychiatric Hospital, Veterans Administration Center
Los Angeles, Calif.

JONATHAN O. COLE
Psychopharmacology Service Center, National Institute of Mental Health
National Institutes of Health
Bethesda, Md.

HERMAN C. B. DENBER
Research Division, Manhattan State Hospital
Columbia University, College of Physicians and Surgeons
New York, N. Y.

KEITH S. DITMAN
Department of Psychiatry, School of Medicine, University of California Medical Center
Los Angeles, Calif.

BETTY G. EISNER
1334 Westwood Boulevard
Los Angeles, Calif.

MORTIMER A. HARTMAN
Psychiatric Institute of Beverly Hills
Beverly Hills, Calif.

MOLLIE P. HEWITT
The Biological Laboratory
Cold Spring Harbor, N. Y.

ABRAM HOFFER
Psychiatric Services Branch, Department of Public Health
Regina, Sask., Canada

CECELIA E. JETT-JACKSON
Medical Department, Sandoz Pharmaceuticals
Hanover, N. J.

SOLOMON KATZENELBOGEN
5312 Pooks Hill Road
Bethesda, Md.

GERALD D. KLEE
Department of Psychiatry, Psychiatric Institute, University of Maryland School of Medicine
Baltimore, Md.

HENRY L. LENNARD
Bureau of Applied Social Research, Columbia University
New York, N. Y.

SIDNEY MALITZ
Department of Experimental Psychiatry, New York State Psychiatric Institute
New York, N. Y.

ROBERT C. MURPHY, JR.
Waverly, Penn.

GWENDOLYN J. NEVIACKAS
The Biological Laboratory
Cold Spring Harbor, N. Y.

T. T. PECK, JR.
Psychiatric and Public Health Departments, San Jacinto Memorial Hospital
Baytown, Tex.

RONALD A. SANDISON
Powick Hospital
Near Worcester, England

CHARLES SAVAGE
Center for Advanced Study in Behavioral Sciences
Stanford, Calif.

C. H. VAN RHIJN
Men's Department, Mental Hospitals "Brinkgreven" and "St. Elizabeths Gasthuis"
Deventer, Netherlands

JOHN R. B. WHITTLESEY
Alcoholism Research Clinic
Department of Psychiatry, UCLA Medical Center
Los Angeles, Calif.

LOUIS J. WEST
Department of Psychiatry, Neurology, and Behavioral Sciences
University of Oklahoma School of Medicine
Oklahoma City, Okla.

THE JOSIAH MACY, JR. FOUNDATION

FRANK FREMONT-SMITH, *Medical Director*
ELIZABETH F. PURCELL, *Assistant for the Conference Program*

THE SECOND INTERNATIONAL CONFERENCE
ON THE USE OF
LSD IN PSYCHOTHERAPY

May 8th-May 10th, 1965

NAME	AFFILIATION
Abramson, Harold A., M.D.	(U.S.A.) Director of Research, South Oaks Psychiatric Hospital, Amityville
Arendsen Hein, G. W., M.D.	(Holland) Medical Director of Foundation Stichting, Veluweland Hospital
Baker, Edward F. W., M.D.	(Canada) Attending staff, Toronto Western Hospital, University of Toronto, Departments of Medicine and Psychiatry
Balestrieri, Antonio, M.D.	(Italy) Professor of Psychiatry, University of Bari
Blair, Donald, M.D.	(England) Consultant Psychiatrist, St. Bernard's Hospital, London
Buckman, John, Dr., M.R.C.S., L.R.C.P., D.P.M.	(England) Senior Hospital Medical Officer, Marlborough Day Hospital, London; now Assistant Professor of Psychiatry, University of Virginia, Charlotteville

NAME	AFFILIATION
Chiasson, John, M.D.	(Canada) Director, Alcoholic Treatment Services, Psychiatric Services of Quebec
Cohen, Sidney, M.D.	(U.S.A.) Chief, Psychosomatic Medicine, Veterans Administration Hospital, Los Angeles
Dahlberg, Charles Clay, M.D.	(U.S.A.) Training and Supervisory Analyst, William Alanson White Psychoanalytic Institute
Eisner, Betty Grover, PH.D.	(U.S.A.) Clinical Psychologist in private practice; Los Angeles
Fox, Ruth, M.D.	(U.S.A.) Medical Director, National Council on Alcoholism
Freedman, Daniel X., M.D.	(U.S.A.) Professor of Psychiatry, Yale University School of Medicine
Fremont-Smith, Frank, M.D.	(U.S.A.) Director, Interdisciplinary Communications Program, New York Academy of Sciences
Godfrey, Kenneth E., M.D.	(U.S.A.) Assistant Chief West Psychiatric Service, Topeka Veterans Administration
Grof, Stanislav, M.D.	(Czechoslovakia) Research Psychiatrist, Psychiatric Research Institute, Prague
Hausman, Col. William, M.C.	(U.S.A.) Deputy Director, Division of Neuropsychiatry, Walter Reed Army Institute of Research
Hertz, Mogens, M..	(Denmark) Assistant Chief Physician, Frederiksberg Hospital, Copenhagen

NAME	AFFILIATION
MacDonald, Donald C., M.D.	(Canada) Psychiatrist, Consultant to Hollywood Hospital, British Columbia
MacLean, J. Ross, M.D.	(Canada) Medical Director, Hollywood Hospital, New Westminster, British Columbia
McCririck, Mrs. Pauline	(England) Psychoanalyst; with Dr. A. Joyce Martin, Marlborough Day Hospital, London
McGlothlin, William H., PH.D.	(U.S.A.) Research Associate, Department of Psychology, University of Southern California
Martin, A. Joyce, M.D.	(England) Senior Hospital Medical Officer, Marlborough Day Hospital, London
Mogar, Robert E., PH.D.	(U.S.A.) Assistant Professor of Psychology; Director of Research, San Francisco State College
Murphy, Robert C., Jr., M.D.	(U.S.A.) Private practice; Waverly, Pennsylvania
Osmond, Humphry, M.R.C.S., D.P.M.	(U.S.A.) Director, Bureau of Neurology and Psychiatry, New Jersey Neuropsychiatric Institute
Pahnke, Walter N., M.D., PH.D.	(U.S.A.) Resident Psychiatrist, Massachusetts Mental Health Center
Rolo, André, M.D.	(U.S.A.) Director, South Oaks Psychiatric Hospital Amityville
Rinkel, Max, M.D.	(U.S.A.) Senior Research Consultant Massachusetts Mental Health Center

NAME	AFFILIATION
Savage, Charles, M.D.	(U.S.A.) Director of Research, Spring Grove State Hospital, Maryland
Servadio, Emilio, M.D.	(Italy) Hon. Professor of Psychology, L.L.D.; President, Italian Psychoanalytic Society, Rome
Unger, Sanford, PH.D.	(U.S.A.) Acting Chief of Psychosocial Research, Spring Grove State Hospital, Maryland
Van Rhijn, Cornelius H., M.D.	(Holland) Psychotherapist, private practice; Enchede
Ward, Jack L., M.D.	(U.S.A.) Staff Psychiatrist, New Jersey Reformatory at Bordentown, Mercer Hospital
Weber, E. S., M.D.	(U.S.A.) Psychiatrist, private practice; Princeton
Wicks, Miss Mary S.	(England) Probation Officer, Kidderminster, Worcester

The Deputy Director
Central Intelligence Agency

Washington D.C. 20505

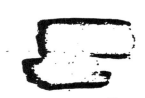

Honorable Leo J. Ryan
House of Representatives
Washington, D.C. 20515

18 OCT 1978

Dear Mr. Ryan:

Thank you for your letter of 27 September to Admiral Turner requesting confirmation or denial of the fact of CIA experiments using prisoners at the California medical facility at Vacaville.

It is true that CIA sponsored testing, using volunteer inmates, was conducted at that facility. The project was completed in 1968. A report setting forth the details of that testing has been released to the authorities at Vacaville and to the public. It is enclosed for your information and review. Also enclosed is correspondence between our Office of General Counsel and T. L. Clanon, M.D., Superintendent of the facility. We have also included correspondence from our Information and Privacy Coordinator to Mr. Thomas K. Dalglish, Chairperson, Committee for the Protection of Human Subjects, California Department of Health. These documents, all of which are now in the public domain, will give you a clearer idea of the nature and extent of the testing, which related to learning enhancement using a well-known non-hallucinogen, magnesium pemoline.

Your letter referred to Donald DeFreese, known as CINQUE, and Clifford Jefferson, both of whom were inmates at Vacaville. In so far as our records reflect the names of the participants, there is nothing to indicate that either was in any way involved in the project. You may wish to contact the authorities at Vacaville for further information.

I trust you will find this information helpful. Please call me if you have any questions or wish additional information.

Sincerely,

/s/ Frank C. Carlucci

Frank C. Carlucci

Enclosures

Approved for Release
Date _____ OCT 1987

24
26

CENTRAL INTELLIGENCE AGENCY

Psychiatrists

The Central Intelligence Agency is seeking full-time board eligible or certified Psychiatrists to participate in a psychiatric program including diagnostic and preventive psychiatry and psychiatric selection. Previous experience such as military service or overseas living is desirable. The ability to participate in a multi-disciplinary psychological and medical group and to communicate psychiatric concepts clearly to non-physicians is essential. Candidates must be available for overseas assignments. Starting salary range begins at $90,000. Coverage by professional liability insurance for line-of-duty medical practice is included. U.S. citizenship is required. Applicants must successfully complete a thorough medical and psychiatric exam, a polygraph interview and an extensive background investigation. Send resume or letter of interest to: Personnel Representative, Dept. 961, Office of Medical Services, Central Intelligence Agency, Washington, DC 20505. We will respond within 30 days to those judged to be of further interest. The CIA is an equal opportunity employer.

254

MEMORANDUM FOR: Director of Central Intelligence

SUBJECT   :   Contingency Plan for Stockpile of
                      Biological Warfare Agents

1. On 25 November 1969, President Nixon ordered the
Department of Defense to recommend plans for the disposal
of existing stocks of bacteriological weapons. (On 14
February 1970, he included all toxin weapons.)

2. On 13 January 1970, the Special Operations Division
of Fort Detrick, Maryland prepared a requested agent inventory, less toxins, and submitted it to the Scientific
Director, Fort Detrick. This inventory was a required input
to assist the Commanding Officer, Ft. Detrick to prepare
a comprehensive plan for demilitarization on site of all
biological agents/munitions which are stockpiled in support
of operational plans.

3. Under an established agreement with the Department
of the Army, the CIA has a limited quantity of biological
agents and toxins stored and maintained by the SO Division
at Ft. Detrick. This stockpile did not appear on the inventory list. The agents and toxins are:

Agents:

1. Bacillus anthracis (anthrax) — 100 grams

2. Pasteurella tularensis (tularemia) — 20 grams

3. Venezuelan Equine Encephalomyelitis virus
    (encephalitis) — 20 grams

4. Coccidioides immitis (valley fever) — 20 grams

5. Brucella suis (brucellosis) — 2 to 3 grams

6. Brucella melitensis (brucellosis) — 2 to 3
    grams

7. Mycobacterium tuberculosis (tuberculosis) —
    3 grams

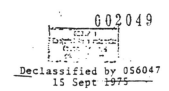

602049

Declassified by OS6047
15 Sept 1975

APPENDIX K
PROJECT OFTEN DOCUMENTS

23 June 1970

MEMORANDUM FOR:

SUBJECT   : Review of EA 3167 Study

   1. In this study, nineteen subjects were divided into three groups which were treated with dosages of ⌐   ⌐units/kg of experimental agent 3167.

   2. In the first group of six subjects, measurements of temperature, blood pressure, respiration, pulse, and pupil size, although showing some variation, did not reveal significant differences which could be related to drug symptomology. In every case, undesirable symptoms were noted, all six subjects experiencing "drowsiness" and "dry throat." Of the three cases of hullucination and mental incapacitation, only one was of a serious nature and this admittedly may have been due to an additional accidental dose of the drug.

   3. The second group (⌐ ⌐units/kg) exhibited a variety of undesired side effects: drowsiness, dry or sore throat, nausea, loss of taste, blurred vision, heaviness in legs, lack of coordination. All seven subjects in this group experienced at least three of these symptoms. Four of the seven suffered severe mental incapacitation accompanied by heightened symptomology. In three of these seven cases a high pulse rate and dilated pupils could be related to drug action though the pupillary response was much stronger. In subjects not strongly affected by the drug, a lower pulse rate sometimes coincided with drowsiness and impairment of coordination.

   4. The group which received the highest dosage proved as variable as the others. Although each subject exhibited the usual symptomology, only two of the six were strongly affected. Those two hallucinated and

10

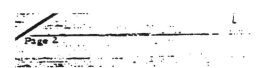

Page 2

dropped to scores of zero on their numbers facilities tests with concomitant increases in pulse rate and pupil size. The four other subjects showed thought hindrance and lack of concentration but apparently as a consequence of extreme drowsiness.

5. In the majority of cases, the side effects appeared within 4 hours after injection. Their duration varied from about 4 hours to 19 days. The desirable primary effects generally did not appear till after the side effects were evident and in every case had a shorter duration, varying from 1 to 90 hours.

6. In the instance of mental incapacitation, the more pronounced effects appeared to be inability to relate to surroundings or time, inability to remember names, and poor performance on numbers facilities tests. Hallucinations were of both visual and auditory nature. Patients would see and hear persons not there and speak to them. Frequent complaints were bright lights or objects on the wall and roaches or flying insects in the room.

7. This study was somewhat unprofessional and a trifle slipshod. The results are inconclusive. Apparently, the drug is not reliable at the dosage levels tested: only nine of the nineteen subjects experienced "desirable effects" (3 out of 6 at ___] units/kg; 4 out of 7 at \units/kg; 2 out of 6 at \units/kg) but all nineteen exhibited undesirable signs and/or symptoms.

13 October 1970

MEMORANDUM FOR THE RECORD

SUBJECT: Visit by Dr.

1. On 30 September 1970, Dr.   Professor
and Chairman of the Department of
                    visited Project Often's screen-
ing facility prior to a subsequent meeting at
Dr.   visit was arranged in accordance with the joint
          steering committee's previously announced plans
to have OFTEN's activities reviewed and assessed by at least
two recognized outside experts in the field of pharmacology
and behavioral science.

2. At the screening facility, Dr.   was given a complete
briefing on OFTEN's objectives, and the methods and procedures
implemented to carry out these objectives. Those in attendance
were Drs.
                    In addition, Dr.   toured
the laboratories where demonstrations were held and representative
data discussed. At   Dr.   reviewed project OFTEN
activities with Drs.   for FY 71, inspected the
computer facility and was briefed on   the file management
program now used to search our toxicological data bank.

3. Dr.   expressed agreement with the design and
operation of the OFTEN project as well as planned activities and
made several suggestions for new agents that have potential as
unique behavior modifiers. These will be screened immediately,
if available, together with other compounds suggested as criterion
agents for standardization purposes.

13 October 1970

4. Finally, Dr.   was invited to join the OF TEN project
on a consulting basis and he accepted the role. It is planned to
have him visit this installation quarterly with opportunity for
more frequent consultation on a non-visit basis. He will also be
present at some meetings of the joint   steering group.
This aspect will be cleared with   in advance.

DRAFT   16 February 1971

MEMORANDUM FOR:

SUBJECT: Transfer of Funds to EARL for ~~Evaluation~~ *Follow-up* ~~Studies in Human Volunteers~~ *Study of Medical Volunteers*

1. This requested transfer of funds is in support of the ███████████████ Project. The goal of this study is to define and quantify the effects in humans of the ██████████ administration of agents belonging to the glycolate class. The study will be carried out within the Medical Volunteer Program at EARL under the direction of Dr. ██████████.

2. Agents of the glycolate class are of interest because of the serious threat certain examples cases of this class present as potential incapacitants. The Soviets are known to be actively working in the glycolate area. Our most effective example item is #3167. This partially investigated item is effective ██████████ in animals and probably also in man, as evidenced by several laboratory accidents. Because the ████████████ of administration are the routes of true potential threat to US. VIP's and other key personnel, it is essential that the present existing data on intramuscular injection in humans be extended to include the ██████████ Simultaneously, information and plans will be developed to implement countermeasures as required.

RELEASED - - APR 1995

26

DRAFT   16 February 1971

Page 2 ;
_____   ____   _ _____

3. Contingent upon the results obtained and evidence of a

clear potential threat, follow-on work at approximately the same

level of effort can be expected for the development of needed counter-

measures.

4. EARL was selected for this work because of their unique

experience with #3167, and because it has volunteer human studies

on-going in a carefully controlled environment. Coordination has

been affected with   and with Dr.

Director of Laboratories at Edgewood.

5. Dr.   will be the

project officer with responsibility for monitoring the execution of

the task. The work will be CLASSIFIED and Agency association with

EARL will be CONFIDENTIAL.

6. The   recommends

the approval of the transfer of $37,000 to Project AD 21 Task 03

(Follow-on Study of Medical Volunteers) at EARL under the direction

of Dr.

12

29 May 1973

MEMORANDUM FOR:

SUBJECT: Summary of Project OFTEN Clinical Tests at Edgewood

1. Funds in the amount of $37,000 were transferred to Edgewood
Arsenal on 17 February 1971 for the purpose of determining the clinical
effects of EA #3167, a glycolate class chemical previously developed
by Edgewood. Analysis of Edgewood file data had flagged this item as
possessing unusual potential as an incapacitant, strongly suggesting
the possibility of

2. The Soviets were known to be actively working in the glycolate
area. Edgewood had partially investigated EA #3167 and found it to be
effective   in animals. In addition, there had been several
laboratory accidents in which the agent had produced prolonged psychotic
effects in laboratory personnel.

3. Since the   were
the routes of potential threat to U.S. VIP's and other key personnel,
it was highly desirable that existing data on
in humans previously acquired by Edgewood be extended to include the
                                  ] Simultaneously, plans were developed to
implement countermeasures as required.

4. Preliminary laboratory work was undertaken to determine the
solubility and   ] of #3167. Additional work was undertaken
to develop laboratory tests to identify the agent in blood. Further work
was carried out on the masking effects of such common medicinals as aspirin,
barbiturates, etc. The agent was found   ] A good
solvent was discovered. A detection test for #3167 was developed, but
barbiturates were found to completely mask its presence.

12

5. Twenty human volunteer subjects, five prisoners (Holmesbury State Prison, Holmesbury, Pa.) and fifteen military volunteers in the Edgewood program were tested. Both the were found to be effective with symptoms lasting up to six weeks.

6. Concerning countermeasures, certain

7. In addition to the above project, in 1967,   established a contract through Edgewood with   for the collection of information on and samples of new psychopharmaceuticals developed in Europe and   The focus was on unpublished data and unusual new developments. Agency support of this action consisted of   in 1967, and   in 1969. The Agency took advantage of a pre-existing contract between Edgewood and   for the collection of information on foreign chemical and pharmaceutical developments. Agency redirection, beginning in 1967, consisted of focusing on psychoactive drugs and on the collection of samples.

8. Agency support of both the clinical testing of EA #3167 and of the collection of information on and samples of foreign develop-ments was terminated in January 1973. The   transferred to Edgewood in 1972 for an enlarged foreign collection effort was with-drawn in January 1973. Expenditures for the human testing program were gradually reduced as subjects were cleared from the program during the necessary post-test follow-up observational and examination period. Agency involvement in the above activities was closely held at all times.

2

6 May 1974

MEMORANDUM FOR: Inspector General

SUBJECT   : Project OFTEN

1. The purpose of this memorandum is to document to the best of my knowledge the activities associated with Project OFTEN. I am writing this at the request of Mr. Deputy Inspector General. I am writing it at this point in time because (a) in a recent telephone conversation with the Office of   it became apparent that there is very little written information available on the project; (b) all of the key people associated with the project are no longer with the Agency; (c) I am resigning from the Central Intelligence Agency on 11 May 1974. I hope this memorandum and attachments will never be needed, but I believe it is in the interest of CIA to have the following information documented in case it should be required.

2. The project dealt with the behavioral effects of chemical compounds (drugs) on humans. Numerous sources of compounds and data bases were used including private industry, other U.S. Government agencies, and foreign sources. An entire research cycle was set up, from the discovery of new compounds or the development of hybrids, to animal screening, to clinical (human) testing. Numerous data bases were acquired to help refine our search for candidate compounds.

3. The following activities were conducted with the Edgewood Arsenal, Edgewood, Maryland. We obtained a large data base from them containing their animal toxicity screen data. They supplied U.S. Army volunteers for testing of our candidate compounds. We transferred funds to them for their efforts. As a result of this testing something called the "Boomer" was developed. After the project was cancelled one more data base was received containing their clinical data on humans. As the project had been cancelled this data base was not exploited but remained in storage. At a recent request of   I visited the   Building to help them determine

the nature of all the stored computer data relating to the project.
Upon examining a listing of the clinical data it became evident that
the volunteers' names were incorporated in the data base. If the
data base contains all of the information described on the forms
used by the doctors at Edgewood, it seems this data base could be
a severe invasion of privacy of these volunteers. One form, the
biographical one, comes to mind immediately. This form contains
questions about the volunteers' sex life, alcohol and drug use,
parents' family life, and numerous personal questions. I believe
the volunteers never intended for this information to leave the
control of the U.S. Army. It should be noted that (to the best of
my knowledge)   had no knowledge of the sensitivity of this data
base until very recently since the data base was not being exploited.
We also obtained their Wiswesser Line Notation (WLN) data base
which contained the WLN notation for the compounds they have
researched.

4. The following activities were conducted with
                          They did all of the benchwork
of animal screening. They took the candidate compounds and ran
them through a series of screens on such animals as mice, rats,
cats, and monkeys. It was a result of these screens that determined
whether to go ahead with further testing in human Edgewood volunteers
It was also through this contractor that funds were used to pay
university professors when needed.

5. Several contractual agreements were made with private
industry to receive new compounds of possible interest to CIA.
These companies include
                                            | and a few
other organizations whose names I cannot remember. Numerous
compounds were received from these organizations and the results
of the screens, in the form of computer reports, were returned to
the sources of the compounds. This was a delicate process because
some of the compounds were under patent consideration by their
companies. Several foreign sources were also used but I did not
have access to which ones.

6. An effort was also put forth to develop our own WLN
data base. Assistance was received from experts at Edgewood
Arsenal and Fort Dietrich.

7. It was my belief that the project had three primary operational purposes. First, it was hoped that new compounds could be derived that could be used offensively. An example would be to come up with a compound that could simulate a heart attack or a stroke in the targetted individual, or perhaps a new hallucinogen to cause the targetted individual to act bizarrely. Second, it was hoped that blockers or even immunizations could be developed for known drugs. Although this would be mainly for use by our people in hostile environments, any progress along these lines certainly would have been welcomed by conventional drug related agencies. Third, it was my understanding that we would use profiles of volunteers who had received known drugs for comparative analysis. For example, if one of our people suddenly started acting peculiarly, a profile of his actions could be run through the data base to see if his particular combination of actions matched any known drug profile. In addition to those three operational goals, other work was being done on a permuted search capability of the WLN data base. There were also plans to develop a file of all known Soviet research in the drug area. The basis for my understanding of these goals was direct conversations with the division chief who had control over the project, the project officer who was running the project, and discussions at which I was present. To my knowledge only one compound was ever perfected. I have no knowledge of it or any other compound being used operationally.

8. I am also attaching a series of Activity Report forms I used over the years to document the progress of my efforts. While these forms represent only my participation in the project, I believe they do give precise information as to the who, when, and where of many of the activities that were involved.

9. If this memorandum or its attachments should raise further questions, I would be happy to assist in any way to get the required answers. However, as I previously mentioned I will be leaving the Agency on 11 May 1974. If I do not receive any queries during this time, I will assume this memorandum and attachments were sufficient so that the Agency will not be caught by any surprises from this project in the future.

Attachments: 2/6

2 6 FEB 1975

MEMORANDUM FOR THE RECORD

SUBJECT: Trip Report/Edgewood Arsenal

1. On 6 February 1975 we visited Edgewood Arsenal Research Laboratories (EARL) for the purpose of clarifying the nature and extent of work conducted by Edgewood for the Agency under Project A021, Task 03 (U.S. Army designator). Certain details of this work are not well documented in existing Agency files, and all personnel directly involved with the research have subsequently left the Agency. The research in question, a part of project OFTEN, was carried out between February 1971 and January 1973. Agency records indicate that EARL was requested to cease work on this project on 4 January 1973 and that charges ceased to be made against the contract after the January-April quarter in 1973. Although $37,000 was originally allocated, the program had expended $27,352 at the time of termination.

2. We met in Dr. ██████████'s office, with Dr. ████, Dr. ████████, and Mr. ████████████, all of Edgewood. The gist of our discussion is as follows. Previous work at Edgewood (not sponsored by the Agency) had involved administration of a substance known as EA3167 to military and prisoner volunteer subjects. In these studies, administration of EA3167 had resulted in delirium and other psychotic behavior lasting three or four days with subsequent amnesia. There were residual effects lasting up to six weeks. Dr. ████████ was positive that no work on human subjects was performed under the contract with the Agency. He indicated that ultimately testing on human subjects would have been a natural conclusion of this research. However, the project was terminated prior to the establishment of the necessary prerequisite analytical and animal experimentation.

3. The purpose of the Agency-funded research was to investigate the potential ████████████ of EA3167 ██████████ from both applications and threat assessment standpoints, since it was known that the Soviets were actively working with similar compounds. Three tasks were conducted for the Agency concerning:

a. Development of analytic methods for detecting low concentrations of EA3167.

b. Estimation of the fraction of EA3167 transferred from various _____ of the chemical to rabbit ___ \

c. Synthesis of _____ EA3167.

4. Development of a satisfactory analytic technique for EA3167 was never achieved. The compound does not present any unique structural moiety which would allow its identification chemically, particularly in the presence of barbiturates.

5. The second task was approached _____ Similar quanti-ties of EA3167

6. Because of the inability to develop satisfactory chemical analytic techniques, an amount of _____ EA3167 was synthesized. This was to have been used in subsequent research, but with the termination of the Agency-funded work in January 1973, the _____ EA3167 was never used. We were told that most, if not all, of the substance is still on hand at Edgewood.

7. We also discussed the sparse documentation of this project. The Edgewood personnel indicated that the work was rather closely guarded at the time and most results had been conveyed verbally. The few reports received by the Agency had been handcarried by Agency personnel. The premature termination of the project also meant that the usual final report and related documentation were never prepared. Dr. _____ did not exactly remember the reason for additional charges to the contract during the first quarter of 1973 but thought that late billings for previous, unclassified work done at other EARL labs was probably the explanation.

APPENDIX L
THE AMES LEAF ROOM

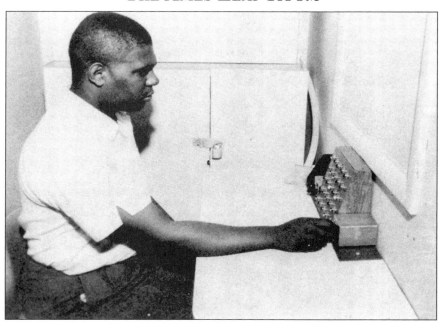

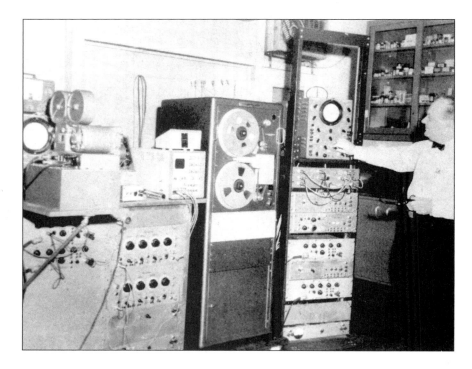

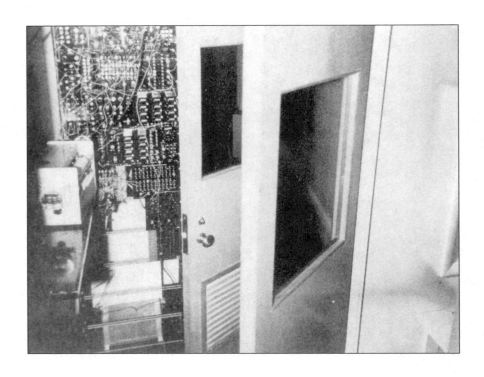

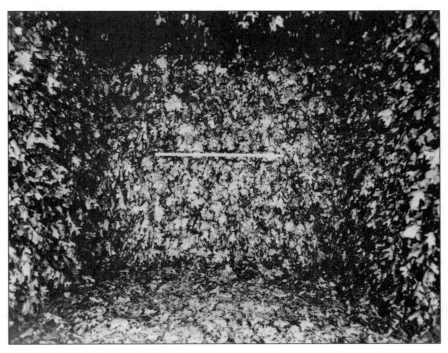

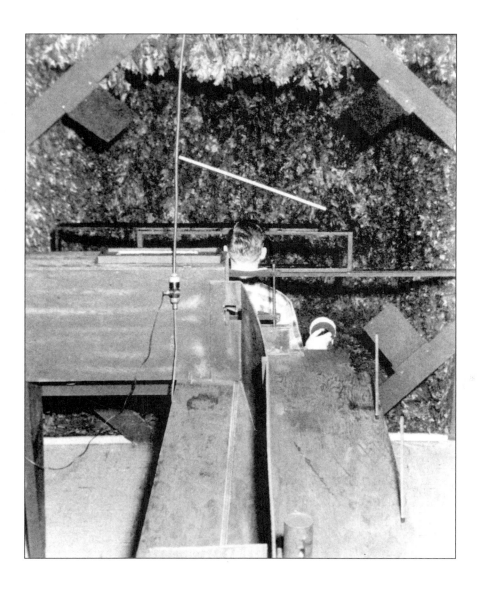